MAN IN FLIGHT

MAN IN FLIGHT

Biomedical Achievements in Aerospace

By
Eloise Engle and Arnold S. Lott

III

LEEWARD PUBLICATIONS, INC.
Annapolis, Maryland

PRINTED IN THE UNITED STATES OF AMERICA

Library of Congress Catalog No. 79-63780
ISBN No. 0-915268-24-8

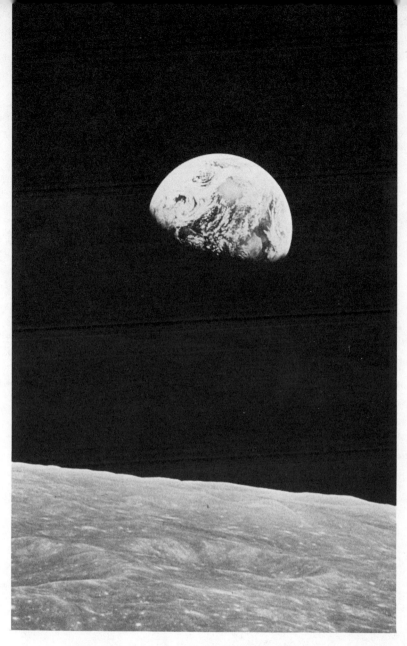

"How brave are those, who with their engine can
Bring man to heaven, and heaven again to man?"

—John Donne

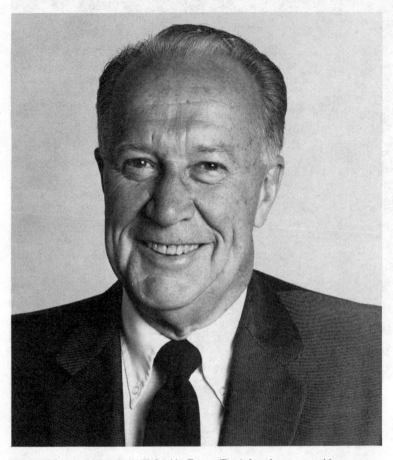

Colonel Robert J. Benford, U.S. Air Force (Ret.) has been an avid aerospace historian and participant in the activities of the Aerospace Medical Association for many years. Following his retirement from active duty as a flight surgeon, he divides his time between Florida and Washington D. C./*Robert J. Benford*

Foreword

Fifty years ago the pioneering founders of the Aerospace Medical Association had no anticipation that their efforts would aid in enabling men, yet unborn, to visit the moon. Such talk about space flight was not part of their deliberations, even in lighter moments. This was an era in powered-flight when the United States government had decided to license airplane pilots and these were the physicians responsible to determine whether the fledgling airmen possessed the physical qualifications to fly safely.

The 60 or so physicians who met in Detroit in 1929, at the invitation of Dr. Louis H. Bauer, to organize a new professional society, believed in the future of aviation. Many were former flight surgeons in the great war that was then 10 years into history. Some even went to France with the A.E.F. They liked to be around pilots, loved to fly. Some were pilots themselves. Each had accepted the appointment of aviation medical examiner (AME) by the Secretary of Commerce, a new responsibiliy in the private practice of medicine.

A Harvard-educated physician of Boston birth, Bauer was a natural leader destined to be a future president of the American Medical Association, and a founder and first secretary-general of the World Medical Association. He would be widely respected and highly honored as a medical statesman. In 1926 he had resigned his Army commission after 13 years of service, the last six as the first commandant of the Air Service School of Aviation Medicine on Long Island, to become the first chief of the medical section of the new Bureau of Air Commerce, an infant appendage of the Department of Commerce.

Founded in 1929 as the Aero Medical Association, the society provided Bauer with the organization he needed to communicate directly with his AMEs in the bureaucratic jungle that even then was Washington. The members' bible was *Aviation Medicine*, the first U.S. textbook on the subject that Bauer had just published. It contained the details of examining procedures developed by the Army and Navy since 1912, along with some early research in flying aptitude. The examiners' goal was to select candidates for licensing with an "absence of organic disease or defect which would interfere with safe handling of an airplane." No easy task. But Bauer had other plans for the continuing medical education of the AMEs—a professional journal.

Prior to the second meeting of the group in Chicago in 1930, the first two numbers of the quarterly *Journal of Aviation Medicine* had been published. From an inauspicious beginning this journal, renamed *Aerospace Medicine* in 1969 and given its present title, *Aviation, Space and Environmental Medicine* in 1975, gained early and sustained interest among scientists. Bauer retired as editor after guiding its policies for 25 years, and lived to see it become the world's oldest, continuously-published periodical—as well as the most influential—in the field of aerospace medicine. Today the journal's international circulation includes subscribers in Soviet-bloc countries, The Peoples Republic of China, and some emerging African nations.

At this same 1930 meeting, there was a significant happening. Bauer, who had been re-elected president of the Association, was obliged in the absence of the scheduled speakers to summarize ongoing research initiated by two Army pilots and flight surgeon David A. Meyers in the first known investigation of the physiology of "blind flying," the often hazardous piloting of an aircraft in reduced or zero visibility. The efforts of these scientists led to the development of simulated flight trainers and modern instrument flight procedures that are now routine throughout the world.

VIII

This milestone was a forerunner of much early study of the effects of flight. The prevention of injury to airmen became paramount as acceleration, altitude, fatigue, noise, speed, temperature, vibration and, eventually, weightlessness began to reach seemingly intolerable extremes. The Association's annual meetings and publications provided wide communication of such investigations—research that in years ahead was to claim the lives of three of its members—by providing opportunities for scientists to be seen and heard and read. Here was the platform and the forum for a new and exciting medical science in support of aeronautics and, soon, astronautics.

The momentum continued. By 1931 the Army Air Corps moved its enlarged School of Aviation Medicine to Randolph Field, the new "West Point of the Air," near San Antonio. Three years later the Aero Medical Laboratory was established at Wright Field, in Dayton, Ohio, and the following year the Civil Aviation Administration opened its first medical research facility in Kansas City. It later moved to Houston, and finally to Oklahoma City where the impressive Civil Aeromedical Institute was dedicated in 1962. And in 1939 the Navy's new School of Aviation Medicine at Pensacola, Florida, accepted its first class of student officers —many of whom were to graduate as flight surgeons with the wings of Naval aviators.

A few weeks after the Japanese air attack on Pearl Harbor in 1941, the growing Association elected as president its first military flight surgeon, Captain John R. Poppen (MC) U.S. Navy. For nearly 10 years Poppen and his colleagues, with the collaboration of Dr. Cecil K. Drinker of Harvard, had been studying pilot blackout in high accelerative forces, and developing and testing anti-g devices—all in strict military secrecy. Unfortunately, by the time these projects were declassified by the Navy, Poppen was accorded little credit for his pioneering work. He was even deprived of the honor of presiding at the 1942 meeting in Indianapolis because by that time he had been assigned to temporary duty in England with the Royal Navy Fleet Air Arm.

In contrast, a spectacular achievement by his successor as Association president, W. Randolph Lovelace, II, M.D., chief of the Aero Medical Laboratory, was widely heralded by the press. On October 25, 1943, just four months before the annual meeting

IX

in Cincinnati, Lovelace plummeted from the bomb bay of a B-17 aircraft nearly eight miles above Euphrata, Washington, in an experimental parachute jump to test bailout oxygen equipment and electrically-heated clothing developed in his own laboratory. It was his first jump!

The mobilization of the country in World War II produced an explosive growth in the aviation medical sciences. Biophysicists, aviation physiologists, flight nurses, bio-engineers, psychologists, anthropologists and human factors specialists joined physicians and established careers in the booming aircraft industry and the air arm of the Army, Navy or Marines. The military schools of aviation medicine doubled and redoubled their enrollments several times. Courses were shortened and curricula reduced to train rapidly the flight surgeons needed in operational units. The Association experienced its greatest period of growth.

With the wartime emergence of the giant aerospace industry, came the rise of the airlines—and their medical departments. In 1936 Eastern Airlines had asked Dr. Ralph N. Greene, a former Army pilot and the first U.S. physician to attain military flight status, to develop a medical service for its flight crews. The following year United Airlines named Colonel Arnold D. Tuttle, a retired Army flight surgeon, its first medical director, and American, TWA and PanAm soon followed with their own services. Today the world's major airlines all have medical departments directed by members of the Association. By 1944, these physicians had developed sufficient mutual interests to form their own professional society, the Airlines Medical Directors Association, which meets annually in conjunction with the parent organization. Other subspecialty groups of members with common interests have also banded together, including a score of recognized constituent and affiliated societies, and several national groups of other countries.

In 1942, the Executive Council created the new membership grades of fellow and associate fellow in aviation medicine, and promptly chose the 11 former presidents as the first fellows. This original group, in turn, elected 15 other distinguished members for this honor, a custom that still prevails. Even in the early years, when election to fellowship was more convivial than scientific, the recognition was held in esteem and is today more highly cherished then ever. In this anniversary year, with the total number of elected fellows approaching 500, selection is still traditionally made from among members who have made "outstanding contributions to aerospace medicine...either in research, in practical usage of research, or by precept and example."

In commemoration of distinguished members, 12 notable awards have been created since 1947 for recognition of excellence in specific fields of achievement. Each includes an appropriate plaque or certificate and an honorarium. In the five years from 1974 through 1978, scientists from Canada, England, France, Mexico, Russia and West Germany have received 11 of these awards.

Other recognition has been accorded members. President Franklin D. Roosevelt in 1940 presented the prestigeous Robert J. Collier Trophy, given annually "for the greatest achievement in aviation in America...during the preceding year," to the airlines of the United States for their high record of safety with special recognition to Drs. Walter Boothy and W. Randolph Lovelace of the Mayo Clinic Aero-Medical Unit, and Captain Harry G. Armstrong, chief of the Wright Field Aero Medical Laboratory. In the same year, Dr. Bauer was the first recipient of the John J. Jeffries Award, given each year "for outstanding contributions to the advancement" of these sciences "through medical research." All recipients of this honor have been members of the Association.

In further tribute to the Association's founder, the Louis Hopewell Bauer Lecture was established in 1955 to bring a keynote speaker each year to the Association's rostrum, often a major figure from industry. Eleven years later the Harry G. Armstrong Lecture was inaugurated as a worthy companion piece to the Bauer presentation.

For many years, even from the earliest days of the Association, the hope for certification of qualified applicants as recognized specialists in aviation medicine never waned. In 1949, after many delays, an interim board of aviation medicine was appointed to undertake the formidable task of petitioning official groups in the hierarchy of American Medicine for such recognition. Finally, in 1953, affiliation with the American Board of Preventive Medicine was approved that permitted this established group additionally to certify physicians as diplomates in aviation (later aerospace) medicine as well as, heretofore, in preventive medicine and public health. Required residency training in recognized schools of public health at Johns Hopkins, Harvard and Ohio State Universities was subsequently established. In the past 25 years members of the Association have been certified as specialists. Aptly, one of the original special requirements for board certification is "regular and frequent participation in aerial flight."

The Association's first "international meeting" was held in New York in 1937, when scientists from Germany and Poland, and several South and Central American countries were guests. Since then, membership has grown to include all nations in which aviation is a part of the economy and defense. The Soviet Union has regularly sent delegations to meetings ever since 1963. In the fall of 1952, a French-speaking Branch presented its first scientific program at the University of Paris. The following year the group met in Brussels, and then in Zurich. These meetings, which attracted scientists from other European countries and the United States, soon became known as the annual European Congress of Aviation (and later Space) Medicine.

Now sponsored by the host country and the International Academy of Aviation and Space Medicine, established in 1956, these congresses have been held in nearly all European capitals, including Warsaw and Prague, and more recently in Munich, Beirut, Tel Aviv, Nice and Johannesburg. As a result of this international scientific fellowship, the spring meeting of the Association and the fall congress of the Academy have become the world's major events in aerospace medicine.

Back in the spring of 1950 a dedicated group of members, who had been aroused and stimulated by a trail-blazing seminar on space medicine at the Air Force School of Aviation Medicine, formed their own Space Medicine Branch of the Association. The Russian *Sputnik* was still 10 years into the future. At the 1952 meeting in Washington—a decade before the first U.S. suborbital flights—this group of pioneers sponsored an historic space medicine symposium that changed the Association's name and its mission. Perhaps things would never be quite the same—even to "a spoofing spaceman" who sauntered among the members like a best-dressed Martian visiting the earth. Space medicine was here even though the nation's space program would not be officially activated for another six years.

This book tells the fascinating story of the participation of medical scientists in the saga of aeronautical and astronautical progress, and the role of the Aerospace Medical Association in its first 50 years.

What's ahead in the next 50 years? The Space Shuttle and further probes of Venus are scheduled. But is that all?

Dr. Robert Frosch, the administrator of NASA doesn't seem to think so. In a recent prediction on the occasion of the tenth anniversary of the epic flights of Apollo XI to the moon, he said:

"There exists in the foreseeable future the very real—although unquantifiable—possibility of contact with other intelligent beings in the universe. Such a contact would transform our lives.

Continued failure to make such a contact, on the other hand, would tend to indicate the temporary nature of advanced civilizations and provide the basis for serious reflections on the character of our own."

Robert J. Benford, M.D.,
Chairman, History and Archives Committee,
Aerospace Medical Association

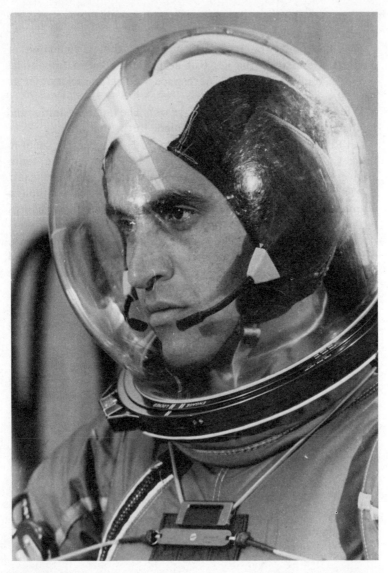

A member of the Apollo 17 mission to the moon, Dr. Harrison H. (Jack) Schmitt was a new type of astronaut—not a military officer, but a qualified geologist. However, he was the lunar module pilot for that mission. He is now a United States Senator from New Mexico./*NASA*

XIV

Introduction

One of the most exciting commitments by the American people in the last decade was the achievement of landing men on the moon. That effort was represented by a unified industry and national ingenuity never before seen in peacetime. The young were caught by imagination, the technical community responded to the challenge, and all over the world people reacted to a new horizon within reach.

The Apollo explorations, and the Mercury and Gemini programs, were man's first halting and clearly personal look at his universe. We have had the audacity to try to understand our place in the universe and in its future, and we have had the further audacity to use that understanding to try to alter the universe and to more fully perceive the earth, using in large measure corrected vision from space.

The technology developed for the space program has provided us with multiple practical benefits. There are applications in agriculture, business, communication, medicine, defense and diplomacy, to name only a few. In the future, that technology will provide accessibility to the new earth orbit resources of weightlessness and high vacuum for manufacturing, medical and surgical procedures and other services.

These benefits could not have been derived from a static technology developed through the exclusive use of the mechanical exploration of space. Man in space means on-the-spot invention, testing, questioning and revision of space technology. The presence of man in space was, is, and shall continue to be vital to the well-being of the space program of the sixties. It is up to man to explore them.

One of the most exciting medical discoveries of the century has been the realization that man can survive extended exposure to the environment of space, and that he can also prosper there. Contrary to many, if not most, expert opinions prior to the beginning of space flight, human beings have so far fully adapted to life in this new sphere of human endeavor. Additionally, human beings have fully adapted to their return to the environment of earth. Realization of these facts means that civilization can indeed move into space and out to the planets.

Many young Americans today are emotionally and philosophically ready for a new long-range space commitment. These young people sense the movement of civilization into the solar system and want to be part of that movement. The Apollo excitement is still there, but now, in the space generations, there is an even stronger sense of continuity and of a future in the universe.

This feeling among young Americans that free men and women must be part of the new solar system civilization overshadows other supporting arguments for space activities. The elements of a national space commitment that appeal to young Americans include:

> The exploration of other planets by Americans within the working lifetime of those now alive, that is, close to the end of the century;
>
> The creation of a near-Earth civilization including space universities, hospitals, factories, solar power plants, and lunar and asteroid mines;
>
> The establishment of a world information system including telecommunications, educational and medical services, resource evaluation, and weather and climate prediction;

The study of stars, the sun and its planets, and to the basic research in physics and space biology that will form the foundation for the "star treks" of future generations.

A commitment to the peaceful exploration of the universe by young Americans is one of the most important investments our generation can make for the future of mankind.

This book commemorates the 50th anniversary of the Aerospace Medical Association. The past achievements of this organization and its members have provided the basis for much of our enthusiastic and innovative exploration of the moon. With a renewed determination to further explore our universe, the future holds great promise for the youth of our nation and of the world at large.

Harrison Schmitt
U.S. Senator

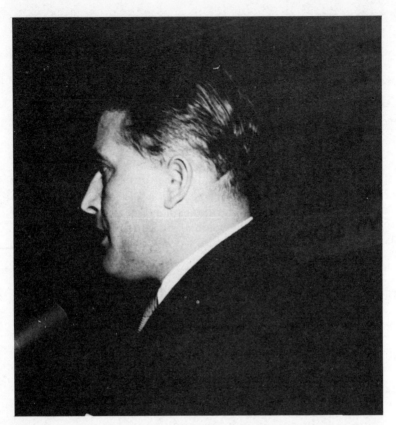

Dr. Wernher von Braun (1912-1977) came to the United States from Germany after World War II ended, and played an important role in the space program. He was one of the world's most renowned rocket and aerospace engineers, and in 1960 became Director of the George C. Marshall Center/*Smithsonian Institution*

"I believe that the time has arrived for medical investigation of the problem of manned rocket flight, for it will not be the engineering problems but rather the limits of the human frame that will make the final decision as to whether manned spaceflight will eventually become a reality."

Wernher von Braun in
Space Medicine, 1951

XVIII

Preface

In narrating the highlights of the biomedical research and development that enabled men to travel to the moon and return safely to earth, an interesting dichotomy was revealed. Researchers not only faced a myriad of problems to which they did not know the answers—they didn't even know what questions to ask. To begin with, available knowledge having to do with space travel consisted of a great amount of miscellaneous information, all of which had to be fitted together like pieces of a puzzle before any final conclusions could be reached. The stumbling block was, no one knew what sort of puzzle they were trying to solve.

The approach to space flight was somewhat like building a brick wall. What sort of bricks are needed? How many? Where do they come from? And with all the bricks at hand, where must the bottom one be laid? "The man who laid the bottom brick is the most important," wrote Dr. James P. Henry. "Then there are all the other bricklayers in between, who sweated out the construction." History is full of the names of men who contributed to the success of space flight; who now can name the one who laid the bottom brick?

Newspaper headlines over the past two decades have tended to name those men who, as it were, put the last brick in the wall—the astronauts who voyaged to the moon—and create the impression that only a few years have passed since man decided to explore the heavens. That is not so. The dream of reaching the moon is older than recorded history. And for more than two thousand years, men have been collecting, bit by bit, the information that finally made possible those four famous words "The Eagle has landed."

Some of the most critical factors involved in the Apollo flights were based on principles discovered hundreds of years ago. Research related to space flight began a century ago. In the past fifty years, people working toward the achievement of space flight have included anthropologists, astronomers, biochemists, biophysicists, engineers, doctors, mathematicians, psychologists, and technicians. The existing literature related to the subject of space flight will fill a large library.

No one book could name all the people who have devoted time and talent to this monumental undertaking. What we have done here is to give some historical perspective to the subject, including all the various disciplines concerned, but to emphasize the contributions, of those skilled in the world's newest science, aerospace medicine, to the success of the space program. In so doing, we have gone to the experts—the doctors, flight surgeons, and specialists in many fields—and derived from their books, articles, unpublished papers, and personal interviews, the material that fills the following pages with an account of how aerospace medicine made it possible for men to fly to the moon in this century and may, in the next, send them out to commence the exploration of the universe.

Eloise Engle
Arnold S. Lott

Acknowledgements

When the authors first assumed the formidable task of chronicling the aerospace medicine highlights that enabled us to put a man on the moon and return him safely to earth, it was clearly understood that a great deal of help from the experts would be needed. Not only was there a requirement to nail down the already reported facts, but new insights of a more personal nature would be sought in order to provide some of the behind-the-scenes difficulties encountered and overcome.

This meant that extremely busy doctors and other scientists would have to make time for this project and explain to the authors just what their roles were during the formative years of the space program. Not only would they tell their own stories, but they would go through their files and memories for leads to other sources.

Stacks of papers, reports and books poured in which covered the historical aspects, the contemporary and future plans for man's ventures into space. The authors can say without exception that the help and cooperation from every single one of the leading scientists approached has been tremendous.

In any research for a project of this magnitude, a great amount of information comes from many sources at many times. So perhaps it would be best to start at the beginning when Brigadier

General Hamilton Webb U.S. Air Force (Ret.) coordinated the actual writing of the book to commemorate the 50th anniversary of the Aerospace Medical Association. It would be a two-year project, the authors were told, and assistance would be forthcoming from whomever was needed.

Immediately Colonel Robert Benford U.S. Air Force (Ret.), the ASMA Historian, began supplying leads, advice and historical papers from his own files. There were meetings during which the book's contents and goals were established. Participants were Captain Merrill Goodwin (MC) U.S. Navy (Ret.), Captain Frank Austin (MC) U.S. Navy, Colonel Roland Shamburek U.S Army (Ret.), Brigadier General Hamilton Webb U.S. Air Force (Ret.), John Marbarger Ph.D., Colonel A. Pharo Gagge U.S. Air Force (Ret.), Stanley Mohler, M.D., Colonel Stanley White U.S. Air Force (Ret.), Colonel George Zinnemann U.S. Air Force (Ret.) and Colonel Robert Benford U.S. Air Force (Ret.). Randall M. Chambers, Ph.D. supplied valuable reports and information on experiments with which he was involved.

From the very beginning, Colonel Paul Campbell U.S. Air Force (Ret.) actively participated in the research. Some of the personal interviews involved considerable travel by the authors; others were obtained by mail and telephone. Those interviewed include Robert Gilruth, Director, Manned Spaceflight Center in Houston, Captain Joe Kerwin (MC) U.S. Navy Skylab astronaut, Charles Berry M.D., Director, Life Sciences; Captain Norman Lee Barr (MC) U.S. Navy (Ret.), Captain Ashton Graybiel (MC) U.S. Navy (Ret.), Colonel Paul Campbell U.S. Air Force (Ret.), Colonel Stanley White U.S. Air Force (Ret.), Colonel Rufus Hessberg U.S. Air Force (Ret.), Captain Ralph Christy (MC) U.S. Navy (Ret.), Major General Harry Armstrong U.S. Air Force (Ret.), Howard Minners, M.D., Colonel William Douglas U.S. Air Force (Ret.), Stanley Mohler, M.D., Lieutenant General George E. Schafer U.S. Air Force, Captain Frank Austin (MC) U.S. Navy, G. D. Whedon, M.D., Captain Walton Jones (MC) U.S. Navy (Ret.) Theodor Benzinger, M.D., Sentator Harrison "Jack Schmitt, Apollo 17 astronaut, (the most *recent* man on the moon) Colonel John Pickering U.S. Air Force (Ret.), Colonel Joseph Quashnock U.S. Air Force (Ret.), Harald von Beckh, M.D., Siegried Gerathewohl, Ph.D., Hubertus Strughold, M.D. and Colonel David Simons U.S.

Air Force (Ret.). It should be noted that the authors have identified the participants in the story by the ranks they held at that particular stage of their careers. Almost everyone listed above as U.S. Air Force (Ret.) is a flight surgeon but the authors have chosen to be technically correct by omitting the "MC" following their names. Doctors Charles Berry and Howard Minners resigned prior to retirement from the Air Force and are therefore listed as M.D.s.

The manuscript has been reviewed in parts and as a whole by specialists outside the editorial board. The authors thank Doctor Duane Graveline, (formerly USAF), and Colonel Jefferson Davis U.S. Air Force for their painstaking critiques. Colonel Charles Wilson U.S. Air Force was very helpful on the environment chapter. The authors are honored that Dr. Hubertus Strughold, General Harry Armstrong, Colonel Paul Campbell, Doctors Theodor Benzinger and Harald von Beckh agreed to examine the manuscript. Earl H. Wood, M.D. Ph.D., at the Mayo Foundation provided very useful material, as did Joan C. Robinette, Scientific and Technical Information Officer at the 6570th Aerospace Medical Research Laboratory at Wright-Patterson AFB. Material and photos also came in from W. R. Franks, M.D., Civil Aviation Medical Unit in Ontario, Canada. William J. O'Donnell, Public Affairs Officer, Office of Space Flight, NASA, and Terry White, in Public Affairs at MSC, Houston, sent along considerable material for the authors' use. Donald J. Sass, M.D., supplied helpful papers, as did Pat Bragg, the friendly and knowledgeable Information Officer in the Office of the Surgeon General, U.S. Air Force. Tim Glasgow at Brooks AFB was most helpful in arranging for the use of eight hours of taping with General Harry Armstrong.

The authors are grateful to those librarians, without whose efficiency and patience all would be lost: Robert A. Hauze, Director of the Library at Trinity University in San Antonio; the librarians at the Nimitz Library at the Naval Academy in Annapolis, the librarians at NASA and those in the Fairfax County system, particularly at the Woodrow Wilson Branch. Librarian Dominick Pisano, at the National Air and Space Museum of the Smithsonian Institution located obscure material which had been forgotten for years, while allowing the authors to plow through papers in that fascinating library. Thanks too, to the interested assistance of Fred Durant, Assistant Director of the National Air and Space Museum, and to Lucy Keister at the National Library of Medicine for securing certain photos. Les Gaver at NASA was extremely helpful in procuring photos from that agency, and Jim Lacy, of the Goddard Space Flight Center, also gave a helping hand. George Catlett, A. Pharo Gagge, Merrill Goodwin, Rufus Hessberg, John Marbarger, Stanley Mohler, Roland Shamburek, Stanley White, George Zinnemann, George C. Mohr, U.S. Air Force, and Robert Benford also deserve mention for their help.

The authors thank Ann Graham in Senator Schmitt's office, who arranged for the Apollo 17 astronaut's extra curricular writing of the introduction, and Mrs. Paul Campbell, Mrs. David Simons, and Dr. Maria Benzinger for their encouragement and hospitality.

Our thanks go also to Professor O. G. Gazenko, M.D., Institute of Biomedical Problems, Moscow, for data and photos of early Soviet pressure suit development.

Eloise Engle
Arnold Lott

Table of Contents

Prologue

Man's first appearance on this earth was a minor event, unmarked and unrecorded in the passing of countless centuries. But man's first departure from the earth was quite another matter; it took place at exactly 3:30 p.m., Eastern Standard Time, on 23 December 1968, when Apollo 8 with a crew of three, at about 194,000 miles from the earth, began *falling up* toward the moon.

The first steps toward that dramatic journey were made by those unknowns who tamed fire, worked metal, conceived the wheel, and developed a written language. Long after them came the great thinkers— Copernicus, Kepler, Galileo, Newton, Michelson and Einstein, on whose mathematical and scientific findings all modern technology is based. And after the thinkers came the tinkerers such as Montgolfier, Watt, Faraday, Bell, Marconi, Edison, the Wrights, Goddard and Post, each of whom achieved some development that helped put man in space.

There is one aspect of space flight that sets astronauts apart from all other adventurers—no matter how fast or how far they go, they do not travel alone. Early explorers sailed off into the unknown for months or years at a time; they were completely on their own until they returned, and until they did return no one knew where they had gone. But man in space flies at the end of a long line of complex communications; his every move is monitored—even his heartbeats are counted—the technical skills of thousands of chair-bound earthlings are at his command, and through the magic of television half the world rides along in the spacecraft.

The first men to leave the surface of the earth did so in a hot-air balloon that carried them aloft for about 25 minutes in 1783. Rockets lifted man above the earth's atmosphere for the first time 178 years later. Then, seven years after that, Apollo 8 journeyed to the moon. The crew of Apollo 8 were not the first Americans in space, neither were they the first men to land on the moon; that crew followed them several months later. But Borman, Lovell and Anders were the first men in history to cross the great celestial divide, the unknown realm in space where the gravitational field of the moon took hold of their spacecraft and they left the earth behind.

The path a spacecraft followed to the moon could be computed, and its performance in flight could be predicted. But as in all the history of flight, the most critical aspect of the operation was the physiological reactions of men placed in an alien environment.

Medical research into the problems related to flight began as soon as men began flying, and has continued ever since, with literally thousands of people contributing to the knowledge that has made space flight successful. Many such researchers never got off the ground, yet without them, no one would have ever reached the moon. Long before men ventured into space, aeromedical research was pointing the way.

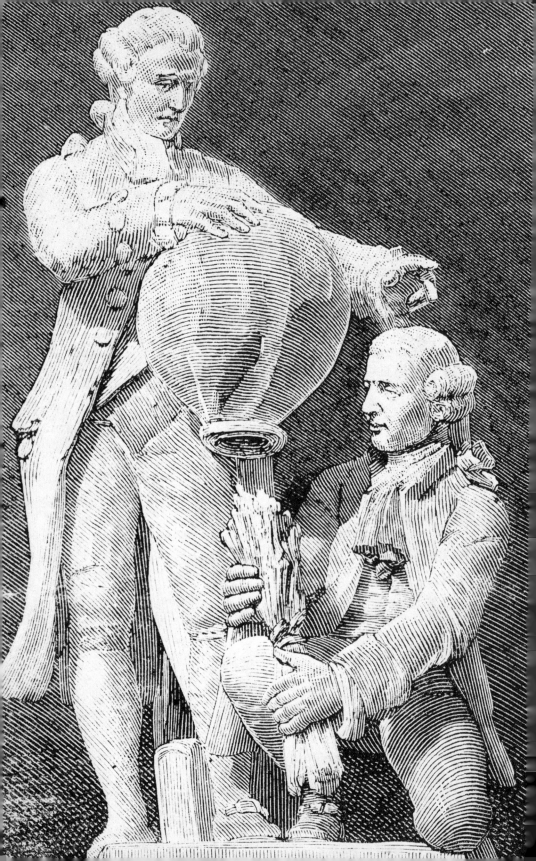

1

From Montgolfier to Stratolab

For untold centuries, men have looked at the moon and dreamed of fantastic contrivances to take them there. Yet the first move in that direction was made less than two centuries ago, in France, when a balloon—basically a paper bag filled with hot air—soared into the sky with the first two men ever to leave the surface of the earth. All previous attempts at flight had been based on aerodynamic, or heavier than air, devices—imitations in one way or another of the flapping-wing system of flight developed by birds. Yet no one—not even that great inventive and artistic genius, Leonardo da Vinci, who studied birds in flight—could perfect a mechanism with power and lift enough to make flight possible.

But such a force existed naturally, and was available to anyone who discovered how to harness it. It was a common fact that hot air rose, even if no one then understood the fact that it rose because heat caused it to expand and occupy greater volume than cold air. And there was the secret—volume for volume, hot air weighed less

This statue in France immortalizes two men, whose imagination and vision changed the world and gave man wings, although they never got their feet off the ground—Jacques and Joseph Montgolfier, with their primitive hot-air balloon. Modern hot-air balloons are still referred to as montgolfiere types./*Smithsonian Institution*

1

than cold air, and the hot air could lift enough weight to make up that difference. All that one needed was the harness.

The Montgolfier brothers, Jacques and Joseph, were paper manufacturers and tinkerers at Vidalon-les-Annonay, France. Like many men before them, they had watched smoke rise in a chimney. But unlike all others, they wondered why. Paper was handy; they filled a paper bag with smoke and saw it rise into the air. They failed to realize that the lift was created, not by the smoke which they could see, but by the buoyancy of hot air, which they could not see. But they immediately saw that the paper bag flew. There was a way for man to fly, and they proceeded to develop it.

First they built a few small trial balloons that flew to altitudes of 70 feet, 600 feet, and finally 1,000 feet. It is difficult to understand how these flights could have been made in secret, yet they evidently did not attract much attention; possibly the peasants could not believe their eyes and kept quiet about the whole thing. Then, on 5 June 1783, the brothers "went public" with a much larger affair, a sphere of linen some 33 feet in diameter, with a volume of 22,000 cubic feet and estimated lift of 490 pounds. The balloon was filled with hot air generated by a fire of straw and wool. Then a handling crew of eight men released the balloon, and to the amazement of everyone, savant and skeptic alike, it swiftly and silently vaulted into the sky until only the keenest eyes could see it, floating 6,000 feet above them. There the balloon rapidly cooled and lost its lift; it came to earth about a mile and a half away ten minutes after take-off, but the sensation it created lasted much longer.

News of the amazing feat reached Paris where the learned gentlemen of the Paris Academy of Sciences arranged a flight of their own. Hot air may have sufficed for the country folk, but in Paris they used hydrogen, a recent scientific development.* Under the direction of Jacques Alexandre Cesar Charles,** another team

*Hydrogen was discovered by Henry Cavendish (1731-1810) who in 1766 determined that it was seven times lighter than air. It was also highly flammable, but this fact did not impress balloonists at first.

**Remembered for *Charles' Law:* If a fixed mass of gas is heated through a given temperature while the volume remains constant, the fractional change in pressure will be the same for all gases.

of brothers, Charles and Marie-Noel Robert, constructed a very small balloon of silk, 12 feet in diameter, made gas-tight by a coating of rubber. Filling the balloon with hydrogen generated by the action of sulphuric acid on iron filings took the better part of five days and nights, a period made remarkable by the fact that no pipe smoker managed to get near enough to the hydrogen to blow the whole operation to bits.

Late on the afternoon of 28 August, with spectators crowding every vantage point around the Champ de Mars, the balloon was released and in a couple of minutes disappeared in a rain cloud. Forty five minutes later it came to earth some 15 miles from Paris where peasants, terrified by the actions of a half-empty balloon wallowing about on the ground, decided they wanted no part of it and demolished it with pitchforks.

From these two pioneering flights there come the terms that still apply to balloons today: A montgolfiere-type balloon is one filled with hot air, while a charliere-type balloon is filled with a lighter-than-air gas. The flights established two time limits in ballooning—a balloon could be inflated with hot air in only a few minutes, while generating enough hydrogen for the job might take days. Modern balloonists use a propane burner to inflate the balloon with hot air and carry it along with them to keep the air hot and thus extend their flight.

Ballooning having caught the public fancy, it was only natural that royalty express an interest; the Montgolfier brothers gave a command performance at Versailles in the presence of Louis XVI, Marie Antoinette, and the Court. For this occasion, they constructed an elaborately decorated envelope with an estimated lift of 1,250 pounds. Five days before their flight was to take place, they tested the balloon, tethered to the ground, only to have a sudden storm destroy it. In the first frantic version of "back-to-the-drawing-board," they gathered a crew, designed and built a new balloon in four days, test-flew it on 18 September, and on 19 September 1873 were at Versailles, ready to go.

Long before the balloon was completed, there were rumors that a man, perhaps a condemned criminal, would ride in it, but the King himself ruled out such a dangerous stunt. Instead, a sheep, a duck, and a cock were given the dubious honor of being the first living creatures to leave the surface of the earth in a man-made

3

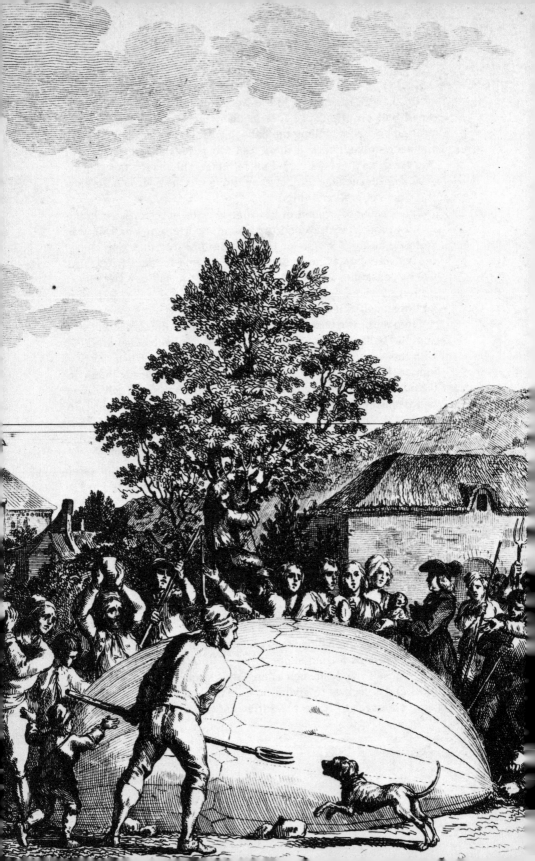

vehicle. On 19 September the balloon was released and reached an altitude of 1,700 feet on an eight-minute flight, before landing in a forest about two miles away.

The first people to reach the scene found all the passengers alive and unharmed by their adventure. It was safe to fly. Furthermore, flying apparently was to be a privilege, not a punishment. Accordingly, about two months later, Pilatre de Rozier, a surgeon, and the Marquis d'Arlandes became the first men in history to fly. On 21 November 1783, they took off from the Bois de Boulogne in a montgolfiere-type balloon for a flight that lasted 25 minutes. After they landed, they folded the balloon and went home. In spite of the excitement of floating free high above fields and woods, the world's first flying surgeon preserved his scientific detachment and noted that flying had no unfavorable effects on the physical system. Curiously enough, while Pilatre de Rozier was a distinguished man of medicine and superintendent of the royal museum of natural history, he is remembered only for his pioneering adventures in aeronautics.

The next manned flight, made only a few days later by the Robert brothers, marked a great advancement in the art of balloon design and operation. The charliere-type balloon they fabricated for that flight established a standard balloon form which remained basically unchanged to 1930. The gas bag—hydrogen filled—was spherical, with an open neck at the bottom through which gas could be added or vented. A flap valve at the top of the sphere allowed rapid release of gas for a controlled descent. A web-like net covered the upper hemisphere of the balloon and supported the car (which eventually became a rectangular basket) underneath the balloon.

The second manned balloon flight in history was made on 1 December 1783, while some 400,000 people watched. One of them was Benjamin Franklin, who had been on hand to witness the first flight. "Of what use is it?" someone demanded, watching the balloon. Franklin replied, "Of what use is a newborn child?"

Filling the charliere-type balloon still took time, as compared to

The first flight of a hydrogen-filled balloon was witnessed by some 300,000 people crowding the Champ de Mars in Paris one afternoon late in August, 1784. But the peasants in whose fields it landed, some 15 miles away, thought it was some monstrous animal and attacked it with pitchforks./*Smithsonian Institution*

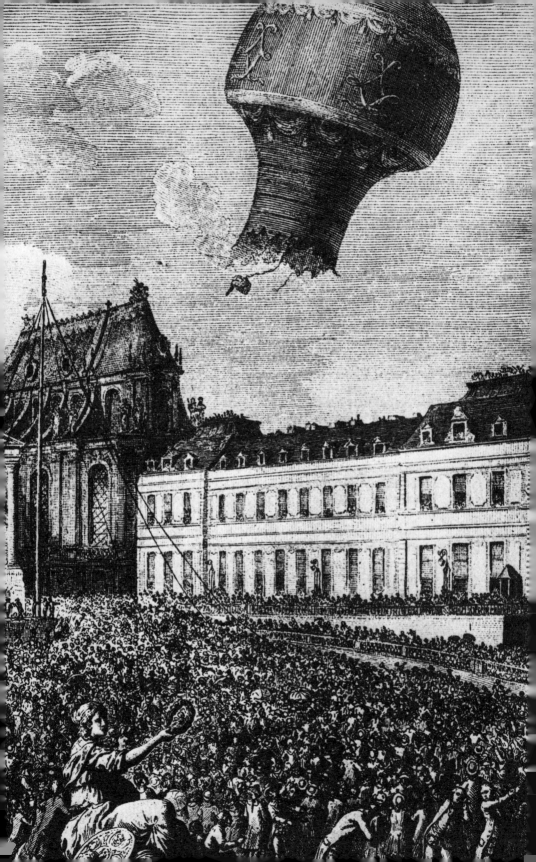

the montgolfiere-type, but once released, the hydrogen-filled envelope rose into the sky with startling speed. The balloonists were airborne for about 25 minutes, during which they flew from Paris to Nesles, a distance of about 27 miles, and reached an altitude of about 9,000 feet. Charles Robert reported the first ill effects of high altitude flight, a sharp pain in one ear, which he deduced as being caused by expansion of air in the inner ear.

Stirred by the spectacle of man-made objects defying the law of gravity, all Paris, it seemed, went balloon crazy. People made their own small balloons, or bought them ready-made, and sent them aloft all over the city. This presented a fire hazard not to be ignored, and finally such balloons were officially banned.

Within a year after the Montgolfiers first flew a balloon, women had also taken to the air. The first ladies of the air age were the Marchioness of Montalambert, the Countess of Montalambert, the Countess de Pondenas and Mme. de Lagarde, who made the ascension in Paris on 20 May 1784, but only in a tethered balloon that rose a short distance above the ground. On 4 June, at Lyons, France, a Mme. Thible accompanied Monsieur Fleurant on a 45-mile flight that reached an altitude of 8,500 feet.

That year, too, the British began launching balloons, and again a physician-chemist, George Fordyce, was the first to do so. However, Fordyce stayed on the ground; it was Vincenzo Lunardi, an Italian, who took off from London the afternoon of 15 September, after days filled with difficulty and confusion in preparing for the flight. He carried a cat, a pigeon, and a dog with him; the pigeon broke loose less than 50 feet from the ground and went home, only to have its feathers plucked out by eager souvenir hunters. The cat and dog survived the two-and-a-half hour trip, despite the cold—they reached 12,000 feet in below-freezing temperatures—and Lunardi was berated by Horace Walpole for risking the cat's life. Samuel Johnson, tired of balloon talk, said he would rather see a cure for asthma.* The rest of London treated

*Nearly two hundred years later, after fantastic sums had been spent to put men on the moon, detractors of the space program said they would have preferred to see the money spent in seeking a cure for cancer. The secret of that cure may be awaiting the biomedical researchers soon to orbit the earth in Spacelab.

On 19 September 1873, the Court of Louis XVI watched a montgolfiere-type balloon make an 8-minute flight from Versailles, carrying a sheep, a duck, and a cock. They all landed safely./Smithsonian Institution

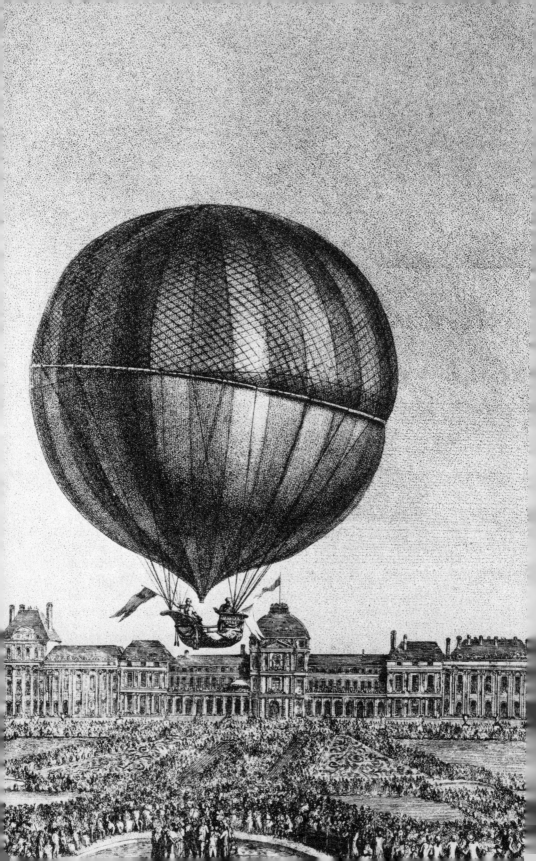

Lunardi with the sort of acclaim Charles Lindbergh received, when he became the first man to fly solo across the Atlantic.

From 1785 on, balloons became as much a part of fetes or celebrations as fireworks, and the state of the art being what it was, balloons sometimes furnished the fireworks. Balloons dotted the skies of Germany, Holland and Belgium. One made a 150-mile flight in France, and one put to sea, as it were, to sail from England to France. That flight was made by a Frenchman, Jean-Pierre Blanchard, accompanied by Dr. John Jeffries, an American physician who paid Blanchard's expenses for the flight—a matter of some 700 pounds sterling.

Another channel crossing got underway from France to England on 15 June 1785, with Pilatre de Rozier and Pierre-Ange Romain using a hydrogen-filled balloon and a brazier to keep the gas hot. The result could have been predicted—fire and hydrogen do not mix—and the balloon exploded at 2,000 feet. The occupants became the first air casualties in history. No matter what caused the disaster, the men died of "injuries, multiple, extreme," the fate of all flyers who finally make the landing they cannot walk away from.

Blanchard was a true professional; he made some fifty ascents, and was the first man to make a balloon flight in the United States. This took place on 9 January 1793, from the Walnut Street Prison yard in Philadelphia, with President George Washington an interested spectator. The flight ended in Gloucester County, New Jersey—15 miles in 46 minutes. Sometimes, even today, the trip takes just as long.

For nearly a century after the first balloons were developed, the state of the art remained about the same; fill the balloon, go up, come down. Almost anyone could do it, and many did. The *Roll of the Aeronauts*, in 1829, named 471 of them. The members of one English family, the Greens, among them made 535 hops. Balloonists rode in open baskets or cars suspended beneath the balloon, and were exposed to the elements and the hazards of the environment in which they flew. This first age of ballooning

On 1 December 1783, Benjamin Franklin was among the crowd of 400,000 who watched Charles and Marie-Noel Robert take off from Paris on a 25-minute flight that carried them to Nesles, 27 miles away./*Smithsonian Institution*

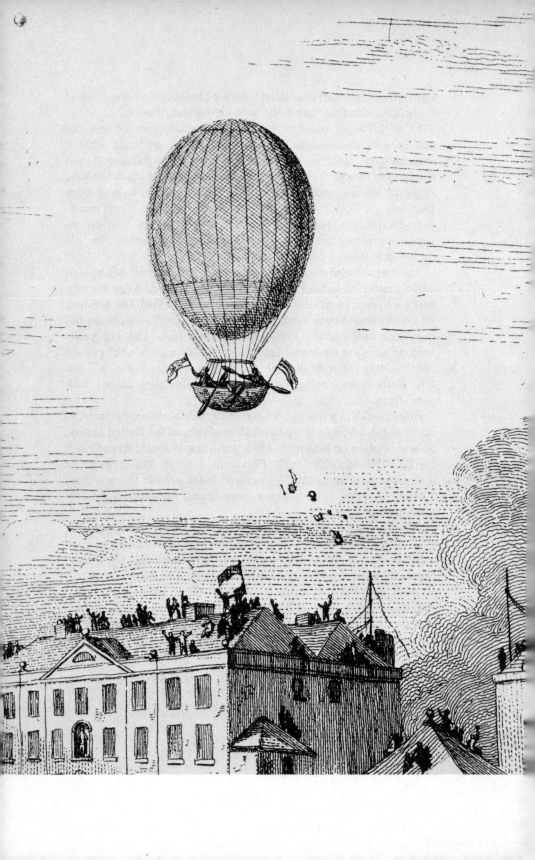

continued into the 20th century, and ended only with the advent of the pressurized gondola.

This—the ancestor of modern spacecraft—was developed by Jean and Auguste Piccard, in Switzerland, and opened the way to stratospheric flight. In August, 1931, Auguste Piccard and Paul Kipfer, riding in a pressurized gondola, reached a record altitude of 51,961 feet over Bavaria. All subsequent high-altitude flights were made under closed environment situations.

However, long before that time, the physiological effects of flight were being studied, some of the hazards were identified, and the first flight protection equipment came into use. At altitudes above 10,000 feet, the human body is subject to the effects of hypoxia, dysbarism, and extreme cold. An early experience with these hazards came in 1804, when on 7 October three Italians, Andreoli, Brasette, and Count Zambeccari, took off from Bologna in a balloon that, due to faulty piloting techniques, first reached an altitude where their hands and feet froze, they vomited and lost consciousness, and then dropped until they were dunked into the Adriatic Sea. Finally hauled out by a ship, all three men suffered from exposure and frostbite, and Zambeccari lost all his fingers as a result.

The history of aerospace medicine may be said to have commenced with the flights of two Frenchmen, Croce-Spinelli and Sivel, in 1874-75. They prepared for their flight by working with Paul Bert, who held the chair of physiology at the Faculte des Sciences in Paris, where they made simulated flights to indicated altitudes of about 23,000 feet in a pressure chamber. But in an actual flight, on 15 April 1875, when they were accompanied by Gaston Tissandier and reached an altitude of 28,000 feet, they failed to use their oxygen supply properly and all three men fell unconscious. Croce-Spinelli and Sivel died, the first victims of aviation hypoxia.

The symptoms of hypoxia—lack of sufficient oxygen in the body—had been described by a Spanish priest, Joseph de Acosta,

The world's first professional balloonist was Jean-Pierre Blanchard, a Frenchman, who made more than 50 ascents in France and the United States. Here he is pictured lifting off from the Royal Military Academy at Little Chelsea on 16 October 1784, on a cross-channel flight to France, with Dr. John Jeffries, an American, as passenger./*Smithsonian Institution*

11

in his book, *Natural y Moral de las Indias,* published in Seville in 1590. The book was translated and reprinted in London in 1604, but because it concerned the natural history of the "Indies," probably no balloonist ever read it. However, what Acosta had encountered in the high mountains of Peru, was acute altitude sickness, the same mysterious ailment that was fatal to some balloonists before men learned what it was and how to prevent it. The symptoms were shortness of breath, headache, impaired ability to concentrate or perform complex tasks, and sometimes nausea and vomiting. Acosta's description is quoted* here; one might wish that all modern biomedical texts were written with such colorful detail:

I thought good to speake this, to shew a strange effect, which happens in some parts of the Indies, where the ayre & the wind that rains make men dazie, not lesse, but more than at sea. Some hold it for a fable, others say is is an addition; for my part I will speake what I have tried.

There is in Peru, a high mountaine which they call Pariacaca, and having heard speake of the alteration it bred, I went as well prepared as I could, according to the instructions which was given me, by such as they call Vaguianos or expert men; but notwithstanding all my provision, when I came to mount the degrees, as they call them, which is the top of the mountaine, I was suddenly surprized with so mortall and strange a pang, that I was ready to fall from the top to the ground, and although we were many in company, yet every one made haste (without any tarrying for his companion) to free himselfe speedily from this ill passage.

Being then alone with one Indian, whom I intreated to helpe to stay me, I was surprised with such pangs of straining & casting, as I thought to cast up my heart too; for having cast up meate, fleugme, & choller, both yellow and greene; in the end I cast up blood, with the straining of my stomache.

To conclude, if this had continued, I should undoubtedly have died; but this lasted not above three or four hours, where all our companions (being foureteene or fifteene) were

*This quotation faithfully follows the old English version, except for the substitution of *s* instead of *f* as appropriate.

much wearied. Some in the passage demaunded confession, thinking verily to die; others left the ladders and went to the ground, beeing overcome with casting, and going to the stoole; and it was told me, that some have lost their lives there with this accident.

I beheld one that did beate himselfe against the earth, crying out for the rage and griefe which this passage of Paiacaca hadde caused. But commonly it dooth no important harme, onely this, paine and troublesome distaste while it endures: and not onely the passage of Pariacaca hath this propertie, but also all this ridge of the mountaine, which runs five hundred leagues long...

And no doubt but the winde is the cause of this intemperature and strange alteration, of the air that raignes there. For the best remedy (and they all find) is to stoppe their noses, their eares, and their mouthes, as much as may be, and to cover themselves with cloathes, especially the stomacke, for that the ayre is subtile and piercing, going into the entrailes, and not onely men feele this alteration, but also beasts that sometimes stay there, so as there is no spurre can make them goe forward...I therefore perswade my selfe, that the element of the aire is there so subtile and delicate, as it is not proportionale with the breathing of man, which requires a more grosse and temperate aire, and I beleeve it is the cause that doth so much alter the stomacke, & trouble all the disposition.

The...mountains...of Europe, which I have seene, although the aire be colde there, and doth force men to weare more clothes, yet this colde doth not take away the appetite from meate, but contrariwise it provokes; neyther dooth it cause any casting of the stomacke, but onely some paine in the feete and handes...But that of the Indies, whereof I speake (without molesting of foote or hand, or any outward parte) troubles all the entrailes within: and that which is more admirable, when the sunne is hote, which maketh mee imagine, that the griefe wee feele comes from the qualitie of the aire which wee breathe: Therefore that is most subtile and delicate, whose colde is not so sensible, as piercing.

Acosta was correct in his assumption "that the griefe wee feele comes from the qualities of the air which wee breathe..."

13

Atmospheric pressure reduces with altitude, decreasing the amount of oxygen available in the lungs, and some people will become acutely ill after several hours at altitudes of only 12,000 feet. Only with the advent of pressurized closed gondolas, and pressurized suits and cabins, was it possible for men to carry with them the oxygen supply that made it possible to reach high altitudes in safety.

No physician, Acosta's experience made him, in the words of Dr. Hubertus Strughold, "the pioneer in the field of altitude sickness and, so to speak, the earth-bound Columbus of the vertical frontier." But although Acosta was first to describe the "mortal and strange pang" caused by oxygen deficiency, two more centuries would pass before men ascertained exactly what it was that was deficient. Again, quoting Strughold, "From the time of the Greeks throughout the Middle Ages, they called this mysterious energy-producing agent in the air 'pneuma' or 'phlogiston' and 'igneo-aerial-spirit,' Finally, around 1800, Joseph Priestly, in England, and Carl Wilhelm Scheele, in Sweden, discovered the element oxygen and its property as a fire substance. Earlier, Antoine Lavoisier, in Paris, recognized its function in respiration and called it the " 'life substance' and 'element of fire.' "

By the end of the 19th century, it appeared that the ceiling for conventional balloons was about 30,000 feet, and that even by breathing oxygen, men could hope to reach no higher than 41,000 feet. Tests by the U.S. Army Air Corps, in 1927, confirmed both the risks and limitations of high-altitude flights.

At Scott Field, Illinois, on 4 May 1927, Army Captain Hawthorne C. Gray took off to establish a world altitude record. Breathing oxygen carried in steel flasks, and wearing a fur-lined suit, he reached 40,000 feet and then 42,470 feet. There he began feeling the effects of hypoxia, and started his descent, but the balloon began to fall out of control and Gray bailed out to make a parachute landing.

On 4 November, Gray made another attempt at the altitude record. At higher altitudes, his log showed the deterioration in handwriting that comes with oxygen deficiency. He reached his previous high—42,470 feet—and started down. But his oxygen supply was exhausted, and he was dead when the balloon landed.

14

Man, a terrestrial animal, evolved and developed at the bottom of an ocean of air. As early balloonists ventured higher into the sky, they soon met the grim barriers—lack of oxygen, and cold—beyond which unprotected flight was impossible. Flight was limited to the troposphere, the layer of atmosphere about six miles deep, and even there the upper reaches were hazardous.

The solution to flight above the troposphere, and into the stratosphere, was simple in concept. The balloonist had to make the flight in an earth-type environment. Like so many other solutions which were simple in concept, but considerably more difficult in execution, there had to be much tedious work of the sort now called research and development (R & D) before the idea was ready to fly. The big step into those remote upper reaches was made possible by Auguste Piccard, who worked out the details of a pressurized cabin with its own self-contained oxygen supply, a system for elimination of carbon dioxide, and heat control.

The first "space capsule" in which Piccard reached into the stratosphere—51,795 feet, on 27 May 1931—was fabricated by a beer-barrel manufacturer, who supplied windows and hatches as directed by Piccard. The capsule was pressurized at one atmosphere—the normal sea-level pressure—and carbon dioxide was absorbed by alkali. Heat control was another matter. It was known that objects exposed to direct sunlight, even in the cold of high altitudes, could grow very hot. Only by actual flight into the stratosphere could the problem of heat control be solved.

On his first flight Piccard had the capsule painted white on one side, black on the other, but it did not rotate as planned, and the interior temperature reached 100°F. Next he tried an all-white capsule, in which temperature dropped to 0°F. Finally the capsule was painted white on top, black on the bottom; this produced an inside temperature of 67°F while the outside temperature was —67°F. In Apollo flights to the moon, comfortable temperature was maintained by passive thermal control (PTC); the spacecraft was set in rotation about its logitudinal axis, one revolution every 20 minutes. Safe stratospheric flight opened the way for high-altitude research in many fields, and for nearly the next thirty years a vast amount of scientific knowledge was brought back to earth by flights that finally reached to the very edge of space.

The flight of the balloon, Century of Progress, was indicative of the trend away from "wild blue yonder" adventure into the fields of pure science. That balloon, constructed by the Goodyear Aircraft Company, took off from Chicago on 20 November 1933, with Lieutenant Commander Thomas G. W. Settle as pilot and Major Chester Fordney, U.S Marine Corps, as scientific observer.

On the flight, they made observations which were vital in the future development of nuclear physics, long before the term became a part of everyday language. Along with cameras, radio, and a quartz spectrograph, they carried Geiger-Muller counter, ionization chambers, and films of cosmic ray studies. In a flight lasting some eight hours, the craft reached 61,237 feet before landing in New Jersey. Its chief value lay in proving that more than 99 per cent of high-altitude radiation consisted of protons from outer space, and that gamma rays produced in the earth's atmosphere were comparatively scarce.

Further cosmic ray studies were made in 1934 and 1935 during the flights of Explorer I and Explorer II, in both of which the U.S. Army Air Corps took part. These were monsters of balloons, with a capacity of more than 3,000,000 cubic feet. Explorer I reached 60,000 feet but the flight was cut short when a gas bag tore. Explorer II, next up, finally reached an altitude of 72,395 feet, and again brought back valuable readings on the levels of cosmic radiation at high altitudes. That flight also succeeded in capturing bacteria and molds at altitudes of 36,000 feet and marked the beginning of space biology.

High-altitude exploration, and especially lighter-than-air development was soon put on the back burner as military build-ups in Europe and the United States stressed heavier-than-air craft with greater speeds and heavier pay loads. Combat effectiveness depended on aircraft design to meet impact and centrifugal force, development of protective clothing, and better understanding of the physical and physiological functions of men involved in combat flying. Aeromedical research became of prime importance (see Chapters 2 thru 4) and by 1953 a Space Biology Branch of the Aeromedical Field Laboratory was established at Holloman Air Force Base under Major David G. Simons, U.S. Air Force.

Rockets, which had been developed by the Germans during World War II were utilized in research at Holloman, but balloons were used by the hundreds; they were less expensive, and had the advantage of being able to remain at altitudes for longer periods, and also of having their flight terminated by radio control. Space biology studies benefitted from many major technological improvements, including those developed away from the Air Force Missile Development Center by private enterprise. In turn, Aeromedical Field Laboratory flight experience was made available to help other balloon operations.

One World War II development—light-weight polyethylene film about 2/1000" thick—greatly advanced the art of high-altitude balloon flight. The film, in transparent bags, has since then made it easier to inspect packaged fruit and vegetables in supermarkets. The first use of such material for stratospheric flights resulted in the Navy's Skyhook program—Moby Dick—all with unmanned balloons. The film was being produced by General Mills, Incorporated, and the idea of using it in balloons was suggested by Jean Piccard, a consultant for that firm. A General Mills engineer, Otto Winzen, who developed the film, took the plan to the Office of Naval Research, where Lieutenant Commander George Hoover saw the possibilities in it. Project Helios was initiated, after which, it might be said, "the balloon went up."

The first Skyhook flight on 25 September 1947 reached 100,000 feet. All Skyhook balloons were unmanned, although some carried mice in cosmic ray research, which proved that exposure to such rays in the stratosphere was in no way as dangerous as feared. Many such balloons were torn apart in the jet streams, a phenomenon existing at altitudes few aircraft had reached.* Other balloons were chased—but never caught—by pilots who sometimes reported that they were after flying saucers.

The development of still larger plastic balloons marked the last stage in balloon flight for research purposes. A 2,000,000-cubic foot balloon, produced by Winzen Research Incorporated, reached an altitude of more than 120,000 feet over South St. Paul, Minnesota, on 18 July 1955, and the next day a similar balloon reached 126,000 feet, a record for the Aeromedical Field Laboratory program and for polyethylene balloons as a class. Such balloons were vital in biological research, as they permitted much longer exposure of individual specimens; in 1954, for example, test laboratory mice had been kept aloft for more than 74 hours on two separate flights.

*The first aircraft to encounter the jet stream was the Winnie Mae, piloted by Wiley Post during his pioneering high-altitude pressure-suit tests of 1934-35.

17

The next step in high-altitude balloon flight represented solid aeromedical research, with an experienced flight surgeon as one of the participants. On 8 November 1956, two naval officers, Lieutenant Commanders M. Lee Lewis and Malcolm D. Ross, took off from the Stratobowl near Rapid City, South Dakota, in Stratolab 1. They wore partial pressure suits, and had electrodes attached to their bodies so that ground stations could monitor pulse and respiration, breathing and heart action. The flight surgeon, Captain Norman Lee Barr, (MC), U.S. Navy, monitored the physiological processes of the balloonists from a chase plane. The artificial atmosphere in the gondola was maintained at a pressure altitude of 17,000 feet, oxygen was fed in through a converter, and a chemical absorption system removed carbon dioxide and water vapor.

Barr, naturally, was aware of the hazard of fire in artificial environments, and had conducted some experiments in extinguishing fires in gondolas. It was determined that if the oxygen concentration in a gondola exceeded 335 millimeters out of a total of 760 millimeters mercury pressure, a fire in the gondola could not be extinguished. In the high-altitude balloon flights, it was standard practice to use a mix of nitrogen and oxygen, with the oxygen content at 150 millimeters. There was always the safety factor of reduced outside pressure—if a fire did start in a capsule, opening any vent to the outside would have literally blown the fire out into space.

In the initial Apollo missions, the spacecraft atmosphere was maintained at 100 per cent oxygen. Unfortunately this condition existed when testing went on for Apollo 7; during a preflight test on the ground, an electrical malfunction turned it into a flaming inferno. Gus Grissom, Ed White and Roger Chaffee burned to death in far less time than the 90 seconds it would have required to open the escape hatch. Subsequent spacecraft were maintained on the pad at 40 per cent nitrogen and 60 per cent oxygen in the cabin. Post-launch, the mix was converted to 100 per cent oxygen.

The Stratolab I flight terminated, after reaching an altitude of 76,000 feet, when the balloon lost part of its helium. The gondola came down at 800 feet per minute, a near-crash landing in which fortunately, the occupants were unhurt. In the next two years Ross

18

and Lewis made three more flights, setting a record of 85,700 feet. It was a quirk of fate that Lewis, who had flown nearly 17 miles high, was killed by a falling piece of hoisting gear while standing in a gondola three feet off the ground. The last flight in that program, Stratolab IV, indicated one use for the Spacelab planned for orbital flight in the 1980s—the gondola carried a 16-inch reflecting telescope and spectrograph for observations of the planet Venus.

In 1956-57 the Aeromedical Field Laboratory and the Space Biology Branch began to cut back on the cosmic radiation program to concentrate on Project Man-High which was planned to explore the environment in which missiles and high-performance aircraft would operate, and to test an effective sealed cabin. Three Man-High ascents were made, with a single pilot riding each flight. It was time, ruled Colonel John Paul Stapp, to put a man up where the monkeys had gone because: "...no amount of training will make a scientific observer out of a monkey, though the reverse has sometimes been true."

The first test pilot for Man-High was Air Force Captain Joseph W. Kittinger, Jr. On 2 June 1957, Kittinger reached the extreme altitude of 96,000 feet. Due to a faulty aneroid flow control connection that let his oxygen supply discharge into space instead of into the capsule, he landed after four and a half hours with his entire 40-hour supply exhausted. At that point his duration of effective consciousness was fast approaching the zero mark. Earlier in the flight, as his blood oxygen content was decreasing and ground control became aware of his condition, there were signs of impaired judgement; ground control ordered him to terminate the flight and he answered "Come and get me."

The Man-High II program was originally planned to study the genetic effects of cosmic radiation, as well as to investigate the effects of cosmic rays on a high altitude pilot. Containers of neurospora mold were carried underneath the balloon capsule, and the pilot, Major David Simons, carried track plates attached to his body as a means of monitoring cosmic ray exposure. Such research could not be conducted under laboratory conditions for two reasons: it had to be high enough above the earth to be nearly on the edge of space where cosmic rays were more numerous, and it had to be in an area of reduced magnetic attraction, as the stronger

19

equatorial magnetic field had shielding effect on cosmic rays. For these reasons, cosmic radiation research is best conducted at altitudes above 100,000 feet and in latitudes above 55°N.

However, as the program went on, and it was recognized that the balloon capsule was an ideal simulator for space flight conditions, investigations were carried on in a wide range of phenomena covering physiological, psychological, and technical conditions. To permit ground monitoring of all flight parameters, a highly sophisticated telemetering system—compatible with rocket telemetry—was developed to record physiological data in ground units: this included respiration, electrocardiogram, galvanic skin response (GSR), and body temperature. Technically primitive at first, by the time the Apollo program ended it was highly sophisticated—a doctor on the ground in Houston could check the pulse of an astronaut on the moon (See Chapter 6).

Temperature control within the capsule was a highly critical problem, as the balloon would operate in long-term exposures of sunlight alternated with extreme cold of night. By contrast, later orbital flights would subject a spacecraft to days and nights no more than 45 minutes long; eventually, craft en route to the moon would rotate on their axis so that "day" and "night" exposures were at times even shorter.

A temperature control system using boiling water as a coolant was pretested at the Holloman Air Force Base and flight tested for the first time on balloon missions in 1953. The effect of high altitude on normal physical laws is that at decreased atmospheric pressure, water boils at lower temperature. At 112,000 feet, the boiling point is a mere 32°F.—the same temperature that at sea level would produce solid ice. Thus, water in a capsule container vented to the exterior would boil at the reduced outside pressure, and as air inside the capsule circulated around the container, heat was carried off to the outside by vapor from the boiling water.

As developed for Man-High II, capsule temperature was controlled by a finned-tube water core heat exhanger. There were no provisions for adding heat, as body heat from the pilot, and heat generated by electrical systems would compensate for any heat loss. At first ethyl chloride was used in the ʻsystem, but finally it was adapted to water, which weighed less and at 100,000 feet

20

would boil in average capsule temperature. The heat exchanger would remove 1600 BTU per hour under normal conditions.

Initial experiments in heat control were made with laboratory mice, and to simplify things Simons measured their heat production in "mouse units." Later, guinea pigs tested out at about 2.5 mouse units, and a small monkey at about 10 mouse units. Considering metabolic output and consumption, an average man checked out at 500 mouse units; by the time Simons had a system that handled 250 to 300 mouse units, he knew it would soon be able to handle a man.

In preparing for actual Man-High II flights, Simons took parachute and balloon training. The object of the flight was to establish a record of 24 hours aloft while reaching an altitude of more than 100,000 feet. At that level, he would be perched on the very threshold of space and pushing the frontiers of feasibility for lighter-than-air flight just about as high as man and material could take it.

Before the first ascent, he underwent a simulated flight in an altitude chamber at Wright Field's Instrumentation Test Section. The simulation involved putting Simons inside his pressure suit, sealing him in, and then putting the capsule inside the test chamber, a worthwhile idea because the capsule developed an oxygen leak and the first simulated flight had to be terminated after six hours.

During the simulated flight, Simons checked out his equipment: a 5-inch telescope, a photoelectric cell to measure the brightness of the sky, and a 16mm motion picture camera and a 35mm still camera. He also monitored the oxygen and carbon dioxide content of the capsule, and watched his own physical condition. It was there that the simulated flight ran into difficulties. After several hours, he began experiencing diarrhea cramps and at the same time his bladder demanded urgent relief. The test finally had to be terminated. Once the chamber pressure was back to normal— ground level—Simons set a new record getting out of a pressure suit.

"Preflight" preparations pointed the way to those physical "indignities" the astronauts would endure a few years later: urinalysis, blood samples, electrocardiograms, temperature, hormone determination, and white blood cell count. Simons went on a low-residue diet for three days—gelatin, fish, lean steak—because, as he put it, the capsule "was not large enough to contain a men's room, and even if it did, pressure suits are not built with a flap in the back." His food supply for 24 hour was not exactly the gourmet quality served in first class passenger cabins twenty years later—it consisted of half a dozen Butterfinger, O-Henry, and Hershey bars, four cans of fruit juice (pineapple, orange, V-8, grapefruit) and four sandwiches (cheeseburgers, ham, and beef). Simons ate the sandwiches during the long truck ride to the launch site, as he was afraid they might spoil in the heat.

The actual Man-High II flight was made from an open iron mine pit near Crosby, Minnesota, on 19-20 August 1957. The tedious preflight routine of later spaceflights became evident in the preparations. Simons was sealed in the capsule, in the Winzen

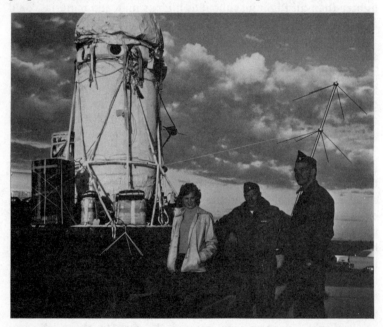

Somewhat resembling an overgrown GI can, the capsule for Man High III, with Lieutenant McClure aboard as pilot, before take off from Holloman AFB. "Ground crew" consists of Vera Winzen, Rufus Hessberg, and David Simons./*Rufus Hessberg*

22

plant in Minneapolis, at 10:43 p.m., the night before the launch and—first example of the "man in a can" role alluded to by later astronauts—was trucked 90 miles out to the launch site while 50 pounds of dry ice atop the capsule, and external air coolers piped into the capsule, kept him from baking in the sultry night.

The process of inflating a 30-story-high balloon was as time consuming as that of fueling a Saturn rocket would be ten years later, and, like the fueling job, could be complicated by a most inconsequential detail. For that flight, it was a plastic band that managed to get itself wrapped around the neck of the balloon after inflation began. This meant that the bottom of the balloon was sealed, and at high altitude reduced air pressure would let the helium expand and explode the balloon. The band was about 30 feet above the ground—impossible to reach. A frantic search around the mine turned up an extension ladder, and while six men held it in place Vera Winzen, who could get dizzy on a kitchen stool, climbed up and cut the band. Having helped in the construction of the balloon, she had the only tool no aviator would ever have thought of carrying—a pair of scissors.

Finally, at 9:22 the morning of 19 August, Man-High II, with the official call letters NCA 38, started its climb into space at the rate of 1200 feet per minute. Four hours later Simons had reached a ceiling of 101,516 feet. The flight terminated at Aberdeen, South Dakota, exactly 32 hours and 3 minutes after lift-off.*

A noteworthy aspect of the flight was the continuous radio link with what later would be termed "ground control," but which for this flight was a van, on loan from the Office of Naval Research (ONR), filled with radio gear. From time to time the van upped-anchor and chased the balloon across the flat landscape of Minnesota and South Dakota, in order to keep within communication and visual range.

The ground control group, headed by Colonel John Paul Stapp, made the difference between success and failure. Instructions radioed from the ground enabled Simons to control the ascent and descent of the balloon within safe limits, and helped him to keep

*The crow-flight distance was about 200 miles. Ground speed was about 6mph. A much faster cross-country flight was made by a Frenchman named Vibert, who in 1871 flew from Paris to near the Zuyder Zee, about 285 miles, at an average speed of 95mph.

23

clear of possibly destructive storm clouds. Also, and most important, ground observers monitoring the physical condition and mental alertness of the pilot were able to recognize sluggish reactions or confused thinking which a man, alone in the vastness of space, might not be aware of. Twice Colonel Stapp had to direct Simons to eat a candy bar to build up his energy.

Temperature control, and the resulting heat exhaustion and fatigue, had been a problem in the Man-High II flight; so also, had been carbon dioxide concentration, or more exactly, lack of understanding of the problem. When Simons reported a four per cent concentration, ground control ordered him down, failing to realize that four per cent at a pressure altitude of 25,000 feet was about the equivalent of two per cent at sea level.

The next high-altitude flight, Man-High III, with First Lieutenant Clifton McClure as pilot, came close to a fatal ending. Among other reasons for being selected to make the flight, McClure had no gray hair on his body. Cosmic rays have the effect of producing gray hairs, on mice and men; gray mice were used in cosmic ray experiments until that fact was realized, after which black mice got the job. Simons had proved an unsuitable subject for cosmic ray research because he already had gray hair before he made the flight.

Man-High III got off to a bad start, although no one but McClure knew it. Weather had delayed operations for a few days in Minnesota, so finally all equipment was trucked down to Holloman Air Force Base. There, on 7 October, as the balloon was being inflated, a breeze came up; soon it freshened, slapped the balloon to the ground, and destroyed it. The ground crew worked all day and night, getting another balloon ready, and by midnight they were ready to go again. About one in the morning, McClure climbed into the capsule, and as he settled in his seat, he accidentally brushed against the restraining pins in his emergency chest parachute, and it opened. He was instantly buried in a hundred yards of parachute nylon.

If the chute had to be repacked out on the ground, the flight would be delayed, and very likely scrubbed completely by oncoming bad weather. For hours, McClure folded and packed the chute, without letting anyone outside know his predicament, and very nearly killed himself in the process. The launch was uneventful, but by the time the balloon had reached 90,000 feet where the outside temperature was -73°F., the internal temperature was 118°F. Worse, McClure's rectal temperature had climbed to 104.1°—firm indication of near physical collapse. As the ground crew considered bringing the flight down, McClure begged to stay up. Before the capsule landed, his heart rate was 180, respiration nearly five times higher than normal, and rectal temperature 106.6°. His body temperature was 108.5° when he landed, but he survived.

Possibly it all boiled down to the restraining pins on the parachute not being tight, or the chute being stowed in the wrong position. McClure's efforts in packing the chute produced more perspiration than the potassium hydroxide water absorbing system could handle, and it heated up. As heat flowed into the capsule, McClure perspired more, and the heat increased; yet despite the heat, he kept cool mentally.

The people at Holloman saw the point. Future capsule ventilation systems would be improved, and future astronauts would be carefully screened for the motivation, emotional determination, and psychophysiological stamina essential to high performance in the strangeness of space. And medical telemetry, as developed in Project Man-High, would be refined to the point where a flight surgeon on the ground in Texas could keep his finger on the pulse of a man on the moon through electronically transmitted physiological measurements.

The slow climb into the skies, commenced by the Montgolfier brothers in France, was picking up speed. Russia put Sputnik into earth orbit on 4 October 1957. Americans would complete many more high-altitude research balloon flights, of which only four manned ascents need mention. In a series of experiments aimed at perfecting a parachute to be used in free-fall from high altitude, the Air Force conducted three Excelsior flights.

The need for improved free-fall techniques arose from the fact that in a high-altitude bailout, a pilot had to drop to 20,000 feet where he had enough oxygen to sustain life, before he opened his parachute. Tests had also shown that in free-fall from high altitudes, a body could be expected to go into a deadly spin rate of up to 465 revolutions a minute.

The project officer for the Excelsior flights was Captain Joseph

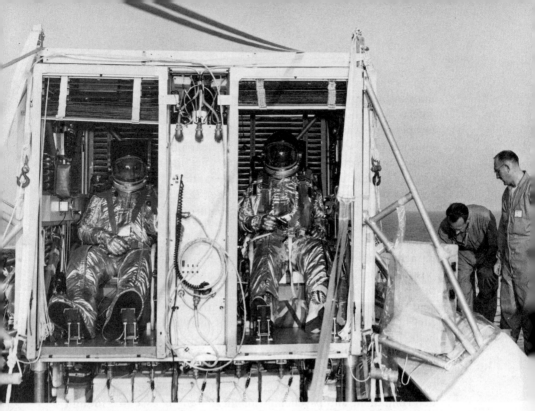

Lieutenant Commander Victor A. Prather and Commander Malcolm D. Ross in the gondola of the Stratolab balloon which set an altitude record of 113,700 feet on 5 May 1961./*U.S. Navy*

W. Kittinger, Jr., and the first flight by Excelsior I was launched on 16 November 1959. Kittinger bailed out at 76,000 feet, with a Beaupre multistage parachute which failed to deploy properly. After falling 65,000 feet—some 12 miles—his reserve chute automatically opened and he landed safely. Kittinger next took Excelsior II to an altitude of 74,700 feet before he bailed out for a successful descent.

Finally, on 16 August 1960, he reached a record altitude of 102,800 feet. Alone in space, with one hand swollen to twice its normal size due to a defective glove, Kittinger described his view of the distant earth and then said: "Man will never conquer space. He will learn to live with it, but he will never conquer it."

Despite his gloomy pronouncement, his jump was successful; he bailed out in a pressure suit and set another record for the longest parachute drop of slightly less than 20 miles. Since then, man has conquered space, to a certain degree. It is hoped that no one will

26

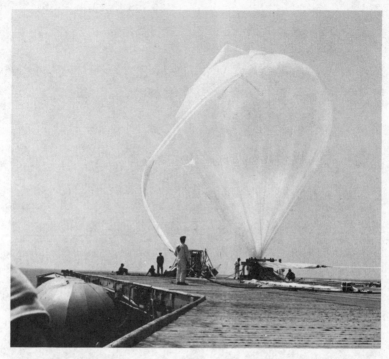

The first balloon flights in Paris were witnessed by vast crowds, but the final high-altitude flights in the United States were made from aircraft carriers, with only a few men on the flight deck to handle inflation of the giant plastic-film envelopes./*U.S. Navy*

ever again have to "hit the silk," protected only by a pressure suit, from such an altitude.

The final test of the full pressure suit was made by Commander Malcolm D. Ross, a naval aviator and balloonist, and Lieutenant Commander Victor A. Prather, a Medical Corps officer, on 4 May 1961. The flight was made in an open gondola suspended from a Stratolab balloon; the balloon, with a 10,000,000 cubic-foot capacity, was the largest ever lofted on a manned flight. At launch, it towered 80 stories high. Because of difficulties with wind effect on such an immense craft, the Navy launched the flight from the aircraft carrier *Antietam* in the Gulf of Mexico; the ship steamed with the wind to reduce its effect to zero speed over the flight deck.

This suits worn by Ross and Prather set the style for those worn

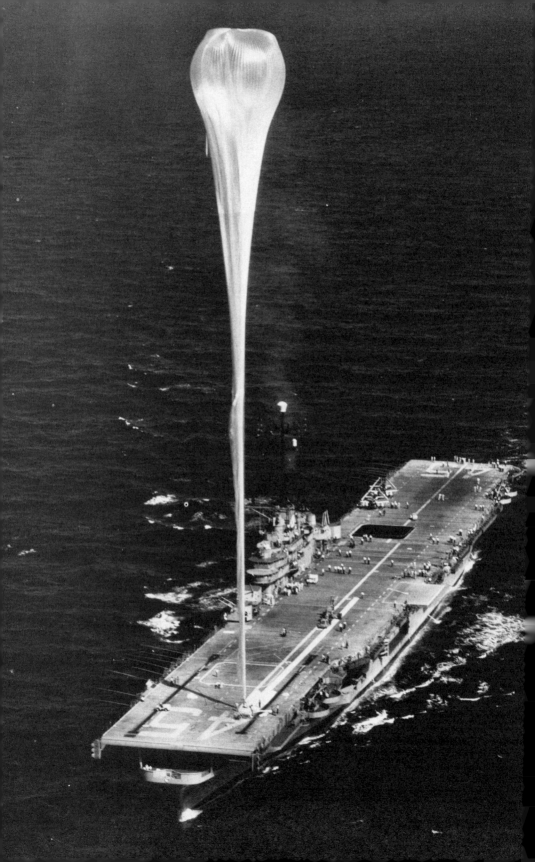

later by astronauts in the Mercury program and proved very effective. At the record altitude of 113,700 feet,* they witnessed the vast blue horizon curve and black sky astronauts would see on their way to the moon. The descent had to be rushed, as oxygen supply was running short, and the gondola splashed down much as astronauts would land later, with helicopters hovering to make the pickup. Then, in an unexplained accident, Prather slipped off the helicopter lifting device and drowned. The frogmen seen dropping alongside capsules in all subsequent splashdowns, ready to recover the returning astronauts, were insurance that such a tragedy would never happen again.

From open baskets to oxygen bottles to sealed gondolas to pressure suits—each development put man one step closer to the moon. The surgeon Pilatre de Rozier, Croce-Spinelli and Sivel, Captain Gray, and Lieutenant Commander Prather, all died in the long process. Some of the smaller mountains on the moon might well be named in their memory.

*The rocket-powered Air Force X-15 exceeded that altitude three times: 246,700 feet on 6 June 1962, 314,750 feet on 17 July 1962, and 354,200 feet on 22 August 1963, but did not *fly* at those altitudes as there was no air to support the craft. It made a trajectory flight out of the lower atmosphere, just as a porpoise gets up speed in the water to leap into the air.

A far cry from Montgolfier's little hot-air paper bag, this Skyhook balloon, with a 10,000,000 cubic foot capacity, towers 80 stories high above the deck of the carrier *Valley Forge* before launching on 30 January 1960./*U.S. Navy*

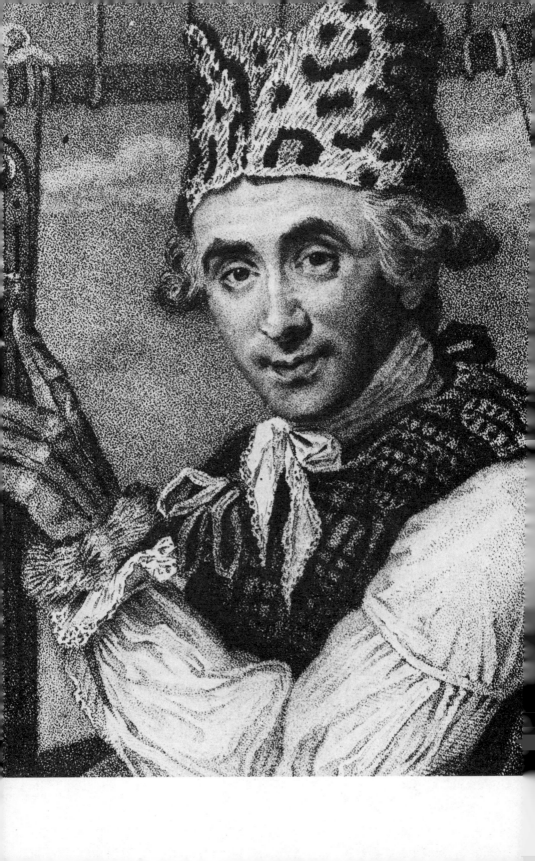

2
Doctors in the Sky

Towering 363 feet into the sky, the Apollo-Saturn spacecraft stood silent, poised for flight. On the morning of 16 July 1969—still less than two centuries after man first left the earth in a balloon—hundreds of thousands of people jammed Cape Canaveral to watch while thousands of engineers, technicians and scientists went through the final moments of the countdown that would send three men to the moon. The command module in which they would travel half a million miles had about the cubic capacity of an average bathroom, and nearly two thirds of that capacity was crammed with highly sophisticated and technical equipment, the black boxes without which no modern pilot, navigator, or astronaut would ever dare to leave the ground. The men had been checked out, plugged in, suited up and strapped down. All systems were go. And with the countdown completed, they went.

The black box and the think-tank experts were confident that the men would reach the moon, complete their mission, and return to earth, despite the misgivings of those doubters who believe that machines were still not to be trusted, and that if men had been meant to fly, they would have been given wings. But the engineers

The first flying doctor was the American, John Jeffries, who, with balloonist Jean Pierre Blanchard, made an ascent over London in 1784, and flew across the English Channel the following year. Jeffries authored the first book on aeronautics./*National Library of Medicine*

31

had reliability factors of 99.999 for their hardware. Their quality control program checked basic components all the way back to their original source as raw ore, traced it from the time it became stock metal, then machined parts, then assembled equipment. Finally whole systems were tested, sometimes to absolute destruction.

But what about the men? There was no way of choosing ancestors for astronauts, let alone selecting the genes and chromosomes that made them tick. While astronauts could be tested, they were not expendable. Their safety demanded the exercise of extreme caution and great dependence on the medical research that had commenced long before most people realized there was a space program.

The complicated process of learning what was "up there" or "what it was like out there" and what the effect might be on humans developed into an involved science that came to be known as Aerospace Medicine. It is new, yet it had its pioneers in the past. In a sense, it is highly specialized with its own procedures and vocabulary; in another sense it is old-fashioned doctoring by people who fly, research, invent, teach, and read science fiction for amusement and relaxation. The one common denominator seems to be a strong curiosity about all things new and mysterious, and this was evident long before the Wright brothers successfully flew in 1903. More than a century before Kitty Hawk, balloons became the vehicles from which physicians could study the physiological problems early aeronauts would face in the upper atmosphere.

But the problems existed long before balloons were invented. "As a science, high mountain physiology is nearly 100 years old." said Dr. Hubertus Strughold.* "Mountain sickness, however, was first described in 1588 by Jose de Acosta. The first inkling of this uncomfortable effect of thin air can be traced back to Greek literature since it was Aristotle who observed that men could not live on the top of the 10,000-foot Mount Olympus in Thessaly without breathing through a wet sponge. So, high mountain physiology, with all its descendants, had its birthplace on a holy mountain dedicated to Zeus or Jupiter."

*Unpublished speech, "From Aviation Medicine to Space Medicine," delivered during the annual meeting of the Aero Medical Association, Washington, D.C., March, 1952.

The first flying doctor was an American from Boston, John Jeffries who became fascinated with ballooning, or "levitation" as it was called in its infancy. He had been practicing medicine in London for several years after the American Revolution, and was impressed by the balloon ascents of that flamboyant Frenchman, Jean Pierre Blanchard, over Paris. On 30 November 1784, he hired Blanchard to take him on a flight over London so that he could make certain scientific observations of the upper air. Jeffries carried a thermometer, barometer, hydrometer, "electrometer" and six glass-stoppered vials filled with distilled water. "...Besides which I took with me a very good telescope, and several yards of very thin light ribbon, colored, which I could occasionally cut into small bits...and had ready in my pocket a sharp strong knife and scissors..." (Jeffries recorded wind currents with his ribbons). During the 81-minute flight over London, the barometer dropped from 30 to 21.25 inches of mercury, representing an altitude gained of about 9,250 feet; the electrometer showed no change, and temperature varied from 51° to 28.50°F. One by one, the water bottles were emptied and air samples collected. These were analyzed by Henry Cavendish, discoverer of hydrogen, with results agreeing closely with modern analyses.

Jeffries also noted the temperature change and the effect of altitude on his ears. "...M. Blanchard now began first to complain of the cold and drew on a thick cap. A little dog which I had taken with me, crumpled himself up at my feet, and began to shake and shed tears with the cold, which I found to be severe, and caused a pain and singing in my ears; on which I followed M. Blanchard's example, and put on a fur cap..."

Jeffries was so elated over his first ballooning adventure he arranged with Blanchard to soar across the English Channel the following year. This feat, along with their earlier ascension over London, marked the first scientific study of upper air composition, the first paid passenger (Jeffries), the first fully successful twosome in the air and the first "airmail" delivery of letters. It also made Jeffries the first American to fly, and the author of the first published book on aeronautics.

There were two other minor "firsts;" the cork vests worn by the pair for overwater survival equipment are not far removed from the underarm life jackets now used in the Air Force. And it was the first recorded requirement for a relief tube for a dual and remarkably functional purpose. This occurred when they ran out of ballast to dump when they were trying to land in France. "...I verily believe, between five and six pounds of urine (were dumped); which circumstance, however trivial or ludicrous it may seem, I have reason to believe, was of real utility to us, in our then situation..."

Jeffries' observations about the cold in the upper air confirmed those made by Jacques Charles who made the world's first flights in hydrogen-filled balloons the previous year. On one flight, Charles reached an altitude of two miles and suffered severely from the cold; it had not yet been established that air temperature decreases about 3.5°F. for every 1,000-foot increase in altitude. It was clear, however, that special protective clothing would have to be developed for aeronauts and later pilots.

Another area of early warning turned up in September, 1784, when the English surgeon, Dr. John Sheldon, made a balloon ascension to study the effects of flight on the human body. He became so terrified that he got sick, and slumped to the bottom of the balloon's basket. This was a clear indication that mental and emotional factors in flight had to be taken seriously.

Of all researchers of early flight, the French physician and physiologist, Paul Bert, made the most thorough and lasting contributions to the knowledge of altitude problems confronting man. Although he was best known during his lifetime for his pioneer work in skin grafting, he later became known as the "Father of Aviation Medicine."

Paul Bert was acquainted with the balloonists of his day and the more he learned of their adventures, the more fascinated he became with the physiology of flight. There was, for example, the flight of Glaisher and Coxwell to 29,000 feet in 1862, during which Glaisher became unconscious due to hypoxia. Coxwell too, nearly blacked out, but was able to pull the balloon's relief rope and valve out gas in time to get them down to an altitude where they could breathe properly again. Bert, who was gathering information on balloonists and mountaineers, wrote in 1869. "I cannot repeat too often that these are reasonings, likelihoods, possibilities at most.

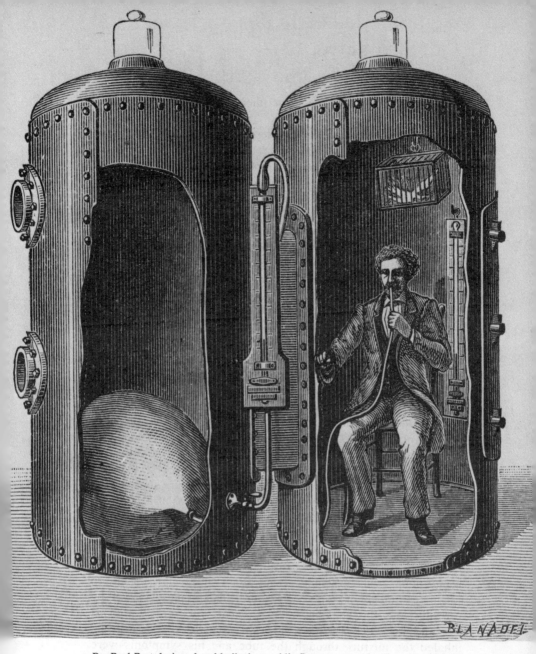

Dr. Paul Bert designed and built the world's first pressure chamber, in which he conducted a number of highly significant experiments in 1874-75. He published the results *La Pression Barometrique, Recherches de Physiologie Experimental* in 1878./National Library of Medicine

When shall we have the experimentation which will bring conviction?''

He began work in his own laboratory, using small animals under bell jars from which the atmosphere was exhausted. He learned that regardless of differences in atmospheric pressure, the partial pressure of oxygen at death averaged 35mm of mercury. Even if the air is enriched with oxygen at the start, 35mm is still found when the animal dies. This means the partial pressure of oxygen is the essential factor in maintaining life in the atmosphere.

Bert then designed and built the world's first pressure chamber which consisted of two adjacent chambers of boiler plate about 6½ feet high and 3¼ feet in diameter. These were connected by a door, and there were portholes through which he could view the subjects in the vacuum created with a steam-driven pump. With this primitive equipment, he could create the equivalent of 36,000 feet of altitude, although most of his experiments were at 28,000 feet. Using large dogs, he showed that with decreased pressure, the heart rate increased as did respiration; digestion was slowed and intestinal gases expanded. Body temperature was lowered and the test subject became dull and listless.

Paul Bert experimented on himself, reaching the pressure altitude of 8,500 feet in 33 minutes. This was not enough to produce hypoxia, but he did notice a slight increase in pulse and gas expansion in his body.

His experiments using pure oxygen at low pressure showed that this prevented altitude sickness. Again using himself as subject, he ran a chamber experiment on 20 February 1874 and reached the pressure equivalent of 16,000 feet of altitude where he remained for an hour and a half (above 11,000 feet). He noted abdominal distention, increase in pulse rate, nausea, and dizziness, and his legs trembled uncontrollably. It was almost impossible for him to calculate numbers in his notebook. But he had prepared himself by carrying into the chamber a bag of air, "extremely rich in oxygen," to which a rubber tube was attached. Periodically he inhaled the mixture through the tube and his symptoms were relieved.

On 10 March 1874, two young scientists, Croce-Spinelli and Sivel, appeared at Bert's laboratory to observe for themselves the "disagreeable effects of decompression and the favourable influence of super-oxygenated air..." Bert took them "up" in the chamber, observing their symptoms at various points. Beyond 20,000 feet, both aeronauts, who had been gay and talkative, became listless and their faces were purple. They had with them the oxygen which they passed back and forth. Croce-Spinelli's dim vision cleared on taking oxygen at 20,000 feet; nausea and other discomforts were relieved.

Bert went into the chamber again on 28 March, going to a pressure altitude of 16,000 feet without oxygen and suffered from nausea and dimness of vision until he inhaled the "super-oxygenated air." He continued to 21,000 feet with no discomfort except intestinal gas, proving that breathing oxygen while ascending (until pressure breathing is required) will eliminate altitude sickness.

Sivel and Croce-Spinelli had been impressed by Bert's experiments and carried several bags of oxygen on their balloon ascent of 22 March 1874. Their balloon, the Etoile Polaire, reached 24,300 feet during the two hour, 40-minute flight, 40 minutes of which was above 16,400 feet. Above 11,800 feet, both aeronauts breathed a mixture of 40 per cent oxygen and 60 per cent nitrogen, and above 19,700 feet, 70 per cent oxygen and 30 per cent nitrogen. Unfortunately neither man realized they should have used the oxygen continuously and their judgement at times was impaired. Although they survived the flight, they became disastrously over-confident during the next feat.

This flight took place on 15 April 1875. They carried a third aeronaut, M. Gaston Tissandier who would increase the drain on their already inadequate supply of oxygen-mix bags. Their goal was 26,200 feet. When they were at 23,000 feet Tissandier who was testing the apparatus wrote, "I breathe oxygen. Excellent effect." The men were so elated they failed to note their pulse increase; certainly they could economize and save their meager supply of oxygen until later. But as Bert had already proved, it didn't work that way. By the time they realized they had to have more oxygen, they could no longer function well enough to obtain it. Tissandier wrote, "Soon I wanted to seize the oxygen tube, but could not raise my arm. My mind, however, was still very lucid...I wanted to cry out, 'We are at 8000 metres! (26,200 feet) But my tongue was paralyzed. Suddenly I closed my eyes and fell inert, entirely losing consciousness...''

When Tissandier awoke, he found his two companions crouched in the basket dead, their heads hidden under their traveling rugs. Like Tissandier, they had been too weak to reach the oxygen tubes when they felt themselves losing consciousness.

Paul Bert mourned at their funeral, "They leap up and death seizes them, without a struggle, without suffering, as a prey fallen to it on those icy regions where an eternal silence reigns. Yes, our unhappy friends have had this strange privilege, this fatal honour, of being the first to die in the heavens."

Some professional contemporaries, not knowing that the young aeronauts had ignored Bert's warning, felt obliged to discredit his theories, based on 670 separate experiments. But time proved he was correct. His monumental work, *La Pression Barometrique, Recherches de Physiologie Experimentale,* published in Paris in 1878, became the basis for high-altitude flight during World War I, 65 years later.

It was a discouraging time for the French high-altitude balloonists, but not for the Germans. They were determined to set a new altitude record, naming meteorological research as the purpose and bringing it under the guidance of the German Association for the Promotion of Airship Travel. Over the years, a number of flights took them higher and higher, with and without oxygen, which added to the physiological data. Conventional balloons of about 70,000 cubic feet appeared to have a top ceiling of 30,000 feet which was not as high as people wanted to go for their weather and physiological studies.

Then, in 1901 the Association was presented with a huge balloon of nearly 300,000 cubic feet capacity, which by using hydrogen could go to 39,400 feet. But could humans tolerate such an altitude, even using oxygen?

The Viennese physiologist, Hermann von Schrotter, whose name stands second only to Paul Bert in the development of aviation medicine, came up with part of the answer. He instructed meteorology professors Berson and Suring in how to recognize the effects of thin air at high altitudes, on pulse, blood pressure and respiration, in his pneumatic chamber. He also supervised the loading of the oxygen equipment in the huge balloon's basket. He wanted face-fitting masks to be used so that if the aeronauts became unconscious they could still get the oxygen. But he was voted down in favor of the glass-tube mouthpieces.

On 11 July 1901, the huge balloon Preussen had a trial flight near Berlin and on 31 July, Berson and Suring were ready for their real attempt. They carried metorological instruments, food and drink, oxygen apparatus and fur flight clothing with fur boots and reindeer-skin jackets.

Within forty minutes of lift off they were at 16,000 feet, breathing oxygen comfortably but distinctly noticing their fatigue. At 33,000 feet, the temperature had dropped from 22°F. to -40°F. But they were beyond the limits of their pipestem mouthpieces. Actually, even with a tight-fitting facemask and 100 per cent oxygen, the arterial blood saturation begins to fall at 33,000 feet. At 34,500 Berson realized he would have to open the valve and descend; as he did so, Suring lost consciousness and Berson collapsed soon after. Luckily Suring revived, put his own oxygen tube in his companion's mouth, then collapsed again. About 45 minutes later they awakened at 20,000 feet; both had headaches, nausea, weakness and drowsiness. They landed safely after their seven-and-a-half-hour flight, and afterwards, Suring reported on the known symptoms of anoxia with von Schrotter's theories.

These theories spelled out in detail the limits to which man could go without oxygen, in what amount, and the upper limit of the use of oxygen. At 16,400 feet, the report stated, a mild oxygen deficiency is noticed, even without exertion; between 19,700 feet to 23,000 feet, it is possible to partially adapt and acclimatize to the thin air, but at 26,200 feet, survival absolutely demanded oxygen for breathing. Suring also pointed out that individual tolerance of altitude did not depend on physical acts such as shallow breathing, but on the oxygen saturation of the blood. And this required a tightly fitted mask which forced the person to breathe the oxygen. A tube with a mouthpiece would no longer be sufficient, "...for in proportion to the general decreases in pressure the partial pressure of the inspired oxygen decreases also, and finally a situation develops where a too-small amount of the gas is delivered to the lungs. Calculations indicate that this will develop at an atmospheric pressure of 116mm, which corresponds to an altitude of about 19,000 feet, but since a further drop in pressure must be taken into consideration with transfer of the oxygen to the blood, the altitude is further reduced, and the top limit to which one may go in an open balloon basket is now established at 41,000 feet, should one desire to break the present altitude record, von Schrotter recommends a hermetically sealed gondola constructed like a diving bell...'' Present scientific knowledge indicates 364.4mm pressure for 19,000 feet.

The flight of Berson and Suring, along with the research of von Schrotter on the effect of reduced partial pressures of oxygen at high altitude, had a profound effect on future ventures. It meant that as early as 1901, von Schrotter was already recommending pressurized gondolas such as those used by Auguste Piccard and later, David Simons. The same principles would be applied to aircraft cabins, and finally spacecraft. These data were accepted for World War I flying and, with further research and modifications, adapted for World War II. Today, military pilots must use oxygen at 10,000 feet; 16,400 feet is considered the "disturbance" zone, and 23,000 feet is the "critical" zone. Von Schrotter's upper limit of 41,000 feet with ordinary oxygen equipment is about what the modern pilot can withstand if he uses 100 per cent oxygen and a tight-fitting mask. And the Viennese physiologist was quite right when he predicted that above that limit, pressurized breathing equipment would be needed to maintain adequate blood oxygenation.

During this period, other problems of aviation medicine showed up. People were experimenting with kites and gliders. In 1896 glider pilot Otto Lilienthal crashed near Stollen, Germany, and died of injuries the next day. In 1899, Percy Pilcher crashed his glider near Stanford Hall in England and died two days later. These accidents foretold the future role of flight surgeons in developing protective and restraining gear for pilots.

Low temperatures, insufficient oxygen at high altitudes, effects of pressure changes on the human body, psychological effects of flight, crash injuries and motion sickness, had all been experienced and recorded before the first powered flight took place. Most of the information awaited scientific interpretation. A sincere attempt was made in 1910 by French medical doctors Rene Cruchet and Rene Moulinier who tested nine pilots during the

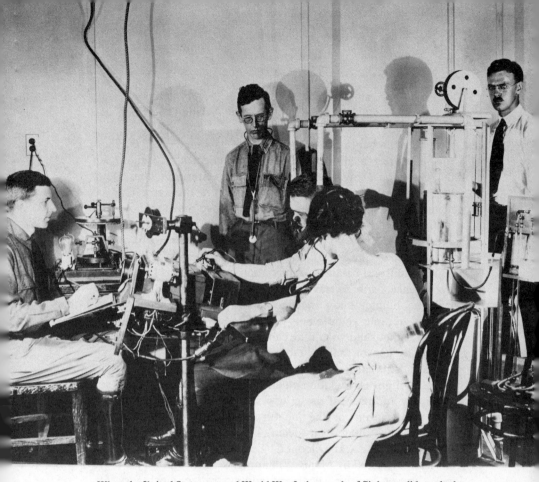

When the United States entered World War I, thousands of flight candidates had to be screened, but in those days, aviation medicine was far from an exact science. This flight candidate is taking the "Altitude Classification Test."/*U.S. Army*

aviation festival of Bordeaux. They measured blood pressure before take-off and after landing and published a paper purporting to describe "aviator sickness," but there were no specifics about the cold, hypoxia, nervousness, fatigue, windblast or confused action. Nevertheless, however ill-defined the disease, a number of problems were recognized as looming.

That same year, the first step in establishing an Air Force medical service came when the Aeronautical Division in the Office of the Chief Signal Officer of the Army was established. A captain, a corporal and a private first-class were charged with "all matters pertaining to military ballooning, air machines and all kindred subjects." In 1914, Congress assigned the Aviation Section the

41

"operation of all military aircraft, including balloons and aeroplanes," and two years later the Aviation Section was established.

This was the beginning of the modern day Air Force. By then airplanes were reaching 20,000 feet with speeds of 125 miles per hour. They would continue to fly higher and faster, but what about the men who flew them? Basically, they were the same kind of people who used to drive stage coaches at five miles an hour.

In the United States, Germany, Great Britain, France and Italy standards were set up for physical examinations for aviation candidates (See Chapter 5), stressing vision, hearing and a sense of equilibrium and balance. But aviation medicine was far from an exact science in those days; people simply didn't know enough about the human body in flight to make value judgements. Problems became acute when the United States entered World War I and thousands of flight candidates had to be screened. It was already known that valuable men and machines were being lost in accidents caused by pilots not physically fit to withstand the stresses of flight. An aviation medical system would have to be set up to study and prevent these losses.

The man chosen for the job turned out to be a remarkably capable and far-sighted physician, Lieutenant Colonel Theodore Charles Lyster, the acknowledged "Father of Aviation Medicine in America." Assisted by Major William H. Wilmer and Major I. H. Jones, he set up the necessary administrative machinery for screening aviator candidates. It was the first time in America that aviation medicine had a sound scientific basis. He accomplished this by forming an Aviation Medical Research Board composed of specialists in various fields; they in turn established the Air Service Medical Research Laboratory at Hazelhurst Field, Mineola, Long Island. Colonel W. H. Wilmer was named Director and staff researchers began work in January of 1918. By the following July, 20 medical research laboratories were in operation throughout the country. In October, a similar laboratory was set up at the Third Aviation Training Center at Issoudun, France, and that same month, the *Air Service Medical Manual* was published.

An important piece of equipment at Mineola was a low-pressure chamber, not too different from the one developed by Dr. Paul Bert. Capable of simulating an altitude of 35,000 feet, the chamber

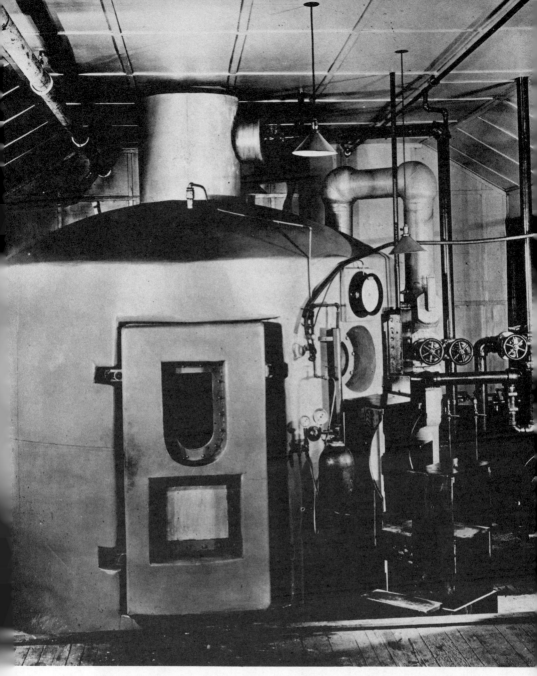

The low-pressure chamber at Mineola could simulate an altitude of 35,000 feet. It was used to test effects of hypoxia and for altitude classification, using a rebreather apparatus and nitrogen dilution methods./*U.S. Army*

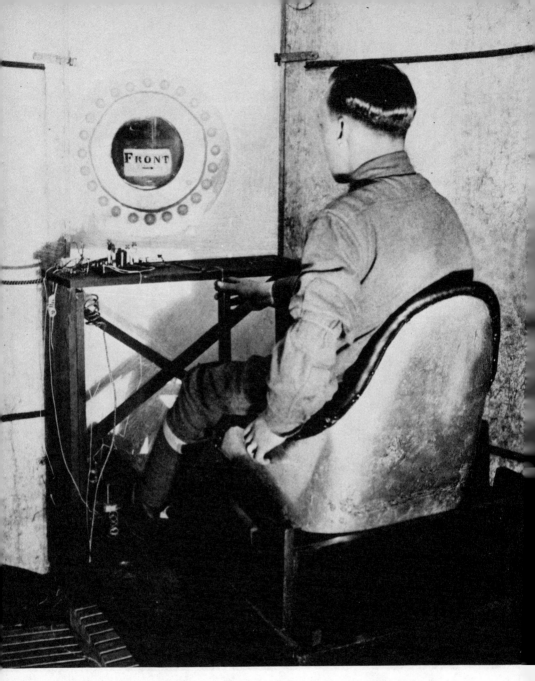

The Air Service Medical Research Laboratory had facilities for testing psychological responses under conditions of low pressure. Instrumentation in the early 30s was both sparse and simple./*U.S. Army*

was used extensively for studies on the effects of hypoxia and for altitude classification tests using a rebreather apparatus and nitrogen dilution methods. Major Edward C. Schneider, who headed the physiology department, developed his Cardiovascular Index which was widely used for years; there were also personality studies prepared by psychologists, neurologists and psychiatrists.

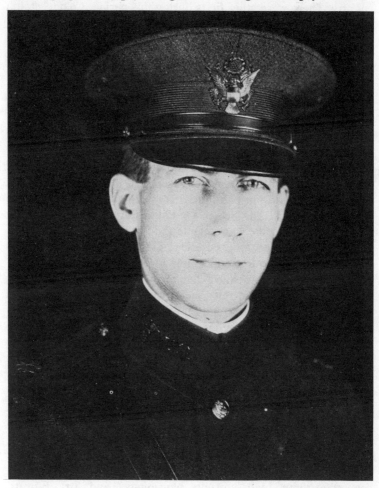

In 1919, Dr. Louis H. Bauer became director of the Air Service Medical Research Laboratory and established the School for Flight Surgeons, the first of its kind in the world./*U.S. Army*

Meanwhile, the concept of the flight surgeon apparently crystallized in the minds of Colonel Lyster and Major Jones while they were visiting aviation groups overseas. When they returned to the Mineola Laboratory they set up a program for the selection and training of flight surgeons. Candidates were selected from among the medical examiners at various airfields around the country. There were other firsts during this period; Colonel Ralph Greene in 1916 became the first medical officer ordered to flying duty, Major William R. Ream was the first flight surgeon killed in an aircraft accident, and on 8 May 1918, Captain Robert J. Hunter was ordered to duty as the first trained flight surgeon. The following year, Dr. H. Graeme Anderson of the Royal Air Force, published the first text on the subject, *The Medical and Surgical Aspects of Aviation.*

In 1919, Dr. Louis H. Bauer relieved Dr. Wilmer as director of the Air Service Medical Research Laboratory and established the School for Flight Surgeons, the first of its kind in the world. Out of his work at the school, Dr. Bauer assembled material for *Aviation Medicine,* published in 1926, the first aviation medical textbook in the United States. The School for Flight Surgeons continued for several years after the war, despite the fire that in 1921 destroyed almost everything at the Laboratory. The school moved to Brooks Field in 1926 and to Randolph Field in Texas in 1931.

Nobody bothered to move the altitude chamber to the new school locations; it was felt that everything was already known about hypoxia and altitude and that the school from then on would concentrate on pilot selection and qualifications. Although not much research was done anywhere for about ten years, history shows that the precedent set by the little institution at Mineola was of incalculable worth; it defined aviation medicine as a science in America

During the 1920s, interest in the subject picked up again in Germany, largely through the efforts of Hubertus Strughold, who became fascinated with balloon and zeppelin flights. Strughold, who took his doctorate in physiology, and then medicine, studied the work of the British researcher Sir Joseph Barcroft, who was concerned with high altitude physiology, and Dr. Edward Christian Schneider, who had a laboratory on Pike's Peak in Colorado. He put together what he called a "cocktail of lectures,"

46

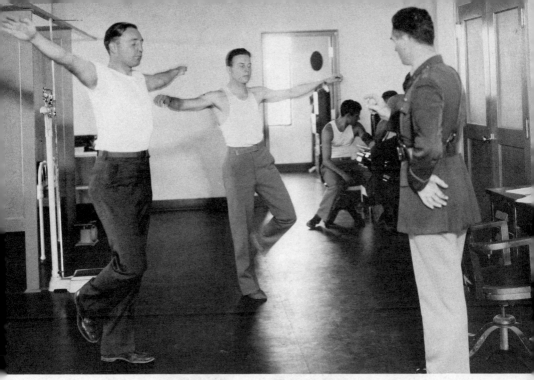

As airplanes were designed to fly higher and faster, doctors at the School of Aviation Medicine kept up with such developments by devising tests to make sure pilot-candidates could handle the stress. These men are not sleepwalking, but undergoing an "Equilibrium Test."/*U.S. Army*

the first *Flight Physiology of Men* for 60 students at the University of Würzburg.

Strughold made a balloon flight out of Würzburg, testing the strength of his muscles with a dynamometer to see how they were affected by 13,000-foot altitudes. He landed near the Czechoslovakian border, none the worse for wear, and scribbled notes on his observations during the return journey. There were no earth-shaking results, save his resolve to delve deeper into the mysteries of altitude.

At the University of Würzburg clinic for metabolic studies Strughold experimented with blowing nitrogen into a low-pressure chamber to simulate high altitude, then entered it for three hours under an oxygen pressure simulating about 7,000 feet and performed various sensorimotor tests on himself. He and his assistant made blood tests at intervals; he noted his violent headaches and other symptoms, the descriptions of which he included in his lectures.

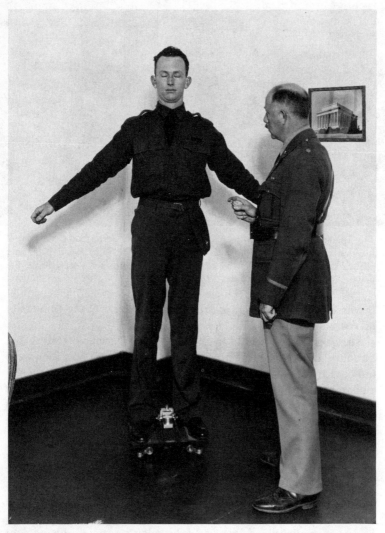

What appears to be an early version of the skateboard is merely a "Wobbleometer," which was supposed to indicate whether the pilot-candidate was susceptible to dizziness and disorientation./*U.S. Army*

But more than simulation was needed; he had to learn to fly in order to do airborne tests. Strughold worked for months to pay for lessons from Robert Ritter von Greim, an ace in the famous Richthofen Squadron. After that came the Rockefeller Foundation fellowship in the United States in 1928-1929 where, at Western Reserve University he studied the effects of oxygen deficiency upon the heart.

Dr. Strughold later came to the United States and became one of the great pioneers of modern aerospace medicine (See Chapter 4). He once expressed his views on how man in the future might see the post-World War I period, pointing out that after 1920 "something of real importance must have attracted the attention of the medical researcher..." That, said Strughold, was the time when a new means of transportation, flight, took men to the " 'top of the world' where normally man could not live." Further, he stated that the widening stream of research would indicate that about 1940 "...a catastrophe must have happened which had already cast its shadow several years before: World War II..." But that was years away and there was a big ocean between Europe and the United States. Billy Mitchell's insistence on airplanes as effective weapons ended with his courtmartial; isolationist America felt that civil aviation was more important than war talk.

In 1926, Dr. Bauer resigned his commission to become Medical Director of the newly established Aeronautics Branch of the Department of Commerce. His job was to set standards for the licensing of civilian airmen and to choose physicians throughout the country who would be qualified to conduct the examinations. On 20 February 1927, Bauer announced the names of 27 physicians selected as the first Aviation Medical Examiners and within two years brought them together to form a specialized professional society, the Aero Medical Association of the U.S.

The group began humbly enough in 1929, meeting once a year to present scientific papers and exchange ideas. There were awards and honors as time went on, friendships were cemented, and a great deal of solid information was circulated in the Association's *Journal of Aviation Medicine.*

The first scientific paper, "The Relation of Hypotension and Aviation," by Dr. John A. Tamisiea, medical advisor of Boeing Air Transport, revealed that the 30 transport pilots he had studied for

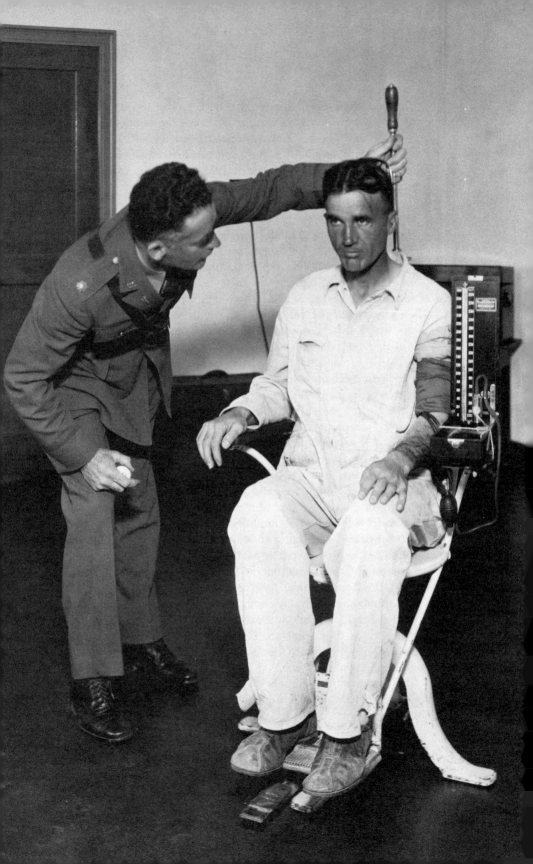

2½ years all had lower than normal blood pressure, a generally healthy sign. To keep them that way, he arranged a program of exercise, established a bowling league, and encouraged the pilots to take up golf and other sports.

The Association's membership grew from a few visionaries to include leading authorities from other countries. Now known at the Aerospace Medical Association, it publishes the journal titled *Aviation, Space, and Environmental Medicine.*

Dr. Bauer received many awards and honors for his innovative work during the early days and for his long years of dedicated service to the specialty of aviation medicine.

The second president of the Association was Ralph N. Greene, the man credited with bringing aviation medicine to the American commercial airlines. He was actually a discovery of Eddie Rickenbacker, general manager of Eastern Airlines, who remembered the young medical corps reservist at work in Issoudun, France, in World War I. Rickenbacker was convinced that Eastern should have its own aeromedical department, believing firmly the principle of constant surveillance of aircraft and engine performance should also be applied to pilots.

Eastern Airlines set the doctor up in his own laboratory in Miami where he could examine pilots, be their family physician, see them frequently and fly with them. At first the pilots were distrustful, but Greene gradually won them over, particularly when his preventive medicine detected signs of hypertension before pilots were aware of what was happening.

Greene flew with a number of the early pilots. He used himself and Eddie Stinson as experimental subjects, taking blood pressure readings, pulse rates, temperatures and examining blood and urine specimens on the ground and aloft. One of his early campaigns was for passage of a Federal law to limit airline pilots to 85 flying hours per month.

Greene published a number of technical reports which he shared with other airlines, several of which ultimately had their own medical departments. In a special research project for Pan

Doctors at the School of Aviation Medicine used the Barany chair in equilibrium testing, and to measure spasmodic movement of the eyes (nystagmus) after turning./*U.S. Army*

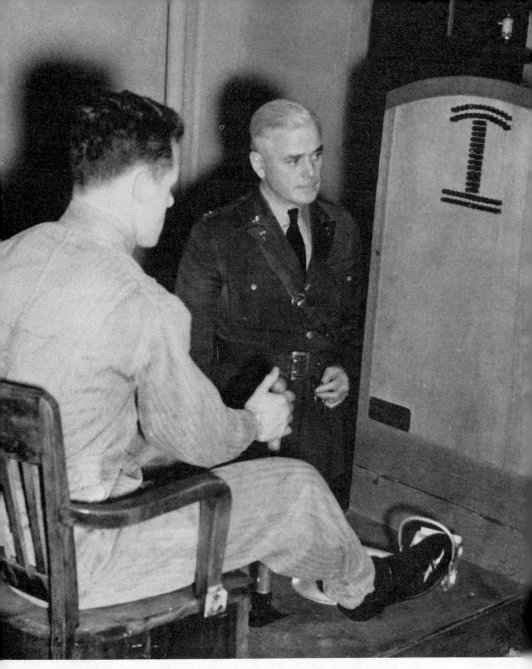

A "Serial Action Apparatus," featured rudimentary stick and rudder controls, but the office chair seemed a bit out of place. It was used to test coordination./*U.S. Army*

American Airlines, Dr. Greene set up a new system for the control and prevention of certain tropical ailments that flight personnel operating in foreign countries were beginning to contract.

Meanwhile, airplanes were being designed to fly faster and higher. During 1927 and 1928, both the Atlantic and Pacific were crossed by air. The North Pole was reached by Lieutenant Commander Richard E. Byrd in 1926; in 1929 he flew across the South Pole. During the 1930s, commercial airlines commenced intercontinental flights.

Air races in the United States and Europe saw records broken by both men and women. Red-faced physicians who had said that women should not fly during the week of their menses had to take another look at their dire predictions, as women took to the air regardless of the time of the month. Among them was Amelia Earhart, who flew nonstop, 2,435 miles from Los Angeles to Newark in 19 hours in August of 1932. She and other women pilots reminded physicians that they still had a lot to learn about the effects of flight on the human body.

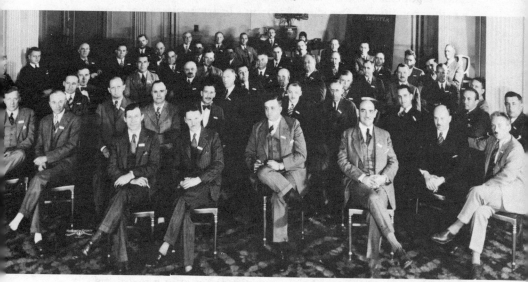

The first annual convention of the Aero Medical Association was held on 7-8 October 1929 at the Hotel Statler in Detroit, Michigan. There were 53 men and one woman present for this historic photograph. Dr. Louis H. Bauer, third from left in front, was elected President during this meeting./*Aerospace Medical Association*

It was not an easy time for flight surgeons. There were no textbooks to describe the flight experiences that pilots reported. Aerobatic pilots began experimenting on themselves with various forms of elastic bandages and anti-gravity belts because experience told them something went wrong with their circulatory systems when they performed certain maneuvers. Pilots of the Pacific Air Transport Service, flying the U.S. mail with their slogan, "The mail must go through," were confronted with fog along the Pacific coast, and without visual references, they found their vestibular systems gave them false information. When Charles Lindbergh crossed the Atlantic in 1927 in the Spirit of St. Louis, he really could not see where he was going. An instrument panel blocked off all forward vision from the cockpit. He either peered out a side window, or through a periscope that gave him a limited view of what might be in front of him.

Pilots did a lot of "blind flying" in those days, and it became the most important phase of aviation research of its day, particularly since mailplanes and commercial transports flew regardless of weather conditions. The idea of trusting instruments rather than the "seat of the pants," or "sixth sense," when pilots couldn't see the ground through the bad weather was not a popular one—yet something had to be devised to determine the plane's attitude in relation to the earth.

The Wright brothers used two primitive flight instruments. One was an eight-inch piece of string knotted at the end, fixed in front of the pilot; when the string was pointing at him, he knew he was flying correctly. The other was an angle of incidence indicator on a strut. Then in 1919 Lawrence Sperry presented William C. Ocker, a young Army air officer, with a set of instruments, a turn indicator and bank indicator which Ocker tested in thick fog, to find he could safely turn 180 degrees, get out of the fog parallel with his course and return to the starting point.

It wasn't until 1926, however, that Captain David Myers, a flight surgeon, convinced Ocker that his vestibular system could not be trusted. He did this by turning him blindfolded on a Barany revolving chair. "Captain Myers explained that after a few turns he had decreased the turning speed, at which time I said I was stopped. Then as the chair slowly came to a stop I reported turning to the left. (Had I been in an airplane in fog and corrected for a left turn I would have thrown the machine into a right hand spin.)''

Ocker's instruments were improved when First Lieutenant Carl J. Crane invented a flight integrator which required little interpretive effort by the pilot and at the same time gave him all the necessary indications of the flight. Years later, Lieutenant Commander John R. Poppen, (MC), U.S. Navy, backed these early pioneers of instrument flying, Ocker, Crane and Myers, in a paper presented at the Eighth Annual Meeting of the Aero Medical Association on 29 August 1936: "I am firmly convinced that in moderate turns and spirals we get practically no dependable information from the labyrinths. I will go so far as to state...that whenever an airplane undergoes evolutions of a rotary nature sufficient to stimulate the normal labyrinth, the information we gain from the stimulation is not only unreliable but actually erroneous...''

He continued, "The keynote of instrument flying is that we must not only disregard our natural feelings; we must deny them...'' Poppen stressed the importance of the location and arrangement of instruments, the illumination of them, the distance, and, "...We should make every effort to reduce eye strain...'' All of these areas of research and development were forerunners of instruments build into today's spacecraft.

As for hypoxia and the effects of altitude that were supposed to have been suficiently understood during World War I—there, too, medical research did an about-face. By 1929, free balloon and airplane ascents were reaching 32,800 feet and in 1931, high-altitude physiologist Hans Hartmann went on an expedition to Kanchenjunga in the Himalayas and climbed to an altitude of 28,200 feet, amassing extensive measurements and data for study. Little by little, tentative conclusions were first drawn, then proven. Paul Bert had shown that the adverse effects of altitude were principally due to the lack of oxygen in the body, that hypoxia at altitude is caused by the decreased partial pressure of oxygen in the inspired air and not by the mechanical effects of the decreased total atmospheric pressure. In other words, the alveoli, which are the air cells of the lung, pick up oxygen easily at sea level where the air pressure is 14.7 pounds per square inch (equal to 760mm

Hg.) but they cannot absorb it so readily at lower pressures. The result is hypoxia—the lack of sufficient oxygen in vital tissues and organs, and the ultimate cause of death from almost any pathological condition.

In the beginning of aeronautics, hypoxia developed slowly with the ascent to higher altitudes. Later, when oxygen was invariably used from, say, 9,000 to 12,000 feet and upward, hypoxia developed suddenly when a pilot's equipment failed or he dropped

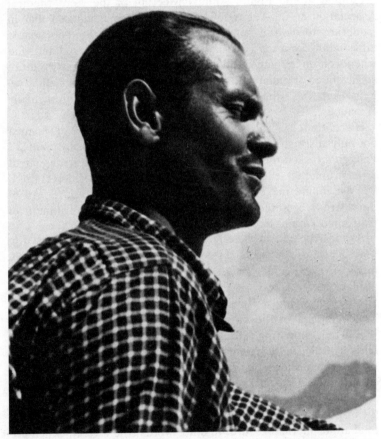

Dr. Hans Hartmann was a member of the German expedition to Kanchenjunga in the Himalayas in 1931, where he spent weeks acclimatizing himself to altitudes of 18,000-24,000 feet. In 1937, in another research expedition to Nanga Parbat he and some others in the party died in an avalanche./*Theodor H. Benzinger*

56

his mask or mouthpiece through which oxygen flowed. The suddenness of the onset depended on the altitude. It also depended on the constitution of the aviator or climber. Condition; fat, thin, robust, nervous habits; cigarette smokers, alcohol imbibers; age; young and not-so-young—are all personal characteristics that affect tolerance to high altitudes. The emotional state of the moment, or anxiety, play a role. The rate of ascent, altitude attained, duration and frequency of exposure must all be taken into account. A relatively fast ascent to high altitude in an airplane or balloon has a different effect than that felt by a mountain climber whose body has a chance to adjust slowly.

By 1933, the altitude record was 45,900 feet and the speed record was 386 miles per hour. Improvement in aircraft propulsion, cruising and climbing speed, operational ceiling, flight duration, radius of action and all the accompanying hazards of vibration, noise and physical disorientation, presented increasing challenges to aeromedical research. If people were going to fly these machines with any degree of safety, there would have to be improvements in oxygen systems; pressure suits would be needed by pilots operating at high altitudes, with the increased speed and maneuverability of aircraft. There would be a demand for g-suits to counteract the effects of heavy gravitational or centrifugal forces.

And there were problems with pilot disorientation when the new low-visibility instruments came into use. By the mid 1930s, more and more flight surgeons were taking to the air to experience the physiological problems at first hand. The Aero Medical Association urged legislation that would put all military flight surgeons on flight status. Their reasoning: "A flight surgeon cannot remain on the ground and theorize about what is going on in the air any more than a doctor can stand outside the walls of a hospital and profit by the experiences taking place within."

One of the early "flying doctors" was Harry Armstrong, a leader in the field of practical research and a genius at getting things going in spite of administrative red tape. During his long military career which culminated in his becoming the second Surgeon General of the Air Force, he established a research laboratory at Wright Field, was instrumental in reestablishing the research program at the School of Aviation Medicine where he

57

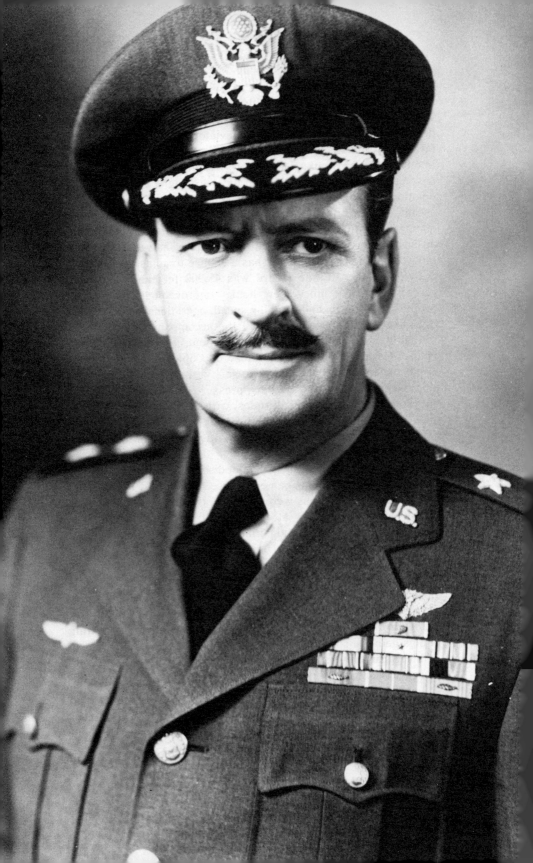

became Commandant, established the department of space medicine and proposed formation of the Aerospace Medical Center.

Dr. Armstrong received a commission in the regular army in March 1930, after taking a course in aviation medicine at Brooks Field in Texas. The following year he was sent to Selfridge Field in Michigan where he was attached to the First Pursuit Group. It was there, flying the 2-seater P-16 aircraft, that he was exposed to all the stress an aircraft was capable of posing, including windblast, noise, hypoxia, vibration, high gravity forces, ear and sinus pain, air sickness and cold.

On one flight to Minneapolis, when the temperature was minus 40°F., the pilot was unable to keep his goggles clear. "He periodically shook the stick, asking me to take control of the plane until he could clear his goggles." This led Armstrong to try to improve the protection equipment of military pilots, because in a combat situation, he figured "...a man would be glad to be shot down to be taken out of his misery."

He wrote to the Air Surgeon in Washington, outlining the problems he had observed, and asked if the people at Wright Field who were responsible for equipment development could do something about it. A month later, Armstrong received orders to report to Wright Field to do the job himself—a disturbing proposition since he had no background in research and development. The Air Surgeon's response to Armstrong's protest was, "You're the one who's complained and you're the logical man to try to solve it."

At that time, Major Malcolm Grow (later to become the Air Surgeon) was the surgeon at Wright Field and had been working on studies of carbon monoxide poisoning in aircraft. He reported that the fumes from the short-stacked engine exhausts of the time went along the fuselage and entered through the rear of the plane—a dangerous situation that had to be corrected. He was also developing winter clothing for flyers and, based on his service in Alaska and his study of Eskimo clothing, advocated reindeer skin.

Harry G. Armstrong, who pioneered aviation and aerospace medicine by self-experimentation and basic research, learned parachuting in order to gain first-hand knowledge of physiological problems of emergency escape. He became the Air Force's second Surgeon General./*National Library of Medicine*

Grow's plan never got very far because of the inadequate supply of reindeer skin, even for peacetime. During a war, it would be even more scarce. In October 1934, Grow went to Washington, D.C., to become Chief of the Medical Section, Office of the Chief of the Air Corps.

Armstrong, who was still assigned to the Equipment Branch, had more frustration and opposition than clout and funds. His was an odd billet and often his line of thinking wasn't at all well received by suspicious engineers. One day the meddlesome doctor discovered a trap door beside his desk—in a building that wasn't supposed to have a basement. He opened the trap door and found a circular staircase so he went down to investigate. There, to his joy, he found the old altitude chamber that had survived the Mineola fire. No one knew it was there, and nobody cared, least of all people at the School of Aviation Medicine who hadn't wanted to bother with the bulky shipment. But for Armstrong, it was a chance to start some studies of his own.

"About six months after my arrival there, I wrote up a proposal to the chief of the engineering section recommending that a medical research laboratory be established. I just addressed it to him and it was sent to Washington where it was approved by the Chief of Staff and orders were issued..."

On 18 May 1935, the Physiological Research Unit, the official beginning of the Aeromedical Laboratory (AML) was established with Armstrong as director. Historical records indicate that the remarkably smooth acceptance of the proposed project had considerable nudging from abroad. That same year France set up an Aeronautical Development and Research High Altitude Test Center, to consider, among other things, "physiological research on the effect of flying at high altitude." The French, in fact, were copying the Italians, and the Germans were busy too, all of which prompted Brigadier General O. Westover, Assistant Chief of the Air Corps, to add to his endorsement, "...it is the desire of this office to continue this development work and to maintain our advantage, already gained, over other countries in this regard."

The beginnings were modest. For the first 18 months, Armstrong had the help of one enlisted man, on loan from the Wright Field Dispensary. They worked in a small basement room where they kept the altitude chamber. The human centrifuge was housed in the balloon loft. For working capital, Armstrong was allotted $600 for experimental animals, $2,500 for the purchase of laboratory equipment and $100 for supplies.

At times it was discouraging. After all, Armstrong was a physician, not an engineer and the idea that a physician was tinkering with aeronautical equipment was not too popular. Often it seemed the two professions were on a collision course: "I had worked for three or four months on a project that I felt was necessary but then I began to wonder if my research was directed along the most important lines. So I went to the head of the engineering section and told him how I felt about it, and asked him to lay out a research program for me to follow. His answer was that he was not a physician and that he felt research in the field of medicine should be my responsibility, that I had a much better knowledge of what the problems were and that I should pursue my own ideas. I shouldn't be too concerned about always getting results because in his experience in R & D if one effort out of a hundred proved successful, that was a very good batting average. And furthermore if I got into difficulty with what I did, he'd back me one-hundred per cent. That gave me a tremendous amount of confidence and encouragement."

But there were negative elements too. The Unit was always short of help and money. These were depression years, and cutbacks were a constant threat, particularly in research where solid achievement was often elusive. Then too, there was a feeling throughout the Air Corps that further research in this area was not necessarily indicated. This was because practically all flying at that time was done under favorable conditions; seldom was there any flying or training of students or combat elements at maximum aircraft performance or at high altitude where hypoxia and low temperatures prevailed. People couldn't foresee what might happen under wartime conditions with the current aircraft, let alone those on the drawing board.

Help did trickle in, however. In June 1936, Dr. J. W. Heim, a Ph.D. from Harvard, joined him and during the next four years there were other professionals; John F. Hall, a biologist from Princeton, and Ernest Pinson, a physiologist from Rochester,

61

New York. The unit also got Private Raymond Whitney, and three other enlisted men.

In those early years, there were never requests from the field for work that needed doing, so Armstrong tackled various investigations on his own. There was, for example, aeroembolism, or the "bends" as it is called by deep sea divers. In 1929 Dr. Jacob Jongbloed, at the University of Utrecht in Holland, described this condition as it affected pilots at high altitude.

Painful, dangerous, and often fatal, aeroembolism is caused by the formation of nitrogen bubbles in the bloodstream when the atmospheric pressure is reduced. As the surrounding pressure decreases, the size of the nitrogen bubbles increase. When the bubbles are large enough, they become trapped in the small blood vessels of the joints. The pain can create a tightening in several joints at once and they become stiff. If one of these bubbles blocks a cerebral artery, death is almost certain.

With deep sea divers, there is too much external pressure. Armstrong suspected that the opposite was true at high altitude and that a decrease in pressure could cause nitrogen bubbles to enlarge and become trapped in the small blood vessels of the joints. Pilots would suffer severe and crippling pain exactly as did a diver.

Armstrong, determined to learn more about this, first used himself as a test subject, taking reduced pressure in his chamber to experience aeroembolism symptoms: "I wound up with the classical symptoms. My hands began to feel stiff and slightly sore and I massaged them, trying to improve the circulation. Then I noticed a series of small bubbles in the tendons of my fingers. I could actually feel them, and by manipulating my finger along my tendon I could squirt these bubbles back and forth. I was certain in my own mind they represented aeroembolism, but it was not positive proof. So I turned to animal experiments to try to actually see the bubbles." This may seem to be a more cautious approach, but on one particular occasion, it wasn't: "I was using a rabbit, and our procedure was to ascend to about 35,000 feet and allow the rabbit to die during the ascent. Then I'd open his chest and abdominal cavity and look for nitrogen bubbles in the blood. We were using a standard altimeter as a guage inside the chamber to indicate the simulated altitude and I had noticed previously whenever we reached 35,000 feet the altimeter failed to record further and I assumed the leakage in the chamber was just balancing the vacuum pumper. So, we let the pump continue to run even after we reached 35,000 feet. On this certain day, I had reached 35,000 feet and was dissecting the rabbit and eventually happened to glance at the altimeter and noticed that we were descending and were at about 20,000 feet. The operator was a private and he was watching me through a porthole and I signaled him to take the chamber back up to the prescribed altitude. I gave him what I considered a very dirty look because he was ruining the experiment.''

"However, the chamber kept descending and when we reached 10,000 to 12,000 feet I noticed that the Post surgeon was also looking at me through the porthole and seemed quite excited. When we reached ground level and I opened the door, he told me I had become unconscious in the chamber, had fallen off the stool to the floor, but during the descent I had regained consciousness, returned to the stool and to my dissection of the rabbit. I was inclined to doubt their story except for the large bump on my head where it hit the floor...''

They later decided the cause of the calamity was Armstrong's ignorance of the kind of altimeter they were using; it stopped registering after 35,000 feet, and with the vacuum pump still running, he probably experienced a pressure altitude of 40,000 to 45,000 feet where just taking oxygen was not adequate to keep him from collapsing.

During this era, Dr. Hans Hartmann, a Strughold associate since 1935, continued to study the effects of high altitude. In 1931 he had been a member of the German expedition to Kanchenjunga in the Himalayas where he spent weeks acclimatizing himself to altitudes of 18,000-24,000 feet. Again in 1937 he went with the German expedition to Nanga Parbat where he and some others in the party died in an avalanche. Dr. U. C. Luft, like Hartmann a Strughold associate, was the only survivor. He continued their work, spending long periods in the Alps to acclimatize himself to high altitudes. He then experimented with a low-pressure chamber for comparison, and deduced that oxygen deficiency would be withstood more easily when one became accustomed to it gradually.

Laboratory researchers sometimes got themselves involved in projects that lacked good common sense. One such project was the development of a liquid oxygen system and its adoption throughout the Air Corps. Armstrong quickly pointed out that Alaska had no liquid oxygen factories, nor did any place else outside major cities in the United States. The answer was to develop an oxygen generator mounted on a truck. When the stratosphere balloon flights were staged in South Dakota the Lab sent a truck-mounted generator out to supply liquid oxygen. The trouble was, the truck had to detour at least 200 miles out of the way on two or three occasions because bridges weren't strong enough to take the weight. It became obvious that the Air Corps had better not depend on liquid oxygen in the event of hostilities, so it was back to the gaseous system, until technology could solve the logistics problem.

During that period, there was no such thing as an oxygen mask in the service. Pilots used what they called the "pipe stem;" the tube from the oxygen simply came up to a wooden stem which they put in their mouth and "smoked"—a highly inefficient system. Then one day Dr. W. Randolph Lovelace and Dr. Walter M. Boothby from the Mayo Clinic appeared at the Lab with an oxygen mask which had been fabricated by another Mayo clinician, Dr. Arthur H. Bulbulian, and asked if the Air Corps would be interested in it.

Armstrong found it totally inadequate. For one thing, it covered only the nose and anybody with a head cold couldn't use it. Secondly, if the pilot forgot to breathe through his nose he could accidentally pass out. The mask had a rebreather bag on it to conserve oxygen and there were metal valves between the mask and the rebreather bag. On testing it, Armstrong found that the valves froze shut. Besides, there was no place for a microphone.

The one feature that had merit was the rebreather bag for conserving oxygen. Armstrong redesigned the whole thing, substituting sponge rubber for the metal valves (should they freeze, the pilot could squeeze the ice out of them). Then he invited the doctors back to go over the whole project. They returned to Mayo Clinic where they developed what became known as the BLB oxygen mask, used for many years by the Air Corps and later the Air Force.

Another important piece of equipment developed during that period was the shoulder-type safety belt, a concept taken for granted today, but for its time, a highly controversial matter. General Grow had visited an accident scene at Bolling Air Force Base about a half hour after the crash. He noted blood on the instrument panel on both pilot's cockpit and rear cockpit. At the hospital, he learned that both occupants were dead from fractured skulls, but were without other injuries of any kind. Grow reasoned that if a way could be devised to keep the pilot's head from hitting the instrument panel, injuries and deaths might be prevented in many crashes. He asked Armstrong to go to work on the problem.

"Everyone said if you restrain the shoulders and you crash, since the head is not supported, you break your neck." Armstrong recalled. "So we rigged up a gimmick in the big hangar. I took an airplane seat and suspended it from the center of the hangar on four chains. They had a tripping device on them, and the seat was equipped with shoulder-type safety belts, so that through a cautious approach (by linking the chain) we would drop the seat a couple of feet. If you got enough bob out of it, and if that didn't hurt, why then we'd hoist it back up and get four feet of chain and let it drop and see how much bob we got. Finally we got a meter that measures the g forces, and we finally knocked that clear through the stop and I never even got a sore neck. You have a powerful leverage in your neck, so I was convinced that if you were going to break your neck you would have bashed your brains out anyway. It was the lesser of the two evils..."

Obviously Armstrong's thesis has been substantiated through the years. But at the time, such Rube Goldberg-type of work by the doctor and his assistants was often opposed, politely tolerated, or openly laughed at. Armstrong remembers a luncheon he attended in 1935 when someone asked at what speed he thought airplanes would someday fly. "I replied they'd fly at the speed of a .45 caliber bullet, and perhaps faster." The statement made headlines in the Dayton newspaper the next day. "And I found myself in serious trouble back at Wright Field from the design engineers. They told me that any such idea was pure fantasy and that a medical officer had no business making a prediction of aircraft performance of the future."

In 1938, Armstrong began writing his book on aviation medicine. When it was ready, he sent it to the publisher who had earlier brought out the book by Dr. Louis Bauer. Armstrong's book was rejected as a money-loser, so he put it aside for a while, then submitted it again. This time it was accepted, went through three additional printings and remained the standard text for over 20 years. According to Dr. Strughold, Armstrong's discovery of the potential boiling effect of the blood above 63,000 feet—"The Armstrong Line"—was one of the most important milestones of the era.

Meanwhile, in August 1937, the first experimental pressurized cabin airplane flew out of Wright Field. Pressurized aircraft entered commercial service in July 1940 with the Trans World Airlines, ensuring the comfort and safety of passengers in aircraft flying at the higher altitudes. But this introduced a new problem to aviation medicine. Emergency oxygen equipment would be needed to ensure the safety of passengers and crew if rapid decompression of the aircraft should occur due to accidental air leakage or failure of the compressors.

Concurrent with Armstrong's pioneering work at the Wright Field Aeromedical Laboratory was that of Heinz von Diringshofen, M.D., a captain in the Luftwaffe. In 1931 he began studies in his "flying laboratories," to measure effects of g forces. His brother Bernd, an engineer, assisted Heinz in developing airborne instrumentation for the acceleration flights. In 1935 in Juterbog, near Berlin, he and his fellow aviators flew the sturdy HE-45 Heinkel biplane in a number of experimental dives, carefully recording the physiological aspects of their daring research.

He worked it out so that after a dive of 2,100 to 2,400 feet from 8,400 feet of altitude, at a speed of 270 miles an hour, a downward spiral could be achieved, sustaining a 6g load or more for 10-15 seconds. For longer than 10 seconds, 5g was tolerated, although vision was lost for a few seconds after the onset of acceleration. Forces of 4 to 4.5, resulted in minor disturbances of vision. In two experiments, they barely tolerated forces of 5.5g, and then only with great effort. He established that full consciousness could be preserved even though vision failed and that the arterial circulation in the eye became insufficient before the circulation in the brain was dangerously impeded.

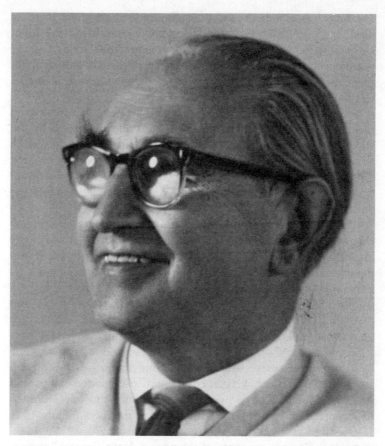

Dr. Heinz von Diringshofen established the world's first "flying" aeromedical laboratory where, beginning in 1931, he measured the effects of g forces. His brother Bernd, an engineer, helped develop airborne instrumentation./*Harald von Beckh*

Von Diringshofen found that the most favorable position was a crouching one, with the chest pressed against the thighs and head straightened up. This improved the limits of tolerance from 4.5 to 5.5, or up to 6.5g. One subject tolerated 7 to 7.5g for three seconds without disturbance of vision.

In 1939, von Diringshofen wrote a unique book, *Medical Guide for Flying Personnel,* the purpose of which was to communicate and explain to the aviator the basic medical problems of aviation.

The book was to help the aviator maintain his health and increase his flying performance. It was also aimed at assisting the flight surgeon to teach and counsel flying personnel in all medical areas pertinent to the flying service. It was widely distrubuted to flight surgeons and flying crews and became a standard item of the German Luftwaffe.

But the book was useful to some Allied aviators as well. It soon turned up in Canada, and was translated and published by the University of Toronto Press in June 1940, nine months after the British Empire and Germany were at war. In all, there were three Canadian printings, a French translation for the exile forces of General de Gaulle and a Rumanian version, needless to say the only one that was not pirated.

Germany during the 1930s had two major research institutes. One was Strughold's, the Aeromedical Institute of the Air Ministry in Berlin (actually established by von Diringshofen in 1935) and the other, founded the year before on 1 March by Dr. Theodor H. Benzinger, was at Rechlin, on Muritz Lake about halfway between Berlin and the Baltic Sea. Rechlin was responsible to the "General-Luftzeugmeister," Ernst Udet, a World War I ace generaly credited with rebuilding the Luftwaffe.

Scientists at both institutes busied themselves with altitude chamber low-pressure studies, including explosive decompression. They worked on oxygen equipment, pressurized cabins and pressure suits. There were acceleration and deceleration experiments on centrifuges, with x-rays of monkeys pulling 12 to 15g, as well as night and color vision studies.

Another German luminary of the period, Hans-Georg Clamann, experimented with pure oxygen in a pressure chamber. As with many of these early experimenters, risks became realities; his associate wound up with a combination pneumonia-emphysema condition while Clamann's lungs became inflamed. Their report, however, concluded that the greatest hazard associated with the use of pure oxygen was fire (See Chapter 8). Clamann's group pressurized a cabin to 30,000 feet and deduced that 100 per cent oxygen is equal to 21 per cent oxygen; pilots need not fear ill effects from oxygen when properly used.

Rechlin was actually the testing center of the German Air Force; the aircraft industry developed prototypes which were then flown

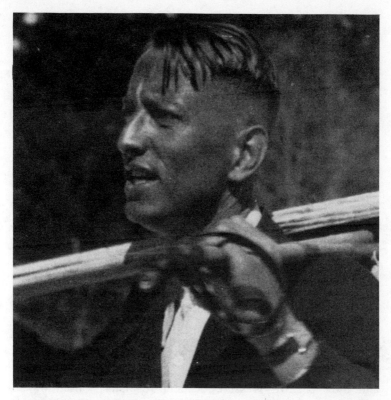

Theodor H. Benzinger, M.D. studied high altitude physiology in the Alps. He was one of the German scientists who came to the United States after World War II to continue working in the space program./*Theodor H. Benzinger*

to the institute where they were tested by Rechlin pilots. Dr. Benzinger's "E med" (Erprobungsstelle der Luftwaffe) was but one of a number of aviation research departments, the others being airplanes, engines, navigation and equipment and armament.

As Benzinger explained his early involvement: "I went there in 1934 as a reservist who couldn't even fly." He had been private assistant in Trieburg to the professor of medicine, Siegfried Thannhauser, a pioneer of research on nucleic acids, the culmination of which was DNA—the "double helix." In Thannhauser's laboratories, Benzinger became a research assistant to Hans A. Krebs, working on uric acid synthesis.

"Well, that same day I said I had no experience in flying but would like to learn so one of the engineers took me up in an old open monoplane with a British engine in it because in Germany we didn't have any engines that could go high at that time. And he took me up to the ceiling altitude in the open cockpit—my face getting very cold—and when he was up there he just turned the nose straight down, turning me around in spins. I got so sick when I got out of that plane you can imagine what happened. I told him it was just marvelous and I wanted to sit at the controls myself and learn to fly..."

This was the beginning of many high altitude flights, both in airplanes and low pressure chambers. Research was exotic as well as humble. An example of the latter was pollution—getting rid of carbon monoxide in airplanes. "I flew them all in a fighter plane with a gallon bottle in my lap. I pulled the stop if the bottle was filled with water, let the water out and the air in. Then I took it home to the lab and with highly sensitive instruments measured the carbon monoxide. It was the first time in my life I was called away from research to do a practical job. It happened again later—I find it difficult to do..."

"E med" doctors developed oxygen equipment in which leakage did not result in air intake, only loss of supply. The solutions found were the "blower," for fighter pilots in the Battle of Britian, and the "positive pressure demand regulator," used by all military planes until the end of World War II. They also wrote the instructions for aviators at altitude (Udet signed them, making them mandatory), and developed the method for testing aviators for premature circulatory failure under lack of oxygen by breathing low oxygen and gaseous mixtures. The equivalent altitudes were calculated by the "alveolar formula." The first continuous measurements of blood pressure (not yet introduced in clinical medicine) were made under "E med's" program. The T-wave of the electrocardiogram was continuously evaluated. Respiratory depth and frequency were measured continuously.

These same German doctors planned and conducted courses for pilots in the European Alps with exercise (skiing) for documented improvement of their altitude fitness measured by time of useful consciousness in the gas test.

There was work on explosive decompression. Said Dr. Benzinger: "I shall dwell a little longer on this because the first self-experiments at Rechlin in the Junkers decompression chamber provided the physiological scientific basis for pressurized cabins in military aircraft for use in combat, and for the development of the pressure suits. The explosive decompression of cockpits or suits is the most vital problem of space operations. No other problem kills so instantly. The suit is the life of man in space."

Explosive decompression kills in two ways—by lack of oxygen so super-acute that it is unparalled by any other causes of anoxia except by cyanide poisoning; and by air embolism which occurs when the airways are not fully open during the explosive decompression. The differential diagnosis between the two, though obvious now, was difficult to determine "after our first experiments went wrong." After Benzinger's first self-experiments he permitted members of his staff to follow. When he extended the team to include the Junkers engineer in charge of pressure cabin work, they had a near fatal accident. "On decompression, he slumped into my lap. After recompression he was put on a stretcher for dead. He came to. He had a hemiplegia and paralysis of speech for a while, but he was all right an hour later."

Dr. Benzinger paid tribute to co-workers Helmut Kind, technician Wilhelm Hornberger M.D. and Helmut Doring M.D. who continued self-experiments with improved instrumentation during his absence in 1940 when he was flying JU-88s in high-altitude reconnaissance missions over Britain. All three experimenters had minor or major incidents of lung over-extensions due to closing vocal chords. They also had, as did almost everybody in Europe, old, inactive calcified remnants of tuberculosis. Kind died; Hornberger developed and recovered from pulmonary tuberculosis and Doring had a surgical turberculosis of one rib and then of a knee which left him crippled.

Explosive decompression, according to Benzinger, "...is anything but harmless but its speed makes all the difference. I do not feel there is a real hazard when a large commercial passenger cabin loses a small window. There is plenty of time. Not so in a suit

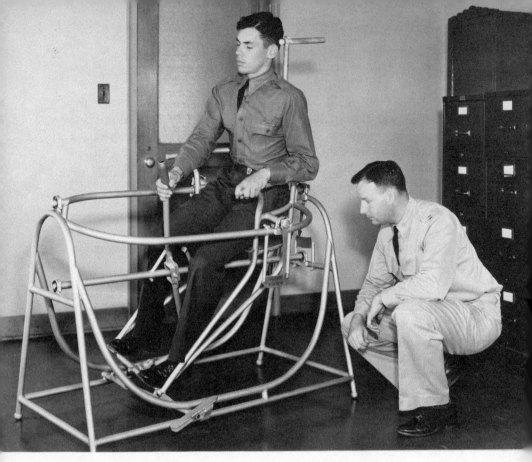

A self-balancing chair, somewhat resembling an early ancestor of the Apollo program's MASTIF (see Chapter 7) was used during the late 30s and early 40s to test pilot candidates./*U.S. Army*

that has negligible air space, or in a small cockpit, or in our experiments…''

And so it was research on hypoxia many years ago that determined time as a critical factor in explosive decompression. The time of useful consciousness for a person breathing air is 15 seconds above altitudes of 43,000 feet.

As problems of explosive decompression were studied, so were the effects of altitude on paranasal sinuses and dentistry. By 1939, flying personnel were complaining of toothaches which doctors attributed to decreased barometric pressure (hollow granuloma) and breathing cold oxygen.

World War II compounded aeromedical problems. Suddenly there was a need for a wide range of experts to come up with

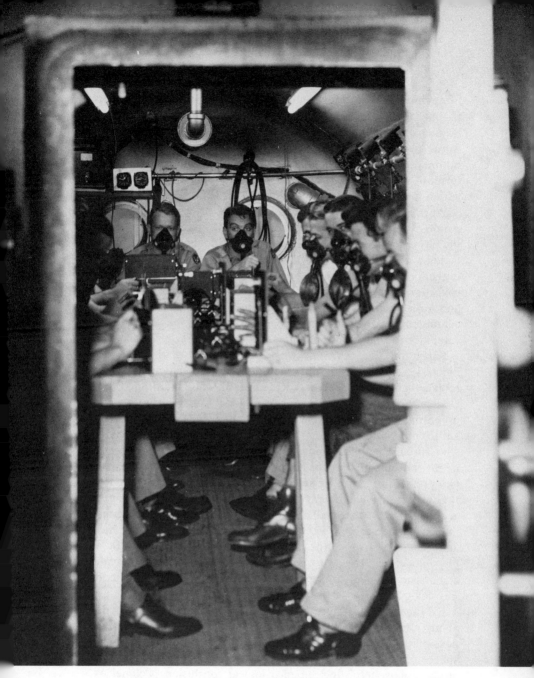

Early in World War II, doctors pushed for high altitude indoctrination for aviation cadets. This chamber was capable of taking 12 subjects simultaneously to simulated high altitudes./*U.S. Army*

lifesaving knowledge for combat pilots. Rations for long distance flights had to be worked out, as well as stimulants to fight fatigue. Studies of oxygen toxicity, carbon dioxide loss and pilot selection were given priority. There was a desperate need for more information on the physiology of acceleration, long term and short term, of wind blast, airsickness, vibration, and ophthalmological variations on color vision and depth.

Work intensified on night vision and the effects of illuminated panels. With the increase in aircraft speed, there were studies of the physiology of reflexes and senses, accidents and contributing factors, or heat, cold, blast and distress at sea. Aeromedical evacuation with trained technicians and nurses introduced the concept of flying ambulances. And in laboratories of both Allied and Axis countries work with experimental animals and humans continued in the decompression chambers, the centrifuges, catapults and parachute facilities.

Early in the war, doctors pushed for a high-altitude indoctrination program that would educate aviation cadets at replacement training centers on the hazards of high-altitude flight. Under the direction of U.S. Army Air Corps surgeons, the programs also determined which cadets had sinus or ear defects of sufficient magnitude to limit their training, and to discover cadets who, through psychic or unsatisfactory neurocirculatory responses might be unsuitable for flight training. Actually it was a two-pronged program for selection and training of suitable pilots.

Low-pressure chambers were procured; aviation physiologists and technicians were trained and by the end of 1942 the altitude indoctrination program was well established in both the U.S. Navy and the Army Air Corps. Young men possessing a Ph.D. in physiology or one of the allied biological sciences were commissioned and trained in five-week courses in Aviation Physiology.

By June of 1943, there was a vast accumulation of knowledge about altitude, yet little was known about emergency escape possibilities from high flying aircraft. Would a parachute opening shock at high altitude be less severe because of decreased density of the atmosphere? It seemed a logical conclusion. Colonel W. Randolph Lovelace, at that time a flight surgeon with the Army Air Corps, decided to find out. He also wanted to test several items of

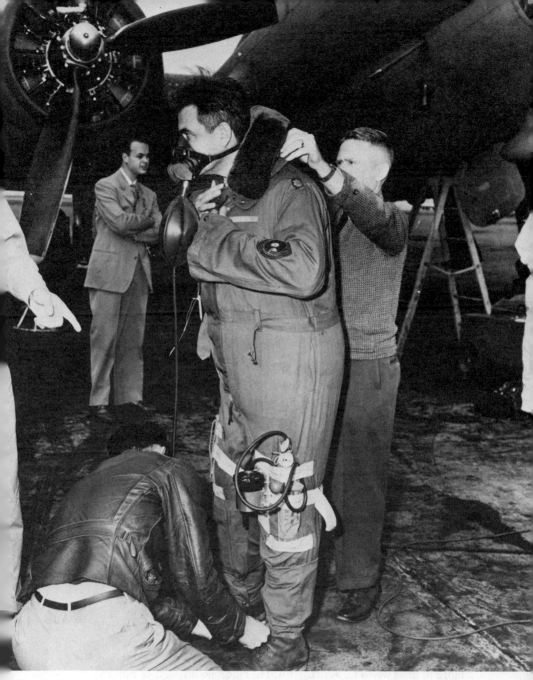

Colonel W. Randolph Lovelace (1907-1965), American aerospace pioneer, preparing for his 40,200 foot parachute jump over Euphrata, Washington, from a Boeing Flying Fortress, June 23, 1943./*Smithsonian Institution*

new equipment, notably a small bail-out cylinder containing about twelve minutes' supply of oxygen for high altitude emergency bail-out.

His jump from 40,200 feet where the temperature was -50°F. turned into a horrifying ordeal. The blast of onrushing air and the severe opening shock of 40g knocked him unconscious. The shock tore the thick outer gloves from both his hands and also snapped off the thin inner glove on his left hand. The bail-out bottle continued to function and gave him oxygen until he reached a lower altitude—with one hand frozen.

A few days later, test pilot Perry Ritchie confirmed the fact that opening shock was greater at high altitude. The only safe escape from the cold, lack of sufficient oxygen and brutal opening shock was a long free fall into a more hospitable atmosphere. In this connection, a number of dummy tests performed in 1944 provided additional data. Then an event took place that changed the entire future of live-testing.

Colonel Mel Boynton, an Air Force physician, arrived one day at the Aeromedical Laboratory with a "warrant" from the Inspector General to do a parachute test jump. His instructions: go high, fall low, and get any support he needed from the labs. Dr. Harvey Savely and Major H. M. Sweeney were on the scene and were uncomfortable about it from the beginning. For one thing, Colonel Boynton "passed out" in the altitude chamber. This was not a good sign for a man about to make a high-altitude test jump. Savely and Sweeney at that time talked him into using an automatic opening device on his reserve chute. To date, this device had never been live-tested but had been successful in many dummy drops.

There were signs of relief after several dry runs were made. But again, all was not well the morning of the actual test. Colonel Boynton showed up without his automatic device and a vow never to use it. "The troops don't have it. I won't use it either."

He jumped from 41,000 feet. Indications were that he was still looking at his stopwatch when he crashed into the earth. According to the estimated time of fall, he would have had about 5,000 feet or more to drop when he actually hit. He made no attempt to pull the rip cord so perhaps inaccurate timing had clouded his judgement. His tragic death remains a mystery.

Colonel Boynton's fate affected live-testing and the policies under which they were conducted for many years. Only in May of 1950, was live-testing resumed in high-altitude escape.

World War II also introduced a relatively new term, "g forces," for acceleration and the problems it caused in bailing out of disabled aircraft. During mass bomber raids of B-24s and B-25s, whole crews were mysteriously lost; they had made no apparent attempt to get out of the disabled aircraft. Could it be that the spinning action of the dropping plane pinned men down so that they were unable to jump to safety?

Before the war, some centrifuge work had been done at the University of Southern California so that there was an awareness of acceleration effects. The spinning turntables and whirling gondolas that would become familiar during the astronaut training programs showed clearly that the reason those men did not get out of their airplanes had to do with centrifugal force.

Advanced piston-engined fighters, the new turbojet-powered P-59 and P-80 and the futuristic rocket-powered German Me-163B and the proposed American X-1 and X-2 all promised speed increases to the point where a pilot could no longer just "get out and walk" if anything went wrong. British wind-tunnel tests had indicated, for example, that at such velocity a pilot ejecting from a cockpit reached the rudder post in less than half a second. He was like a cigarette ash flicked out the window of a speeding car.

Dichotomies began to appear as doctors wrestled with complex problems at the Naval Air Crew Equipment Laboratory in Philadelphia and the Aeromed and Equipment Laboratory at Wright Field in Dayton. Before long, Holloman and White Sands, Patuxent, Edwards and El Centro would all be involved. Labs at Pensacola, Johnsville and top civilian industries would all pursue answers to the myriad physiological problems of sending man into the air and space.

World War II brought droves of highly distinguished researchers from civilian life into the military. Three Navy doctors, made significant contributions during this period. Ross McFarland from Harvard University pioneered the medical support of Pan American Airways and researched the physiological effects of altitude and developed pilot selection criteria. His *Human Factors in Air Transportation* was published in 1953. Joseph L. Lilienthal,

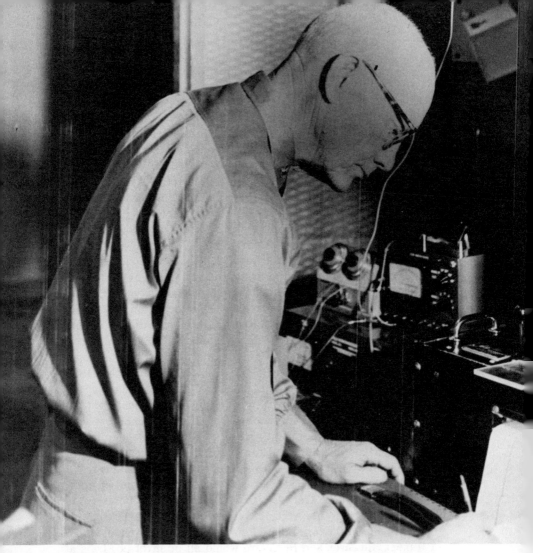

Captain Ashton Graybiel (MC) U.S. Navy, explored problems of weightlessness and vestibular function. He is shown here at the control panel of the slow rotation room at Pensacola./*U.S. Navy*

from the staff of the Johns Hopkins University School of Medicine, worked on the effects of reduced barometric pressure, carbon monoxide and air sickness, as well as selection criteria for aviators.

Ashton Graybiel, over the years, became involved with almost every aspect of research. He was director of research after World War II and retired as a captain. He continued working in medical research and is presently head of the Biological Sciences

Department at the Naval Aerospace Medical Research Laboratory—a direct descendant of the original Navy School of Aviation Medicine.

Another doctor, Eric S. Liljencrantz, who had headed Pan American's medical facility in San Francisco, went on active duty as a lieutenant commander. He was killed on 5 November 1942 near Pensacola while on an experimental research flight.

In 1945, a fundamental study of the anatomical and physiological factors in engineering design was begun by the Aviation Branch, Research Division and the Naval Medical Research Institute. The project was aimed at standardizing aircraft cockpits for the benefit of pilots rather than engineering convenience. "Human Factors in Engineering Design," so dear to the hearts of flight surgeons and other aeromedical specialists, became an accepted practice.

By the end of World War II, a number of more or less independent fields of aviation medicine were recognized: high altitude research, aircraft accident medicine, aeromedical pathology, medical investigations of the effects of weapons, temperature and climate research, the aviator's diet, physiology of reflexes and of the senses—including optical problems, physiology of aviation, flying fitness (physiological), special medical care for flying personnel and related subjects. It was a good beginning. Aviation Medicine was a respected specialty. As for Space Medicine, that was like developing a cure for a disease that did not exist. The very word, "space," was used guardedly by a few visionaries. "Atmospheric space equivalence," worked for a while, like a fig leaf covering the unmentionable on the sober stage of science.

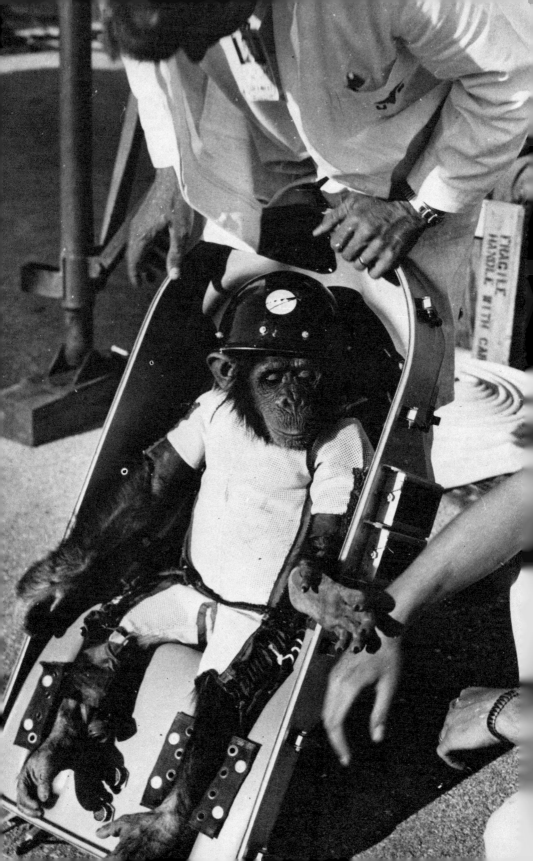

3

Apes, Fruit Flies, and Flying Mice

At 10:17 a.m. on 29 November 1961 a Mercury-Atlas-rocket lifted off the pad at Cape Canaveral in a tower of flame, thundered into the sky and disappeared down range. Tracking stations soon reported the bird on course, and in earth orbit at 17,500mph. Signals transmitted to the ground receiving stations indicated that the lone passenger was carrying out his prescribed tests exactly as planned. However, on the second orbit the spacecraft began to tumble and flight director Christopher C. Kraft, Jr., decided to bring it down after two orbits instead of the scheduled three. At 1:28 p.m. the capsule splashed into the Atlantic some 200 miles south of Bermuda and a boat from the destroyer *Stormes* soon had it aboard the mother ship.

The capsule was opened, and out hopped "astrochimp" Enos (known as *Anthropopithecus* in scientific circles), a little groggy from the interior temperature of 106°F. He soaked up some fresh air for a moment, and then went around shaking hands with all the sailors on deck, for it was a historic moment—Enos was the first chimpanzee to have orbited the earth. He had operated in a condition of no weight for 181 minutes, had experienced

Ham, the nation's first space-ape, made history on 31 January 1961 with his sixteen-minute sub-orbital flight. Trained at Holloman Aeromedical Laboratory, this chimpanzee initiated the U.S. space program with a 156-mile flight into space./*NASA*

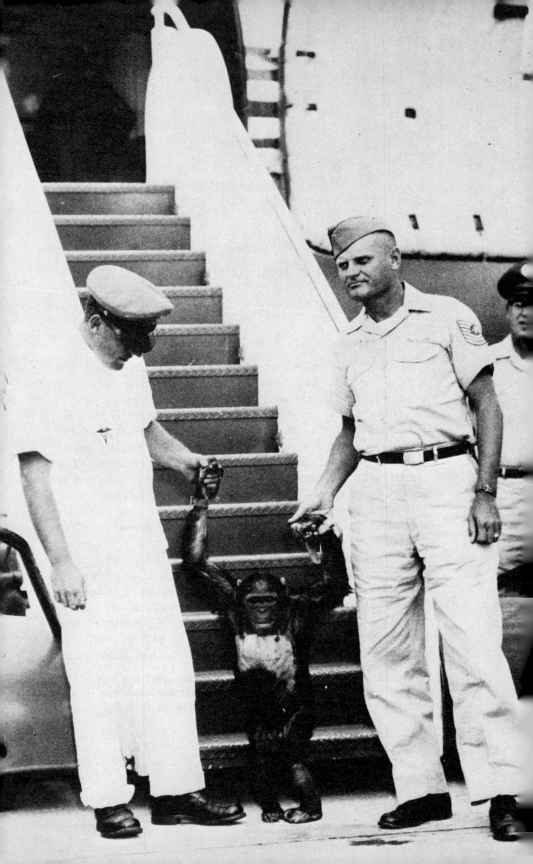

deceleration forces of 7.4g, had suffered no adverse effect of motor functions or visual acuity, and had been able to eat and drink in flight.*

In subsequent press accounts, and some of the space literature of the period, Enos got top billing, yet it was a fellow ape, Ham, who deserved even greater praise, for Ham was the first chimpanzee ever to go into space. Ham (who obviously was attached to the Holloman Aeromedical Laboratory) made his historic space hop on 31 January 1961, lifting off from Cape Canaveral in a Mercury-Redstone rocket. He flew 414 miles in 16.5 minutes and reached an altitude of 156 miles. Ham sipped water, munched on banana-flavored pellets, and pulled levers in his spacecraft as directed by flashing lights on the dashboard, proving that it was possible to operate under conditions of zero gravity.

During the launch, the Redstone booster built up too much speed and the capsule landed 130 miles farther down range than planned, which left Ham bobbing around in the Atlantic for two hours before he was picked up. But his capsule was watertight, and aside from getting rather warm, he suffered no ill effects from his historic journey into space. Ham's respiration and body temperature were monitored during the flight—a first beginning for biomedical telemetry from space. Pre-flight training for Ham—219 hours—showed he had high tolerance to acceleration, and he displayed excellent psychomotor performance and physical reaction during the flight. Enos, whose flight was a more complex affair, had trained for 1263 hours before he went into space.

Ham's flight, short as it was, marked a great step forward in the development of manned spaceflight. Only the Russian dog, Laika, had preceeded him into space. But Ham was a primate, closely related to man, and his reactions in space were of far more value to biomedical research than those of a dog. It might be said that Ham opened the door to spaceflight, Enos stepped through, and proved it was safe, and only then did the astronauts follow them.

*Enos died of *Shigella* dysentery at Holloman Air Force Base on 4 November 1962.

Enos, first chimpanzee to orbit the earth, made his historic flight on 29 November 1961. For 181 minutes, he was literally out of this world—to prove that weightlessness was no problem for a well-trained ape./*NASA*

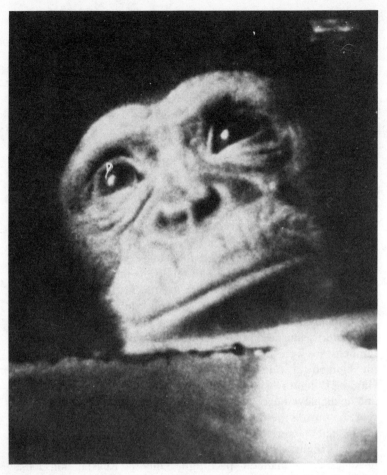

One can only speculate as to what sensations passed through the brain of this serious-faced space traveler, during his historic flight. Ham was making 5,000 miles an hour when this photograph was made./*NASA*

It is fitting to point out here that somewhere in the Miocene age, about 25 million years ago, one of Enos' remote ancestors, a shaggy fellow called *Pliopithecus*, climbed down out of a tree and set out on the long experiment in evolution that would result in *Homo sapiens*. Now *Homo sapiens* was about to set out on another long experiment, so it seemed sensible to call on that still somewhat closely related primate, the chimpanzee, to go see if it might be safe for *Homo sapiens* to venture to the stars.

Man has depended on "all creatures, great and small," ever since Cro-Magnon man sent his dogs into what he hoped was an empty bear's den to make certain it was safe for him to enter. Before men first left the earth in balloons, nearly two centuries ago, to sail the great reaches of the sky where unknown danger might lurk, they again sent animals, to make certain, as it were, that the bear's den was still empty.

Three times, back in 1783, Frenchmen had watched balloons soar into the blue sky and return safely to earth. But what was it *like* up there? Might the rapid rise cause a man to lose his senses? If a man dared to look down from such a height, might he become dizzy and fall to his doom? Long before guinea pigs became the furry symbol of laboratory research, King Louis XVI established the precedent for "Let's guinea-pig it." At his order, a balloon sent up from the gardens of Versailles carried a sheep, a duck, and a cock, whose only apparent reactions to their 8-minute flight was that they had got behind on their eating.

Dogs were frequent passengers in early balloon flights, probably because a spare dog was always handy where any excitement was going on. The logical candidates for all flight and space experiments are, of course, humans, and until the development of high-altitude balloon flight, and the first rocket experiments, all flights were made by men—and a few women. But as flight performance crept up into the unknowns of height and acceleration, trained pilots became the one non-expendable factor of all experimental high altitude flight. The new guinea pigs had to be smaller than a man, bigger than a mouse, smarter than a dog, adaptable and trainable. Primates were the answer, more so because their opposable thumb made it possible for them to perform manual functions in a space capsule, and their reaction time was only two-tenths of a second slower than that of humans.

There were other factors favoring the "chimps" as logical candidates for the honor of preceding man into space. The animals are friendly, easily trained—as the "eggheads" of the animal kingdom they outrank orangutans, gorillas, monkeys, dogs, cats, raccoons, elephants, pigs, mules and horses in intelligence—and

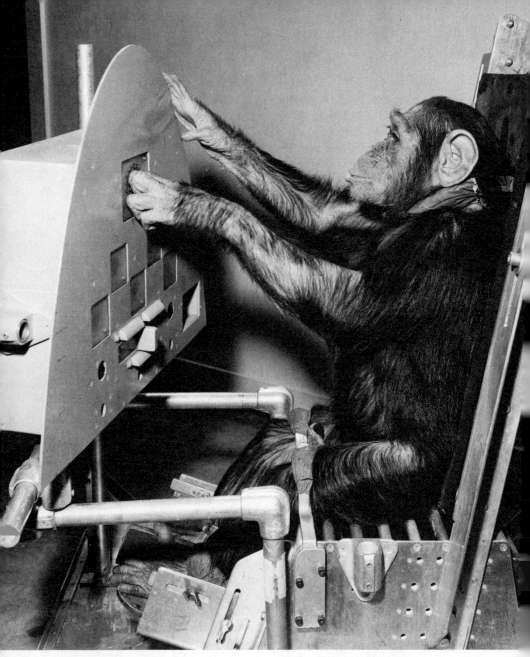

A chimpanzee's opposable thumbs and long fingers made it easy for him to manipulate laboratory equipment, as this willing worker demonstrates. By the very nature of things, there were more apes than astronauts involved in the space program./*Dynalectron Corp.*

are large enougth (115 to 120 pounds, four feet six inches tall) to closely resemble a human body.

In April 1958 President Dwight Eisenhower signed the National Aeronautics and Space Act which created NASA and initiated the national space program. The Air Force had previously initiated a manned space program under the title of Man-in-Space-Soonest (MISS); it was proposed to start test programs with animals about 1958-59, and follow with a manned flight in late 1959. Some 500 military pilots entered the selection and elimination program for Project Mercury which would eventually produce seven astronauts, one of whom, John Glenn, would orbit the earth early in 1962. However, the best way to get into the space program at that time, it appeared, was to be a chimpanzee.

The Aeromedical Research Laboratory at Holloman Air Force Base began training chimpanzees in 1958 in a program initiated by Lieutenant Colonel Rufus R. Hessberg with Major John D. Mosely and Lieutenant William Ward directly responsible for the chimps. Hessberg believed that chimpanzees could be used as a good surrogate of man in terms of testing out the "human consumption" aspects of the Mercury capsule. The idea was chosen by NASA for use in the early demonstration flights of the Mercury program—to test the environmental system with a live load and to test sensory, motor and performance capacity in spaceflight. The idea was in working with chimpanzees, it was possible to start with an entirely new model and train the animals without forcing them to "unlearn" anything—the chimps, born in the Cameroons of West Equatorial Africa, arrived at Holloman when only a few months old, and probably retained only dim memories of their jungle days. They lived with people, worked with people, and performed the experiments in which people were not yet to be committed. Before man finally landed on the moon, chimpanzees had taken part in innumerable experiments and at times made headlines, just like any other astronaut. The chimps proved that they could maintain sensorimotor functions and mental acumen during spaceflight. Man could be expected to perform these same functions during weightlessness and later during the lunar missions.

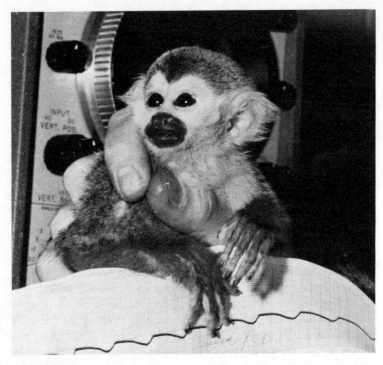

Squirrel monkeys, such as bright-eyed Miss Baker, flew long before chimpanzees got into the air, because their dimunitive bodies fitted into early rocket models. Note the handler's thumb and finger around Miss Baker's neck./*U.S.Navy*

Small *rhesus* monkeys and squirrel monkeys, as well as mice, were sent into space before the chimpanzees were flown—the monkeys because their size made it practical to fit them into earlier rocket nose cones, and mice because they multiply so rapidly that the effect of cosmic radiation on heredity could be quickly determined. Bears and hogs, too large to fly, also took part in deceleration and acceleration tests. But many smaller creatures have been lofted in rockets, or utilized in ground-based research of many types; the space research zoo includes cats, rats, mice, dogs, hamsters, sparrows, turtles, frogs, fruit flies, guppies and spiders. Each in their own small way, the members of this menagerie provided inceased confidence that man's successful performance in space was possible.

Research in many aspects of biomedical science advanced slowly in the early years, and in some cases, because of technical difficulties, the projects never got off the ground. If a line of research commenced in Vienna in 1931 had been completed, headlines some thirty years later would have informed the world that the first astronauts from earth to land on the moon would have been, not men, but mice.

The "Moon-Mice Investigations" began with a chance meeting in the cafeteria at the University of Zurich when Constantine D. J. Generales, Jr., a third-year medical student at the University of Berlin, shared a table with another young fellow who turned out to be Wernher von Braun, from whom, for the first time, Generales heard of Herman Oberth and Robert Goddard and their experiments with rockets. Even then, von Braun was enthused about space travel and the possibility of sending a rocket to the moon. Generales saw at once that space technology would be highly dependent on medical science, and advised von Braun "If you want to get to the moon, it is better to try with mice first." Spaceflight, to von Braun, meant linear propulsion and linear acceleration, and Generales suggested that experiments with mice in a simple centrifuge would show their reactions to high-g forces.

The first centrifuge was a prime example of much of the make shift research that went on later in the space program. Generales pulled a wheel off his bicycle, rigged it on a stand, and put mice in small bags around the rim of the wheel. Within a week, the primitive centrifuge was producing forces as high as 220g, far in excess of what mice could tolerate. Dissection showed displaced heart and lungs, and bleeding in the thorax, abdomen, and cranium. If men were going to the moon, they had to learn to contend with g forces and understand their limitations in that respect.

Unfortunately, the first centrifuge experiments were cut short by an over-fastidious landlady. The two men did their work in von Braun's room, until a mouse flew off the centrifuge at high speed to become a bloody splatter on the wall, and the first biomedical research fatality, all at once. One more mouse on the wall, ruled the landlady, and the police would be there.

Thirty years later, in Rochester, New York, Generales made a somewhat poorly received proposal to the Medical Society that a "Moonbeam Mouse Project" be set up to investigate how terrestrial life would react to lunar conditions, to detect possible lunar micro-organisms, and to study the effects of such captive hosts on terrestrial germ-free rodents. The plan was to launch mice in a rocket that would land them on the moon where a special capsule would bore at least ten meters under the lunar surface, with a two-week life support system and through multiple-channel telemetry return extensive biomedical data to earth.

Although a microbiologist of the Rockefeller Institute and a rocket engineer with NASA favored the project, it was turned down in 1960 by NASA because no one could see "how mice could survive in the moon's environment." Twelve years later mice actually flew to the moon. Two turtles made the trip too, in 1968, aboard a Russian unmanned vehicle that made a circumlunar passage. The mice—five of them—were pocket mice (*Perognathus longimembris*) from the California desert, who made the 13-day trip aboard Apollo 17. They remained aboard the spacecraft, in an experiment designed to assess the degree to which exposure to cosmic ray particles might endanger astronauts. Four of the mice survived the trip, but one had trouble walking on return to earth; it was found to have suffered hemorrhage in its middle ear cavities during the flight. The five mice were hit by a total of 80 cosmic ray particles during their flight. The conclusion was that the lack of demonstrable lesions in their brains left unresolved the degree of vulnerability of brain tissue to radiation. Animal flights alone had all the risks and problems of spaceflight, but without men available to take action in case of a malfunction. Men undoubtedly would have gone to the moon, whether or not apes and mice preceeded them into space, but there may have been some small comfort in the thought that anything an ape or a mouse could do, a man could do better.

The short-lived centrifuge experiments by Generales and von Braun were not the last, fortunately, in the effort to simulate conditions of angular and linear acceleration incident to spaceflight. Nor were they the first. Erasmus Darwin, an English physician in the late 18th century, tried a simple centrifuge for its therapeutic value in producing sleep or reducing heart activity. German experiments later resulted in better understanding of centrifugal force on both respiration and circulation. The German Air Ministry in the mid-30s began operating a centrifuge, as did the American Interplanetary Society. The most sophisticated centrifuge for its time was that engineered by the Navy Aviation Medical Acceleration Laboratory at Johnsville, where the experimental subjects were usually human, although chimpanzees have been used. The chimps were supplied by the Aeromedical Field Laboratory and subjected to forces as high at 40g for up to 60 seconds. The animals survived, but developed electrocardiogram abnormalities. Autopsies performed by the Armed Forces Institute of Pathology showed that they had suffered internal injuries. The tests, aimed at determining re-entry capsule configurations, showed that a subject in a completely supine position was relatively unharmed.

During the foreseeable future, astronauts will probably do much of their work in pressurized suits, but the suggestion that they could withstand far greater forces while immersed in a fluid has resulted in experiments with small animals. At Pensacola, the Navy's School of Aviation Medicine has subjected mice to a force of 1300g for 90 seconds. Guppies have survived up to 10,000g—while submerged, naturally—and the micro-organism *Euglena gracilis* has survived up to 212,000g for four hours. The average man subjected to such a force would have an apparent weight of about 1850 tons.

American experiments in space biology began with the Air Force firing of captured German V-2 rockets at the White Sands Proving Grounds. These experiments were sponsored by the Aero Medical Laboratory at Wright-Patterson Air Force Base, where Dr. James P. Henry was head of the Acceleration Unit of the Biophysics Branch. The intricate and sophisticated spacecraft that put men on the moon had its beginning then, as Dr. Henry, Captain David Simons, and others sought to devise a pressurized capsule in which a small monkey could ride in the nose cone of a V-2 rocket to the upper limits of the atmosphere. The merits of sending a monkey up first soon became apparent, because, while scientists and engineers gained valuable experience, the flights

91

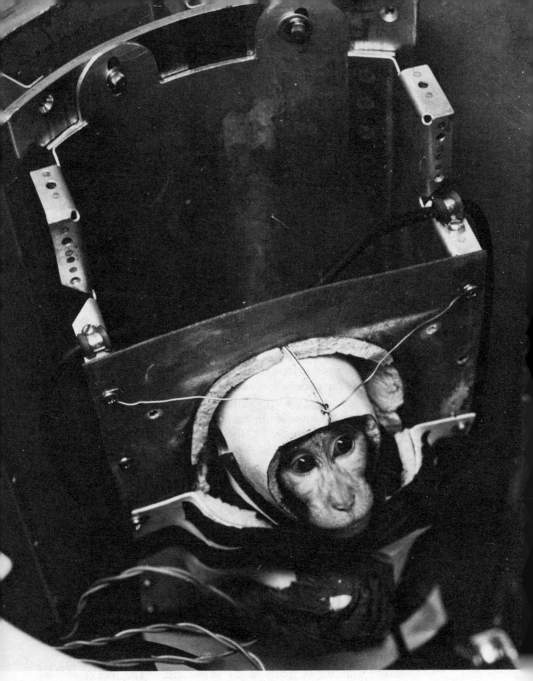

An American-born rhesus monkey, named Able, is suited up for a 9g ride on the centrifuge, during which his physiological reactions were recorded./*U.S. Army*

were hard on the monkeys, who justly deserve mention in some simian hall of fame for their small sacrifices in the space effort.

The first V-2 flight was made on 18 June 1948, with a nine-pound rhesus monkey named Albert as the passenger. Albert was anesthetized, which was as well, because he died as a result of breathing difficulties before the rocket got off the ground. There were many operational failures; the equipment for transmitting respiratory movements malfunctioned before launch, and the parachute recovery system failed, so Albert would have been killed on impact if he had lasted that long. A year later another rocket with a redesigned capsule lofted Albert II; that one worked a little better; Albert II won the short-lived fame of having survived a rocket launching, and ascent, to 83 miles. But again the chute was defective and the high-speed descent to a crash landing proved fatal.

A third time, a fourth time, a fifth time the Aero Medical Laboratory people watched a V-2 rocket blast off into the sky. The animals survived peak forces of 5.5g during acceleration, they withstood up to 15g when the parachute recovery system opened, and they survived the period of zero-gravity and sub-gravity—but the parachute always failed and none of them survived impact.

In 1948-49 operations shifted to Holloman Air Force Base, where an Aerobee test facility had been established as a part of the Air Force missile program. The first aeromedical Aerobee flight went up on 18 April 1951. The recovery capsule for the flight, extensively redesigned, was fully instrumented. Ground recordings indicated that the monkey had normal respiratory and circulatory conditions, and that acceleration, deceleration, and weightlessness did not affect him. He survived everything except the impact due to a faulty parachute. At that point, it was apparent that nothing less than perfection in all aspects of a flight had to be achieved before a man ever rode a rocket into space.

The next flight, on 20 September 1951, proved that at last the system had been perfected. A monkey and 11 mice were lofted to the extreme height of 263,000 feet, and returned to earth alive. The parachute worked. The capsule landed safely. But the ground crews *could not find it* for an hour, and the baking desert heat killed the monkey. The mice fared better, and proved that after flying in a state of weightlessness they suffered no disorientation or incapacitation of physical dexterity.

The Aerobee flight series ended on 21 May 1952 when two rhesus monkeys named Patricia and Michael and two unnamed mice rode another rocket to an altitude of 36 miles and returned safely to earth. The mice were placed in a rotating cage and photographed during flight. One, with a paddle to cling to, remained oriented during sub-gravity; the other, with nothing to cling to showed temporary disorientation during the period of weightlessness—which was too short to allow any firm conclusions. The monkeys, one seated upright and the other in a supine position, showed no adverse physiological effects of the flight. They "retired" from biomedical research and went to lead a quiet life at the National Zoological Park in Washington.

As might be expected, people of the "if man had been meant to fly he would have had wings" school of thought and certain animal lovers complained strongly against the V-2 and Aerobee aeromedical flights. In contrast, many people volunteered to ride the rockets. They were not all headline hunters; some were hoping to pay some debt to society by gathering scientific information at considerable personal risk and inconvenience. One of the volunteers wrote from a state penitentiary, possibly on the assumption that any change in his status would be for the better.

The Russians, too, utilized animals in research, and it is probable that they launched an animal-bearing rocket as early as 1951. But as they were inclined to keep quiet about unsuccessful ventures and publicize only those that paid off, it was not until they orbited Sputnik II, with a dog on board, on 3 November 1957 that the world learned of their biomedical research in space.

The dog, named Laika, was a Siberian husky, weighing about 13 pounds. The space capsule carried a life-support system adequate for a week—air conditioning, temperature control, and food. Through telemetry, the Russians were able to monitor the dog's respiration and heart rate, as well as blood pressure and electrocardiogram. There was no attempt to recover the satellite—after a week in space the dog was "put to sleep" by asphyxiation.

94

The episode aroused animal lovers everywhere, who were concerned about the dog, hurtling through space in silence and loneliness. Actually, the dog had been well trained for her mission, and after adjusting to the condition of weightlessness, probably became bored and spent much of her time sleeping, as any dog would. At that point, there was nothing animal lovers could do about a Russian dog that passed over the U.S. once every 103 minutes at an altitude of some 100 miles. There was not nearly so much objection to the use of chimpanzees in U.S. space experiments, despite the fact that biologically they were man's first cousins—dogs were man's best friend.

At least, after Russia's first astro-dog died, no one had to go out and bury her. Laika remained in space for over six months, during which she made 2,470 orbits of the earth; she finally returned to earth as a "shooting star," trailing fire and smoke, to splash down into the Caribbean south of the Virgin Islands on 14 April 1958.

The Laika flight was unique in the field of subgravity studies, although results would have been more conclusive if the dog had been recovered, or photographic records had been made. However, there was no evidence of disabling ill effects as a result of lengthy subgravity exposure.

The first animals to return from space were two dogs named Strelka and Belka, sent aloft by the Russians on 19 August 1960 in Sputnik V. They were accompanied by a pair of white rats, a couple of dozen black and white mice, and several hundred fruit flies, as well as some plants and various biological and bacterial specimens. The animals spent 24 hours in space, during which they orbited the earth 16 times. The Russians had equipped Sputnik V with biomedical telemetry to furnish physiological data on the dogs, and equipment to monitor the life-support system of the spacecraft. They also fitted the capsule with television, which showed that the dogs appeared uneasy and alarmed during the launch. At that time their normal heart beat rates of from 75 to 90 climbed to 150 to 160, and respiration went from 24 to as high as 240 per minute. But once in orbit, they ate, showed irritation from time to time, and slept.

In general, the dogs and rodents all withstood the forces of acceleration and deceleration, and the condition of weightlessness, with no adverse effects.

Subsequent Sputnik missions put several dogs, and one rabbit, into earth orbits. Only one flight failed—Sputnik VI, with Pschelka and Mushka on board, burned on re-entry in December of 1960. A dog named Chernuska landed on 9 March 1961 after an orbital flight in Sputnik IX. Later that month, the world's only known space rabbit, Zvezdotchka, returned safely from an orbital flight aboard Sputnik X. Russian scientists kept five of their space-dogs under careful observation for 18 months after their flights, during which time none of them showed any pathological effects of their ventures into space.

Project Mercury, for which Hessberg began collecting chimpanzees at Holloman Air Force Base, was the first American program in which man was able to test his physiological capabilities to withstand the effects of the extra-terrestrial environment for more than a few seconds. To that point in aviation history, earth-bound research had been able to acquire only limited information on many problems affecting spaceflight; weightlessness, subgravity, radiation, potential disorientation, toxic hazards, and acceleration, deceleration, and impact forces. However, NASA management was concerned with the entire spectrum of life sciences, which included ecology, exobiology, and the projected application of space medicine. What had been known as aviation medicine became, with the initiation of Project Mercury, space medicine. Later it became known as aerospace medicine.

But in Project Mercury, and in other areas, research went on in many other aspects of spaceflight; design of seats and capsules, environmental control of capsule interiors, telemetry, and re-entry, that critical part of the spaceflight when return to earth depended on prompt deployment and operation of the parachute that took a capsule to splashdown. The complete list of interrelated disciplines grew longer almost daily, yet in all such work, from cosmic radiation to subgravity, chimpanzees and other animals played a most useful part.

Early high-altitude balloon flights almost always carried experiments in cosmic ray research, and insects—especially fruit flies—provided good subjects because of their rapid reproduction rate. During the Moby Dick series of flights, fruit flies were sent up in packages of 600 each. But the flights were too long to allow effective tracking, small packages were difficult to locate when they returned to earth, and only a few of them were returned to Holloman where the flights originated. Generally, ground heat killed the flies before they were found—out of several thousand sent aloft, only 12 flies came back alive.

Another cosmic ray research project, carried aloft by Commanders M. Lee Lewis and Malcolm Ross on a flight from 26 to 27 July 1958, set a sort of record for the most passengers ever carried in a balloon and offered some rather itchy prospects if anything went wrong, as they carried a lively crowd of 10,000 small laboratory subjects, from fleas to honey bees.

While cosmic ray studies had been conducted at Holloman Air Force Base for several years, with insects, monkeys and other small animals being sent aloft, some time passed before it was felt safe to launch a manned flight for such purpose. There was valid reason for the delay; it was easy enough to put an experimental subject into space, but getting him down intact, and finding him, was another matter, as the fruit flies proved. The first cosmic radiation flight made after David Simons took over the Space Biology Branch in 1953 involved seven hamsters which landed, in a sealed capsule, after a 90,000-foot-high, long duration flight, at a naval air station in Florida. The Navy, somewhat understandably reluctant to open something about which no one knew anything, telegraphed the Aeromedical Field Laboratory requesting disposition of the packages. A communication foul-up at headquarters kept the message on ''hold'' for six days before it was delivered. A priority telephone call to Florida saved the unhappy hamsters from starvation, although one died the next day and another was eaten by his hungry friends.

The use of animals in space research—and a prediction of the sort of fate that overtook the Holloman hamster—was described, long before the space age, by Jules Verne in his classic account of lunar adventure, *From the Earth to the Moon*, published in 1865. Before the actual ''moon shot,'' Verne's technical expert staged an experimental shot with a 32-inch mortar, to determine impact force. The passengers were a cat and a pet squirrel. The projectile reached an altitude of about a thousand feet before it splashed down in the bay. Within five minutes it had been recovered, and opened, and the cat, healthy as ever, hopped out. But, according to Verne, there was no trace of the squirrel: "They had to face the truth: the cat had eaten his traveling companion."

Space experts may praise Verne for his understanding of the celestial mechanics involved in a moon shot, but cat lovers will have to fault him on his knowledge of cats; a cat will play with his catch for a long time before he eats it, and the hungriest cat in the world would not eat fur and bones under any circumstances.

Even plain backyard-type radish seeds and hen eggs were used in experiments on the effects of cosmic radiation. The Aeromedical Field Laboratory at Holloman Air Force Base sent the radish seeds aloft, then watched their germination in order to detect any resulting effects. They also tried the same trick with eggs but gave up on that one—nature had never designed eggs to become test subjects. Fruit flies exposed to cosmic radiation were returned to the laboratory for mating—but aside from the insects themselves, according to Simons, the experiment was of interest only to pilots "in terms of morale."

Possibly the most unique experimental research in subgravity was conducted in Argentina where Dr. Harald von Beckh worked with water turtles as the subjects. Dr. von Beckh who later joined the Aeromedical Field Laboratory, discovered that a turtle whose vestibular function had been accidentally injured outperformed other turtles in coordination and orientation during an aircraft subgravity flight. The turtle had evidently learned to compensate visually for the lack of normal gravitational cues. Even normal turtles, exposed to subgravity in vertical dives lasting as long as seven seconds, adapted to such conditions. Later, human subjects were used and in a series of eye-hand coordination tests, reacted as did the turtles, by first over-reaching during subgravity, but later improving. These experiments also showed that when a plane entered subgravity by a maneuver causing high acceleration forces, the recovery from acceleration-induced blackout took longer than normal.

While astronauts might reasonably be expected to be as sure-footed as cats, it came as some surprise to researchers in

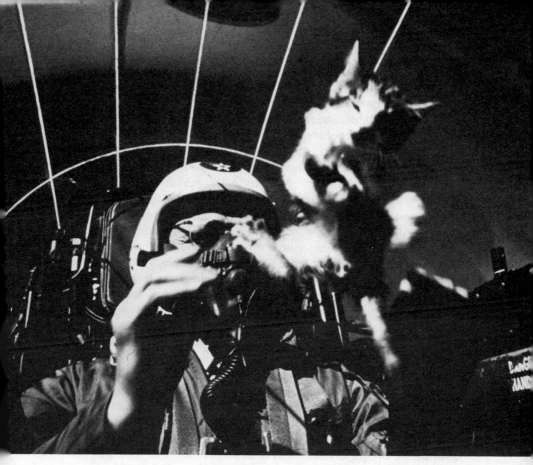

This high-flying cat, not worried about which way the pilot is sitting, instinctively goes through bodily contortions in order to get right side up./*NASA*

subgravity to find that cats did not make good astronauts. Experiments at the Space Biology Branch of the Aeromedical Field Laboratory, commenced in the mid-50s under the direction of Captain Grover J. D. Schock, utilized domestic cats in subgravity research. Cats were known to have a highly developed vestibular function, and a reflex ability to always land on their feet even when dropped from an upside down position. Surprising enough, cats dropped upside down in subgravity lost their sense of which way was up. Some cats with part of their vestibular apparatus removed were equally confused; on the other hand, those cats with all vestibular apparatus removed and accustomed to "navigate" without it remained fully oriented and displayed normal reflex actions when dropped—unless they were blindfolded. Once again, the critical importance of visual orientation was confirmed.

Let there be no misconception about chimpanzees being "suited up" for rocket flights, and treated with soft drinks at governmental expense, as some sort of inspired Air Force monkey business. The Mercury-Redstone flight on 31 January 1961 in which Ham reached an apogee of 156 miles and a range of 414 miles in about seventeen minutes, and the Mercury-Atlas orbital flight of 29 November 1961 in which Enos flew around the earth twice, were in effect dress rehearsals for the similar, subsequent sub-orbital flight by Alan Shepard (apogee of 115 miles in 14.4 minutes), and orbital flight of John Glenn (three orbits in 4 hours 56 minutes).

The animal test program at Holloman was established to provide animal verification of a successful spaceflight prior to manned flight, collect data on the physical and psychological demands which were to be encountered by the astronauts during space-flights, conduct dynamic test of operational procedures and training of support personnel in handling the biomedical program for manned flight, and evaluate the spacecraft environmental control system and bioinstrumentation under flight conditions. The ultimate purpose of the program had been simply stated in 1959 by Colonel Don Flickinger: "In preparing for the first manned orbital flight, the factor of crew reliability and safety is one of major importance...we are faced with the prime requirement of insuring the complete attainment of mission objectives, including the safe return of the astronaut—and on the first try."

The "chimponauts" trained for their flights by spending many long hours restrained in a laboratory model of the flight couch. The animals were trained in the use of a psychomotor flight programmer, an intricate electronic package in which flashing display unit symbols or colored lights had to be responded to in an exact, timed sequence for a reward of food or water. Incorrect response resulted in either a blackout of display board, or an electric shock.

Setting the style for later manned flights, both pre-flight and in-flight medical and physiological aspects were monitored. Pre-launch physiological data were recorded direct; flight data were recorded and taped in the capsule, then telemetered to ground stations or recorded by in-flight aircraft. Measurements were made of ECG, respiration waveform, and rectal temperature. Heart rates and respiration rates were also measured. In the first

100

minutes of flight, heart and respiration rates, and rectal temperatures were lower than measured when the animals were tested on a centrifuge. During re-entry, heart and respiration rates went well above those recorded in the centrifuge.

The flights showed that the noise and vibration of a rocket launching did not affect work performance of the chimps, nor did exposure to weightlessness. It was possible to eat and drink normally in the weightlessness state, and visual and temporal response processes and continuous and discrete motor behavior were not affected by weightlessness. The one great hole in the spread of information gained by the ballistic and orbital flights of chimpanzees was that which could only be furnished by trained pilots communicating their reactions and observations to ground observers to settle that century old question: What's it *like* up there?

Ever since Isaac Newton established the law of gravity, man had been content in his belief that what went up must come down. But rocket-powered flight offered two unpleasant alternatives: without proper guidance, a rocket that escaped earth orbit would never come down and any spacecraft returning to earth would subject its occupants to heavy and possibly fatal deceleration and impact forces. (The Apollo II astronauts, on returning to earth, were moving at more than 24,700 miles an hour on re-entry, only 11 minutes before splashdown.) Experiments to determine the effects of such re-entry forces were conducted at Holloman commencing in 1953, under the direction of Colonel John Paul Stapp. Again, chimpanzees were frequent, if not always willing, participants —after a 600mph ride terminating in a shattering stop, one could understand why a few of them "went ape" the next time they were brought out to the rocket sled.

In the Holloman tests, subjects rode a rocket-powered sled, known as Sonic Wind Number 1, developed by Northrop Aircraft Corporation, along a 3500-foot track. As usual, a chimpanzee went first, on 28 January 1954. Three months later Stapp rode the sled which reached 420mph, then came to a sudden stop measured at 22g. Later the track was lengthened to 5,000 feet for higher performance; in 1957 a chimpanzee took a force of 247g for one millisecond, then came to a stop measured at 22g. After more chimpanzee runs at speeds around 600mph, Colonel Stapp rode the sled on 10 December 1954 in a memorable experiment that made him in fact "the fastest man of earth"—the sled reached a maximum speed of 937 feet per second—more than 10 miles a minute—and actually passed a T-33 aircraft flying overhead. Stapp experienced a windblast effect of more than 1,000 pounds per square foot, and when water brakes brought the sled to a stop in 1.4 seconds, deceleration commenced at 600g per second. The effect was the same as driving a car into a solid wall at 120mph.

Another dozen chimpanzee runs with Sonic Wind Number 2 reached top speeds of just under 1,000mph. Then tests moved to China Lake in California, where Captain John D. Mosely was in charge. An Astrodyne rocket motor called "Megaboom" developed a thrust of 1,000,000 pounds in 10 seconds to drive a sled down the new 35,000-foot track, the longest in the world, at mach plus 2. The first test run there, designed for windblast, was made on 13 April 1957. The chimp wore a special flying suit devised by the Aeromedical Field Laboratory, and a helmet, but the headrest broke before the sled reached supersonic speed and the helmet failed, jerked, and broke his neck. In further tests, helmet and clothing failed; the subjects received second and third degree burns from windblast. Even so, chimpanzees held up better than guinea pigs: in one test, two guinea pigs attached to the sled with nylon net and a third riding in a metal container with a 1X2-inch opening simply vanished in terrific windblast.

None of the high-speed sled runs determined a precise tolerance limit for windblast, much less the point at which it would become fatal. The tests helped in designing better protective clothing, and also helped point the way toward development of an ejection seat for supersonic aircraft, and an escape capsule to eliminate windblast.

The Sonic Sleds were unique vehicles, designed for one use only, and their passenger list was a select group—a dozen or so chimpanzees and a few Air Force officers. An even more unusual facility was developed at Holloman under the prosaic title of Task 78503—the Holloman Short Track. A mere 120 feet long, it was designed to fire a test sled by compressed air, as did the Daisy air rifle, and so became known as the Daisy Track, even though for several years before the compressed air system was operational,

102

the sled was fired by gunpowder charges used in seat ejection catapults.

The sleds carried couches in which a subject lay on his side in a seat that could be rotated in all directions at 15-degree increments. Its purpose was to test animal and human reactions to dynamic linear forces of 50 to 5000g per second at rate of onset, 10 to 200g magnitude, and durations of 10 to 100 milliseconds, in all phases of body orientation.

As usual, a chimpanzee went first, followed by Lieutenant Wilbur C. Blount on 17 February 1956. Other officers and enlisted men assigned to the Biodynamics branch rode the sled, as did Colonel Stapp, but the most unusual passengers on the Daisy Track were bears and hogs.

Bears were used because their pelvis is similar to that of humans. Only four were used at a cost of only $150 each, but they created great excitement among that portion of the national press which makes big news stories out of small leads. After tests were run, the animals were "expended" in laboratory examinations. A few hogs were also used in Daisy Track experiments, which led to a request for Colonel Stapp to explain things to a Congressional subcommittee: "You wonder why I use hogs and chimpanzees? Well, man is somewhere between the hog and the chimpanzee. Some people are more like hogs; others are more like chimpanzees."

Nothing was said about humans and rats, but one Daisy test showed that rats had their worth. In an all-time record run, on 16 May 1958, Captain Eli J. Beeding, Jr., seated upright and facing backward, took a force of 83g for a duration of one-tenth second. He went into shock for a short time, but recovered. Two rats rode the sled on the same run. One, protected by an "anti-g platform," showed no shock effect at all. The other was unprotected and much the worse for wear.

In 1962, a couple of nameless bears took part in the first supersonic tests of ejection seats. In March a bear was ejected from a B-58 at 45,000 feet, at a speed of 870mph and the following month another bear was ejected at 1,060mph. The animals were not pets, but laboratory subjects pure and simple; they were anesthetized before the tests, and autopsied afterward to evaluate the physiological effects of high-speed ejection.

It may come as some surprise to biomedical researchers and test pilots, whose background in astronomy might be limited, to learn that the nameless bears they expended in working out details of spaceflight already have their own monument in space. Since the time of Ulysses, the constellations of Ursa Major and Ursa Minor—the Great Bear and Little Bear, but better known as the Big Dipper and Little Dipper—have circled the Pole Star. And long before rockets boosted dogs into orbit, the dogs, too, had their celestial monuments—Sirius, the most spectacular star in the northern sky, marks the constellation of Canis Major or the Great Dog, and Procyon marks the constellation of Canis Minor, or the Little Dog, Even the fruit flies that were expended by the hundreds in cosmic ray research have their name in the sky; down beyond the Southern Cross is a dim constellation of seven stars, called Musca—the Fly.

The first "flying fish" in the space program were common goldfish, sealed in common goldfish bowls and taken on brief zero-g flights in Keplerian trajectories during experiments at Brooks Air Force Base in 1960. Goldfish did not care for the heavy g forces of acceleration and deceleration, but during the brief intervals of zero g they swam sideways, belly down, or belly up, with apparent disregard of which way was really right. Astronauts on the Apollo moon flights found out that the goldfish were right. In space, up is merely the direction from a pilot's feet toward his head.

Long after the Apollo series of flights terminated, animals still were active in space research. Two notable participants in space research were a couple of common spiders named Anita and Arabella, who made the 59-day mission in the first American space station, Skylab, from 22 June to 25 September 1973. The spiders were taken aboard at the suggestion of science-minded teen-ager Judith Miles in an experiment to determine how their web-spinning capability would be affected in a zero-gravity condition. The spider named Arabella was allowed to spin webs at once, but she had difficulty until she adjusted to weightlessness. Anita was not allowed to commence a web until she had adjusted to zero-gravity, at which time she went to work just as she used to back on earth, to spin a perfect web on her first attempt.

104

Along with the spiders went what might well be termed the worlds highest-flying fish, some Mummichog minnows—certainly no other fish had ever flown 270 miles above the earth. The minnows at first had trouble in their zero-gravity world, and swam in tight loops until they had learned the secret of no-gravity navigation. But the secret was readily learned. Some Mummichog minnow eggs were also taken into space. When they hatched, the tiny space-fish, having adjusted to zero-gravity while still in their eggs, swam exactly as their ancestors had on earth, regular minnow fashion. Weightlessness, whether experienced by men or minnows, is not the hazard it was once suspected to be. When men set out on the months-long voyage to Mars, the Mummichog minnows will cheer them on the way.

Of all the animals that took part in the space program, the ones that might have seemed most removed from anything having to do with space or the moon in any aspect were *Crassostrea virginica*, better known as oysters. No oysters went to the moon, but after the Apollo flights, numbers of them had lunar material injected through small holes in their shells, to ascertain if it contained any viable or replicating agents capable of infecting and multiplying in animals. If the experiment proved anything, it bore out the truth of that light-hearted variation of "Murphy's Law," known as the "Harvard Law of Animal Behavior," which states that under carefully controlled conditions, organisms behave as they damn' well please. The oysters that got lunar material brought back by Apollo II and 14 curled up and died in large numbers, while those that got the stuff brought back by Apollo 12, remained, one might say, as happy as clams.

The successful completion of the Apollo missions, and the subsequent Skylab flights, proved the immense value of using animals in testing out capsules, restraining devices, protective clothing, re-entry techniques, cabin environment, and biomedical telemetry. Only a few of the primates and dogs were given names; most of them were laboratory subjects, numbered for record purposes, and they were so "expended." As momentous as it seemed, man's first small step on the moon was made possible only at the expense of countless lesser creatures.

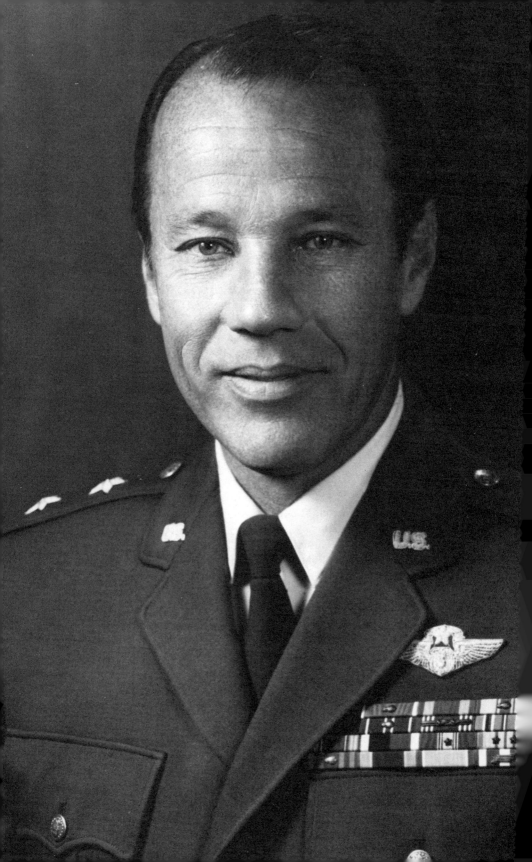

4

Who Did What and Why

The emotions men feel on leaving this green earth for the dark voids of space have been described many times. Each astronaut who has made such a journey has had a unique and highly personal reaction. One of the men who most recently walked on the moon, geologist-astronaut Harrison H. Schmitt, considered his experience in a highly philosophical light, and expressed himself with sensitivity well worth reading.

"...we see the earth only as we prepare to leave it. First, there are the basically familiar though expanded views of earth from the now well-traveled orbits: banded sunrises and sunsets changing in a few seconds from black to purple to red to yellow to searing daylight and then back in never-ending progression; tinted oceans and continents with structural patterns wrought by aging during four-and-one-half billion years of time; shadowed clouds and snows ever-varying in their mysteries and beauty; and the warm fields of lights by night and of homes by day created by men but not seen without the boundaries in their minds."

"But then, as we leave what is familiar, the strange new perspective is that of the earth filling only one window and

George Schafer was the first American flight surgeon assigned to a jet squadron, where he sought to ease pilot concern over possible damage to virility by experiments with rats. He recently retired as Surgeon General of the Air Force and was a former President of the Aerospace Medical Association./U.S. Air Force gradually, not even doing that. The disquieting thought is that it is no longer the earth of our past. It is only a fragile blue globe in space.''

"There is no apparent purpose in the cyclic wandering of our ship through its own universal sea. The forces that hold us to this invisible course have been long explained but never understood. There are waves that we do not feel, there are storms we cannot see, and there is history we have not read. Only the hope of continuity has always been reality during our voyage around the sun and through the galaxy.''

"Again, like childhood's home which we now only visit, changing in time but unchanged in the mind, we see the full earth revolve beneath us. All the tracks of man's earlier greatness and folly are displayed in our window in the course of a single day. The Roman world, the explorers' paths around the continents, the trails across old frontiers, and the migrations of peoples are accented in their significance by our own act of seeing.''

"Then, with some of the disappointment felt as loved ones age, we see the gradual change with each revolution as the full earth changes to half and then to crescent and then to a faint moonlit hole in space. The line of night, like time itself, masks but does not destroy beauty.''

Schmitt was a new kind of astronaut—a civilian. By the very nature of things, all U.S. flight operations from World War I on had been conducted by the military services with military pilots. But the space program was conducted by NASA, which is not a military organization, and with the inception of the Apollo program, it became evident that qualification as an astronaut did not necessarily require a military background. Civilians Walter Cunningham and Russell Schweickart had preceded Schmitt into space, and others would follow him. The new trend was reminiscent of the change in status of flight surgeons who, up until World War II, performed most of their duties on the ground.

Following World War II, the profile of the flight surgeon changed considerably and many were flying as pilots. Lieutenant Colonel Burt Rowen who would later act as flight surgeon for the

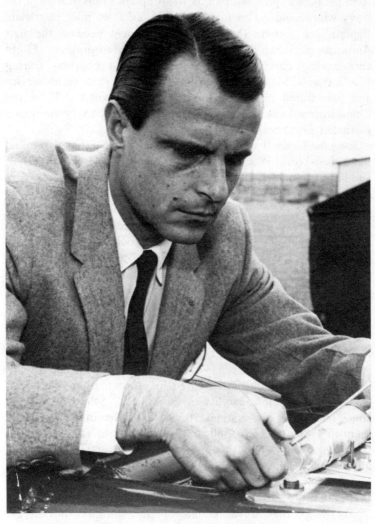

After World War II, Harald von Beckh, M.D. left Germany for Argentina. At the invitation of Colonel John Paul Stapp, he came to the United States to investigate weightlessness problems, acceleration and deceleration. He is now Director of Medical Research at the Naval Air Development Center in Warminster, Pennsylvania./*U.S. Air Force*

X-15 pilots, was jet qualified, as was Captain Frank Austin of the Navy who would go on loan to NASA as a jet pilot physician. Captain Joe Kerwin (MC) U.S. Navy would become the first American physician astronaut during the Skylab program. Flight surgeons took part in balloon and parachute test programs. During World War II, Major Don Flickinger formed a Pararescue service and parachuted to rescue survivors of a downed C-47 in the China-Burma-India theater. Among those rescued was the famed journalist Eric Sevareid.

Surgeon General of the Air Force, General Schafer recalled those post-World War II days: "It was a very interesting period, and I think a lot of aviation medicine had to do with people's fears as opposed to reality. For example, a man was supposed to blow up if he broke the sound barrier...That was the time (1947-48-49) that we were first getting into jets. There were theories about such things as, "jet illness," and that men would become impotent because of jet flying. Literature came out of England describing cases of jet illness; one turned out to be multiple sclerosis and the other was central nervous system syphilis."

General Schafer was the first flight surgeon assigned to a jet outfit—the Fourth Fighter Squadron. An early problem was to get the men to stop worrying about their virility. "...so we manufactured an experiment. And I can remember so well it was probably the sloppiest thing ever done, and perhaps had a little bit of chicanery in it, but we wanted to prove to them that they wouldn't lose their capability to reproduce." Schafer wheedled some rats out of the National Institute of Health and air-lifted them in F-80s (the old P-80s). "As a matter of fact I kept the rats in one of the squadron ops and the guys mixed up a couple of girl rats with some of the boy rats and we had babies before we were supposed to. It messed up our data..."

Eventually, Schafer wrote a report of this experiment along with other things that were related to the so-called physiologic problems of jet flying. He was told by the Strategic Air Command Surgeon that he should present his findings to the National Research Council, which he did with some trepidation. "I started out by saying this is not controlled, it may be of no value but it's the only thing we have right now. An old physiologist out of

110

Harvard wanted to know if I had taken the rectal temperatures of the rats. He criticized me vehemently for not doing that..."

The story ended well, however, with the pilots' fears being allayed. The only harm done occurred during a temporary duty assignment when he was weathered in at Maxwell Air Force Base for seven days. "I finally got a message delivered to me one night at the officers club, "Return at once. One of the female rats just bit the old man!"

Backache was another problem with the first squadron of jet pilots. There was considerable conjecture as to the causes at the time; the solution proved quite simple though probably unscientific by today's standards. "Pilots were sitting on their old parachute seat packs in the bucket seats. The seat pack would eventually slip out a little bit from under them and they'd wind up sitting in the hiatus between it, and they'd really be sitting on their lumbar spine half of the flight. So I wrote this up, sent it in and said all we have to do is put a face on the seat so the seat pack won't move. I got all kinds of criticism for that because I didn't use the right forms or submit the right reports and so we eventually went out and put in wood blocks. Just bolted them in. Wood blocks. Eventually that was corrected but it wasn't for some time..."

Meanwhile, in Europe following World War II, there was tremendous interest in German rocket technology. Even as rocket-launched missiles rained death and terror on London, it was clear that a means had been developed for literally reaching into space. The Russians wanted everything they could get in the way of records, prototypes and most important, the scientists themselves. So did the Americans, and they were the more successful in recruiting the top German scientists to the Allied cause.

The Germans came to America in a program called "Operation Paperclip," because those selected had paperclips attached to their personnel record folders. These people were invited to the United States for six months where they would be debriefed, interrogated and asked to write reports on whatever their province was. Among them were Dr. Wernher von Braun, Dr. Walter Dornberger. Dr. Krafft Ehricke and more than a hundred other

111

rocket experts who had developed the V-2 at Peenemuende. Von Braun went to work immediately as technical advisor and project director on U.S. Army rocket programs at White Sands Proving Ground, New Mexico and Fort Bliss, Texas, before being named chief of the Guided Missile Development Division at the Army's Redstone Arsenal in Alabama. Dr. Dornberger, whose V-2 rocket bomb became the model for all space rocket research became design consultant to Bell Aircraft Corporation where he worked on the Rascal air-to-surface missile and the Dyna-Soar manned space glider program. Dyna-Soar was dropped, but the concept was revived in the space shuttle program. Krafft Ehricke, aeronautical research engineer, worked on advanced V-2 programs and jet propulsion and was involved in many space shots including the first Atlas flight on 17 December 1957. Others went to various military and civilian research centers, private industry and learning institutions. Most of the scientists elected to stay in the United States and become citizens.

Along with the scientists came equipment and gadgets of interest to flight surgeons and researchers. Before long the Aeromedical Laboratories at Wright-Patterson Air Force Base were humming with activity, testing various kinds of German flight equipment, parachutes, automatic opening devices, oxygen equipment, ejection seats, g-suits and related items.

Even as the rocket experts were being wooed, so were German flight surgeons. Brigadier General Malcolm G. Grow, Surgeon of the U.S. Strategic Air Force in Europe, conceived the idea of inviting scientists who had knowledge and experience in high altitude aviation and rocketry to get together at the Kaiser Wilhelm Institute for Medical Research in Heidelberg.

By September of 1945, the Institute was receiving "recruits," each of whom was told to prepare a chapter or section for a book, giving the results of his wartime research in aviation medicine. The project, under the direction of the Commanding Officer, Colonel Otis O. Benson, included the works of 56 authors which resulted in the two-volume *German Aviation Medicine, World War II*. It was published in 1950 by the Superintendant of Documents under the auspices of the Surgeon General of the Air Force.

Behind the scenes of this obviously worthwhile and successful venture was the difficulty of pulling it all together in post-war

Germany. Dr. Anthony N. Domonkos, at that time a young captain with the Air Corps was surprised to receive orders to report to General Grow at the Headquarters in St. Germain in France. There were several reasons why he was selected for that assignment: he was first of all a flight surgeon, had attended medical school in Budapest (he was of Hungarian parentage), was familiar with Europe geographically and spoke German. General Grow, he soon learned, was convinced that German aviation medicine was far ahead of what the Americans had accomplished in this field. Said Domonkos, "Dr. Hubertus Strughold had been to Wright Field in earlier years and when he returned to Germany, Hitler provided the necessary funds for research." Furthermore, "Hitler was in a hurry to develop the Luftwaffe..."

Domonkos' unprecedented duties first took him to London for duty with British intelligence experts. Timing was of utmost importance. He arrived in Frankfurt the morning after it had fallen and immediately headed for the hospital to collect information. It was soon apparent, however, that interviewing people for an hour or so and gathering various articles of equipment was not the way to go about it. Besides, much of the German scientists' work was still in the experimental stage. For example, Dr. Siegfried Ruff, developing ejection seats, had researched the amount of force needed to throw a pilot over the tail of a plane flying at 900mph. "This had not been compiled and I felt this was important."

Such observations were reported to General Grow and by the beginning of August 1945, following a meeting of a dozen American flight surgeons, Grow wrote to the Commanding General of the Air Forces in Europe, proposing the establishment of the laboratory in Heidelberg.

There was some difficulty in putting the plan into effect, Colonel Harry Armstrong recalled: "When I arrived in Berlin, the aeromed lab had been abandoned. There was no one around; the few people I knew who had been assigned there had disappeared and no one knew where they were. The problem was that because the victorious Allies were picking up and jailing Nazis throughout the country, anytime an American asked a German if he knew where somebody was, they'd assumed they were to be arrested and punished. They'd either plead ignorance or tell you a bald face lie. So for several months I was not able to locate anyone."

Colonel Armstrong finally located Dr. Ulrich Luft at the University, and Luft helped him find others. "But I still had difficulty because they weren't sure where all the people had gone. They'd scattered all over the countryside. Two of them who had been working on artificial limbs, I found in the Bavarian Alps in a chicken coop, doing more research than most of us do in a laboratory."

Armstrong tried to get research reports but most of them were hidden in a convent. "I was able to get copies of those by getting gasoline for the individual's automobile which he used to go back and forth to the convent."

It was a difficult time for the Germans coming to America. They had just lost the war and to many Americans, anybody who had a thick German accent was a Hitlerite. Working at poverty level salaries, they were without families for the first six months and were systematically debriefed and interrogated. At the end of this time, they had their choice of returning to Germany or sending for their wives and children.

Altogether, 34 German scientists, "came over." Among the leaders who went to the U.S. Air Force School of Aviation Medicine at Randolph Field, Texas, were Doctors Hubertus Strughold, Heinz Haber, Ulrich Luft, Fritz Haber, Hans-Georg Clamann, Konrad Buettner and Siegfried J. Gerathewohl. Dr. Otto Gauer, Dr. V. K. Henschke, Hanning von Gierke, Hans Oesteicher and others went to the Aeromedical Laboratory, Wright-Patterson Air Force Base, Ohio. Dr. Hermann Schaefer, Dr. D. Beischer and others went to the Naval School of Aviation Medicine at Pensacola, Florida and Dr. Theodor Benzinger went to the Naval Medical Center, Bethesda, Maryland.

"That was the most marvelous experience of my life," Benzinger recalls: "I had lost a war. I was an enemy or had been an enemy of the American people so to speak. I came to Washington D.C. and the commanding officer called me in and he said, 'Tell me what sort of research you want to do.' The manner of this man [Captain Albert Behnke, (MC) U.S. Navy] this civilized and highly polished Navy style...the kindness in his voice was absolutely marvelous. I was overwhelmed..." Benzinger felt badly about not wanting to continue his research on blast which was what the Captain had hoped for. Instead, Benzinger wanted to

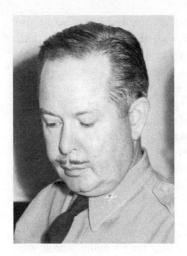

Colonel Paul Campbell, who acted as chairman of the first meeting of the new Space Medicine branch of the Aero Medical Association in 1951, was an early enthusiast of the specialty. Over many years he acquired an extensive aerospace library which he recently donated to Trinity College in San Antonio, Texas./ *Paul Campbell*

Dr. Hubertus Strughold, another German who came to the U.S. after World War II, was named director of the Department of Space Medicine at the U.S. Air Force School of Aviation Medicine. A linguistics historian, he designated the new speciality as "Aerospace Medicine."/*Hubertus Strughold*

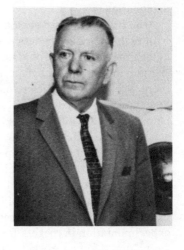

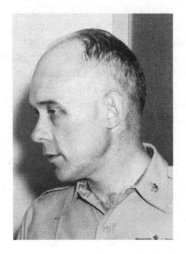

Dr. David Simons, who participated in the Man-High balloon flights, presented a paper on his experiences at a meeting of the International Astronautical Federation in Barcelona, Spain. He was somewhat over-shadowed because at the same time the Russians put Sputnik I into earth orbit./*David Simons*

115

research heat, and the effect of heat on the temperature of the human body. To his amazement, he was allowed to do just that, and later was deeply involved in stress testing of the Mercury astronauts.

Time healed the wounds of war, particularly when pink-cheeked, cherubic German children appeared in base school yards and local chapels. Resentments softened, then disappeared as German wives shopped the commissaries, joined clubs and worked on charity drives. The doctors settled down to pursue their research and stimulate their new colleagues in the field that was yet unnamed. The Russians wound up with "Cosmic Medicine;" the Americans with "Aerospace Medicine," a Strughold designation.

Armstrong, who had seen aviation medicine race unsuccessfully with technology and aviation engineering for so many years, was determined that this would not happen with what he believed was the inevitable reach of man into space. The V-2 said it all, and there were now American and German brains gathered together. Space travel was coming, and the medical community had better be prepared. On 12 November 1948 he organized a panel to meet at Randolph Field, Texas, to discuss the daring subject, "Aeromedical Problems of Space Travel." Dr. Strughold reviewed the international status of this intriguing subspecialty. Dr. Heinz Haber, an astrophysicist and one of the world's great authorities on space spoke about some of the medical problems of spaceflight. General Otis Benson stressed the desirability of animal experimentation in rockets for biological information before there were any manned rocket flights, and Colonel Paul Campbell emphasized the fact that there was no society of space medicine in the U.S. "Such a society," he said, "could assist and advise the armed forces on problems in this field. It could function as a liaison between universities, the aeronautical industry and federal agencies..."

A few months later, on 9 February 1949, Armstrong's scheme to establish a department of space medicine at the School of Aviation Medicine became a reality. It was interdisciplinary from the beginning, with the four founding members being a medical doctor, a physicist specializing in astronomy, an engineer and a

116

bioclimatologist. Heinz Haber, astrophysicist, who would normally have no business in a medical laboratory, and his brother Fritz, an engineer who had been chief of the design group at Junkers Aircraft Company in Germany and had worked with the French government on jet engines, were in on it from the beginning. So was Dr. Konrad Buettner, who brought his special knowledge of bioclimatology, a unique field allied to meteorology. Strughold was named director the following year. Armstrong's idea was that even in the face of budget cutbacks, studies should be made which would define the problems man would be confronted with in space. What precisely were the hazards, and what could medical people do to protect man during a trip to, say, the moon?

Elsewhere during the 40s, information was being collected that would be used as building blocks to space. Pilots were going ever higher and faster in the rocket-powered aircraft of the X-series and flight surgeons began to think of spaceflight as a logical extension of high-altitude flight. In October 1947 when test pilot Charles E. "Chuck" Yeager, then a captain in the Air Force, flew the rocket-powered X-1 faster than the speed of sound, a new milestone had been passed.

In 1945-1948, Captain John Paul Stapp did some extraordinary scientific investigation on the problems of deceleration at Edwards Air Force Base in California. During this period, ejection seats were tested at Wright-Patterson Air Force Base. Warrant Officer Larry Lambert, in 1946, made the first live ejection test in the U.S. from a P-61 Black Widow night fighter. His comment, "Man, whatta whoomp!" and the fact that seat separation and parachute opening were done manually indicated the creaky state of the art at that time. His seat was based on the German He-162. The U.S. Navy favored the British Martin-Baker seat, which was standardized and installed in all new service jet aircraft. The work of production and installation was put in hand for Meteor, Attacker, Wyvern, Canberra and later the Sea Hawk and Venom aircraft.

Features of this first seat were the two-cartridge gun, the stabilizing drogue, withdrawn by a drogue gun, the face screen for firing, and an adjustable seat pan allowing pilots of varying body length to be accomodated without increasing the height of the seat, and integral thigh guards and adjustable foot rests. The first

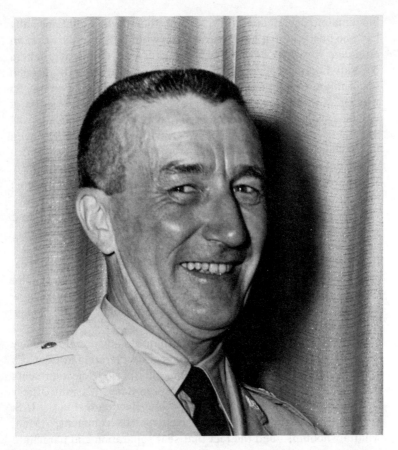

Brigadier General Don Flickinger, who retired from the Air Force after 27 years of service, was awarded the Distinguished Service Medal on retirement, for his contributions to the spaceflight program, and for being instrumental in solving many early organizational problems/*U.S. Air Force*

person to save his life in an emergency with this Mark I ejection seat was Mr. J. O. Lancaster, a test pilot who blasted himself to safety on 30 May, 1949.

Live testing of ejection seats called for considerable skill and bravery on the part of the subjects. All, of course, were trained parachutists, but "human factors," were frequently evident. Major Edward Sperry, who tested the downward ejection seat for the B-47, B-52, B-66 and F-104, recalls: "I will never forget the

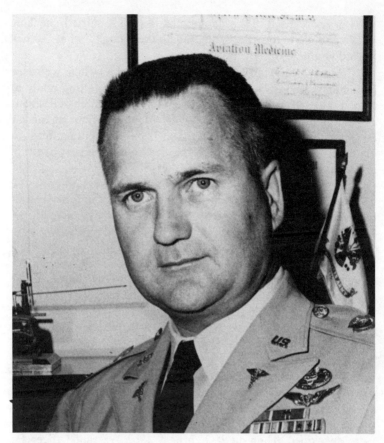

Major General Spurgeon H. Neel, MC, U.S. Army, is a Fellow and Past President of the Aerospace Medical Association. In 1977 he received its Theodore C. Lyster Award for "Outstanding achievement in the general field of aerospace medicine," based largely on his direction of the program for developing and testing helicopter air evacuation techniques used successfully in Korea and Vietnam. He was the first Army physician certified in aerospace medicine; the first Chief of the Aviation Branch in the Office of the Army Surgeon General; and the first physician inducted—as the "Father of Army Aviation Medicine"—into the U.S. Army Aviation Hall of Fame./*U.S. Army*

tower as I am afraid of heights. I used to go up 60 or so feet and then sit very still, afraid the ratchets or the track would break. The hardest of all was to climb up and hang wires of instrumentation. Those climbs were hell..."

.

"I never realized it was dangerous till people started sneaking back up to me to retie the string (again the thought, what the hell am I doing here?)"

"Colonel John Paul Stapp came by one day when we were installing the downward ejection test tower and getting ready to ride it also. It had a brake that grabbed a center rail about two-thirds of the way down and an air bag decelerator at the far end which was stuffed with styrofoam. Then, last, but not least, a big concrete wall. Stapp came by the day before the first live ride and asked, "How do you stop this thing?"

"When I explained the series of stops culminating at the concrete wall, he said, "Only suggestion I've got is hook that air bag to an organ and when you hit it, play 'Nearer My God to Thee.' Then he stomped off."

Ejection seats were developed for jet fighters, but in order for them to be "sold," live demonstrations had to be made to prove that they worked. On 31 May 1945, at 10,000 feet, while flying at 555mph over San Pablo Bay, north of San Francisco, Captain Vince Mazza successfully ejected. He also tested a new automatic parachute-opening device. All systems worked perfectly. Two months later, the U.S. Navy's first emergency jet escape occured near Walterboro, South Carolina. Lieutenant J. L. Fruin of VF-171, using a McDonnell seat, successfully ejected from a crippled F2H-1 while traveling at a speed of 597mph.

Low level ejection and ejection through the canopy underwater were developed. Then on 28 February 1962 Warrant Officer Ed Murray, U.S. Air Force live-tested a 700-pound aluminum escape capsule from a B-58. The capsule and occupant were flown to 20,000 feet and, at a speed of 565mph, were blasted 250 feet in the air. Propellants were two rockets with 10,000 pounds of thrust with Murry experiencing vertical acceleration of 13g. Murray's comments, on being retrieved by Air Force doctors and engineers: "I feel fine. No sweat."

In the immediate post-war years dozens of prominent university and military scientists became more involved in biological experiments that pointed toward spaceflight. Tests covered such exotic factors as the effects of radiation upon living organisms and the behavior of animals at zero gravity. The first of these

120

experiments was undertaken with captured German V-2 rockets at Holloman Air Force Base, New Mexico. In 1946-47, Harvard biologists, in cooperation with scientists from the U.S. Naval Research Laboratory, recovered seeds and fruit flies after flights at altitudes up to 100 miles. In 1948 Dr. James P. Henry of the Air Force joined the group, and during the next few years it launched successful flights with mice and monkeys as passengers.

Paralleling these activities after 1950 were biological experiments in unmanned balloon flights culminating in the Man-High experiments in which the human subject went aloft just before Russia launched the first Sputnik. This laid the groundwork for biological experimentation prior to high-altitude manned flight and spaceflight. Also important was the development of the X-12, X-15 and the proposed Dyna-Soar, all of which were concerned with testing human factors and providing basic knowledge upon which the first U.S. space program would be built.

But generally, these activities attracted very little public attention. The general news media, the politicians and much of the scientific community were more concerned with the atomic bomb and the thermonuclear breakthrough which produced the hydrogen bomb.

Politically, the cold war was escalating and by 1950, the United States was involved in the Korean conflict. Defense funds went for armed hostilities rather than Buck Rogers-type research. Television swept the country, as did computers, and Professor Norbert Wiener of MIT called both developments "...harbingers of a whole new science of communication and control..." which he promptly named "cybernetics" from the Greek word meaning steersman.

About that time, in August 1949 at the annual meeting of the Aero Medical Association in New York, two papers having to do with spaceflight were carefully slipped into the agenda. By deleting the word "space," General Armstrong dared present his paper, "Some Aviation Medical Problems Associated with Potential Rocket Flight," and Dr. Paul Campbell camouflaged his with "Cybernetics and Aviation Medicine."

Then came the event that illustrated that space travel was not as unpopular as many people supposed. General Armstrong and Dr.

Andrew C. Ivy of the University of Illinois co-sponsored a symposium on the "Biological Aspects of Manned Space Flight," on 3 March 1950 at the Medical College of the University of Illinois. It was a stellar cast, with Armstrong on "Space Medicine in the United States Air Force," von Braun on "Multi-stage Rockets and Artificial Satellites," Strughold with, "Physiological Considerations on the Possibility of Life Under Extraterrestrial Conditions," Heinz Haber, "Astronomy and Space Medicine," Paul Campbell, "Orientation in Space," and Buettner, "Bioclimatology of Manned Rocket Flight."

Such an array of exotic subjects was expected to interest a small select audience; instead, the auditorium was packed with people, many of whom were students who had arrived in their new Volkswagens, having skipped the TV presentation of "Kukla, Fran and Ollie" to hear the discussions. Afterwards, Dr. John Marbarger, who then headed the Environmental and Aviation Medical Laboratory, mimeographed the papers and distributed them to the participants. Several weeks later, he arranged with the University of Illinois Press to publish the symposium in book form. The result was *Space Medicine*, which sold out the first three printings before the participants received their copies. The biggest buyers were space-minded young people.

During this period a few members of the Aero Medical Association felt they needed a forum within the Association's framework through which they could meet and discuss space matters. Colonel Paul Campbell and Dr. John Marbarger wrote to about twenty-five people, inviting them to get together during an annual meeting of the Aero Medical Association. The date was 31 May 1950 and in Dr. Strughold's opening remarks it was clear that such an organization was badly needed.

Said he: "In the beginning of aviation, Aviation Medicine lagged behind technical development. As General H. G. Armstrong has recently emphasized, this must not be allowed to repeat itself in the field of rocket and spaceflight. A review of literature, however, reveals that the very same danger is imminent. Fortunately, in the United States, the first Department of Space Medicine has already been established by General H. G. Armstrong at the School of Aviation Medicine at Randolph Field in 1949. Since its establishment, this Department has published nine

122

papers. Several more papers have come from other institutions in the United States. In Europe (England, France and Italy), as well, the first papers in the field have recently been published. It can be predicted that rocket and spaceflight are in the same state of development as was aviation in 1920, whose field of research, including the medical sciences, experienced an explosive development in the following decades. It appears that the space sciences will develop along similar lines. In order to enable the medical faculty to keep pace with the presumable technical development, it is mandatory to place Space Medicine on the broadest possible basis, and in this manner, effect a rapid and extensive development. One means to this end would be the founding of the Space Medical Society..."

Such talk produced quite a few smiles and a certain amount of criticism among the non-enthusiasts. Getting things into perspective, the October 1950 issue of *The Journal of Aviation Medicine* ran an editorial comment which said in part, "In order that space medicine will have the same meaning for all people, the term must be defined and the field of interest delimited. The word "space" to most people probably implies the "boundless void" beyond the earth's atmosphere. Actually, space can be variously defined; it is as difficult to pin down as the word "fatigue" and is at about the same level of abstraction. The following definition is gratuitously offered with the full realization that it may not be acceptable to all: *Space medicine is concerned with the medical problems involved in modes of travel which are potentially capable at least of transporting us beyond the earth's gravitational field; and it is also concerned with special hazards encountered in the upper part of our atmosphere and beyond.*"

The editorial explained further: "To escape the earth's gravitational field, a single-stage rocket must attain an initial speed of 25,000 miles an hour. It is inconceivable that such a rocket could be manned, even if it could be built. However, the greater the reduction in initial velocity, the greater the power requirement, and for this reason, the technical design of the first space ships will probably represent a compromise between the engineer and biologist; the magnitude of the medical problems involved here requires no emphasis..."

The first meeting of the established organization, the Space

Medicine Branch took place at the annual meeting in Denver on 17 May 1951 with Colonel Paul Campbell acting as chairman. The organization had taken only a year to arrange its first official meeting; this was more than six years before Sputnik I was launched, almost seven years before Vanguard I and seven and one-half years before the National Aeronautics and Space Administration (NASA), appeared on the scene. The Space Medicine Branch of the Aero Medical Association was the first organization of its type in the world.

Being first, however, did not bring on a round of cheers and applause. Even space enthusiasts were skeptical of man's role as traveler. "Why send man into space and to the moon? Instead, send instrumented vehicles and computer-driven lunar landing machines. So who needs space medicine anyway?"

The skeptics had some pretty good arguments that were hard to refute at the time. The main complaint was that man was not worth his weight in black boxes; you couldn't miniaturize him like you could a piece of equipment. His reaction time is slow compared to a machine; he tires and gets bored. He seldom does the same thing twice in exactly the same way. He's easily distracted and can't usually do or watch many things at one time. And there's all that worry about his emotions, his health, his safety, "It's just not worth it, at least not for many years to come."

An instrumental package is something else. It can be built to withstand more shock, acceleration, heat, cold, and vacuum than any human could endure. It would not need life-support and atmosphere-maintaining systems, pressure shells, space-suits, food, water, air-conditioning or training. Such packages could stay in their hostile environment for a couple of years, and report findings back to earth. There need be no worry about their recovery because they would not have to be brought back when their work was done. Instruments were expendable.

Those arguments were soon proved to be invalid. Man was a good machine builder, but he wasn't perfect. Machines and monkeys couldn't correct a botchy job midway through a mission, but an educated, experienced astronaut could.

So, shortly there was a positive look at man. Certainly he is primarily a sea-level, low-speed, 1g, 12-hour animal and represents the weakest link in aerospace development, but he is flexible and can exercise independent judgment. If he makes a mistake, he can correct his action next time. No amount of gadgetry can get a craft out of trouble the way man can; no instruments have man's serendipity, finding things they are not looking for. As an observer, man can, with one sweep of the eye over the lunar landscape, do a more valuable job than dozens of instruments, and can write detailed accounts of his experience afterwards.

During this pioneering period, special experimental research, preceded or accompanied by theoretical analysis, was concentrated upon three major areas: the g-pattern which included a large range from zero g to multiples of g; the study of the biological effect of cosmic rays and the development of a closed ecological system as represented by a cabin to be used in space or even as low as 70,000 to 80,000 feet.

An important step in the exchange of knowledge on spaceflight was the first international symposium on "The Physics and Medicine of the Upper Atmosphere." Forty-four speakers from various countries appeared on the program which was held in San Antonio, Texas, in November 1951. This symposium was organized by Brigadier General Otis O. Benson, Jr., Commandant of the School of Aviation Medicine (SAM) at Randolph Air Force Base and Dr. Clayton S. White of the Lovelace Foundation, Albuquerque, New Mexico. Seven years later, in November 1958, at the end of the Geophysical Year, a second international symposium was sponsored by the SAM, and organized by the Southwest Research Institute of San Antonio. The latest findings in the exploration of space by means of research satellites, the latest and future types of rockets, the medical problems in space operations, and the conditions on the moon, Mars, and Venus were discussed by the world's leading physicists, astro-physicists, rocket engineers, physiologists, psychologists and medical doctors.

Space medicine papers began appearing in a number of publications in addition to the *Journal of Aviation Medicine* (edited by Dr. Robert J. Benford). The American Rocket Society, the Institute of Aeronautical Sciences, and the American Astronautical Society printed medical articles. In 1955, at the annual meeting of

125

the American Rocket Society, the first paper on the medical problems in satellite flight was given. In 1956, the society formed a special Space Flight Committee with several medical doctors as members. Medical problems of spaceflight were also discussed at the First International Symposium on Health and Travel in 1955 in New York City. A human-factors panel was included in the program at the first Symposium on Astronautics, held in San Diego in March 1957. It was organized by the Consolidated Vultee Aircraft Corporation and sponsored by the Office of Scientific Research of the Air Force.

In 1954 space medicine was included in the annual meeting of the International Astronautical Federation, an organization comprising 25 national member organizations. Technical magazines devoted space to medical topics; *Missiles and Rockets,* begun in 1957, had a regular column on space medicine.

Meanwhile there were stepped-up programs in education, with the SAM's primary, advanced, refresher and review courses in space medicine, aimed at familiarizing medical students and physicians with problems of the future. The subject was also on the program of two lecture series: one on satellites offered by the Massachusetts Institute of Technology in 1956, and the other on space technology given at the University of California in 1958.

In May of 1958, two representatives of space medicine appeared before the special House Select Committee on Astronautics and Space Exploration in Washington, D. C. to testify about the medical aspects and prospects of spaceflight. With the creation of a Division of Bioastronautics of Air Research and Development Command under the direction of Brigadier General Don D. Flickinger, U.S. Air Force, it was clear that space medicine would play an increasingly heavy role in the "man in space" program of the newly created National Aeronautics and Space Administration.

Paralleling the Air Force's stepped-up research and development program, was the work going on in the U.S. Navy. The Naval School of Aviation Medicine, established in 1939 at Pensacola, Florida did considerable research under joint Navy and National Research Council sponsorship. Captain Ashton Graybiel, (MC), U.S. Navy, Director of Medical Research, explored problems of weightlessness and the vestibular function. Scientists at the school were also involved in biological research projects for the Army, thus helping to build the capability for manned flight. The school's special facilities included low-pressure chambers, low-level alpha-radiation laboratories, an electrophysiological laboratory, a slow-rotation room and a human-disorientation device.

The Aviation Medical Acceleration Laboratory, located at the Naval Air Development Center, Johnsville, Pennsylvania had installed the largest human centrifuge in the world. It was used extensively in the X-15 and Dyna-Soar programs, and later in the Mercury Program.

In Philadélphia, Pennsylvania, the Naval Air Crew Equipment Laboratory, established in 1942, conducted basic research in the biological, psychological and human engineering aspects of aviation medicine as applied to personal and safety equipment. Their special facilities included underwater test facilities, a complete liquid oxygen laboratory, and an escape-system recovery net capable of recovering ejected free-flight seats and capsules. This lab, too, would make important contributions to manned spaceflight.

With so many people involved in research in such wide ranging fields in such distant places it was almost impossible to avoid duplication and a certain amount of inter-service rivalry. Add to this the lack of popular public support and it's a wonder so much serious basic work was accomplished during those years. What kept progress on course, however, was the spirit of the scientists involved. Most had almost zealous faith in their mission; they published papers, gave speeches, participated in symposia, cemented personal and professional friendships and generally kept their knowledge and findings circulating among those who had a need and desire to know.

And then came Sputnik—the world's first artificial satellite— launched by the Russians on 4 October 1957. It was small, only 22 inches in diameter and weighing 184 pounds, but it was a real shocker to a world scientifically involved in the 18-month International Geophysical Year (IGY). Sputnik I, which would orbit for three months, was joined a month later by Sputnik II carrying a living passenger, a dog named Laika.

These spectacular feats had tremendous political and military implications. A potential enemy that had usually been considered inferior to the U.S. in technology was suddenly playing leapfrog, jumping ahead into the next century. America's prestige was at stake, and reporters did what they could to fuel the flame of terror. Unhappily, few of them knew much if anything about space except for what they could hastily lift from encyclopedias. Editors assigned political, crime and straight news reporters the task of writing highly technical stories about Sputnik's journey. At the Smithsonian Astrophysical Observatory (SAO), the ladies' lounge became the "Astrophysical Press Association" literally a classroom for scientists to explain just what was happening. *Life* magazine wanted to know where to send an airplane in order to photograph Sputnik. Cost was no object. Dr. J. Allen Hynek of the SAO later said, "If I had said Tierra del Fuego, within minutes the *Life* crew would have been dispatched there..."

There was also confusion within the Russian press corps. When Dr. Strughold, accompanied by Dr. David Simons, arrived in Wiesbaden after attending a meeting of the International Astronautical Federation in Barcelona where Simons had presented a paper on his Man-High balloon flights, a Russian correspondent cornered Strughold with: "Now professor, since Sputnik has been launched, do you not agree that all the medical problems of spaceflight are solved?"

Strughold replied, "Not a single one."

Needless to say, those members of the American military services who had done the bulk of the space research and development were exasperated that they were not first in space. They could have been, they said, had it not been for political constraints on the use of military rocketry. Furthermore, they were well into plans of manned spaceflight.

It was particularly upsetting to the Air Force because three months earlier at a conference in Los Angeles, General Don Flickinger and Dr. Albert Hetherington reported that given vehicular reliability, no additional life-sciences knowledge was needed for normal orbital flights. Environmental control and other factors could be accomplished within 18 months. Most of the discussion centered on the vehicle itself; should it be a purely ballistic type with a drag configuration for re-entry, or should it be a "lifting body" configuration that would reduce the re-entry g-load?

Shortly after Sputnik, General Bernard A. Schriever, Commander of the Ballistic Missile Division, of the Air Research and Development Command (ARDC), brought together 56 leading scientists and engineers, headed by D. Edward Teller, to make specific recommendations as to Air Force space requirements. General Flickinger recalled Dr. James P. Henry to head an ad hoc committee on life sciences. In essence, everyone agreed that the Air Force could place a man in orbit within two years. Such a flight would add to national prestige and advance science and technology.

The earlier plan, presented in May 1958, called Man-in-Space (MIS) was superseded a month later by an accelerated plan known as Man-in-Space-Soonest (MISS) which proposed test programs with animal flights as early as 1959-60 to be followed by the first manned flight in October 1960. Subsequent flights would lead eventually to a lunar landing by 1964.

Meanwhile, the Army in January 1958 proposed a tri-service man-in-space program which was called Project Adam. The carrier would be a modified Redstone thrust unit and an instrument compartment as used in satellite and re-entry firings. The human passenger would travel in a reclining position, as suggested by Maxime A. Faget, to keep acceleration effects at a minimum. Biomedical aspects would include almost all of the data that finally wound up in Project Mercury.

The Department of Defense formally requested that the National Academy of Sciences establish an Armed Forces—National Research Council Committee on Bioastronautics to study all facets of manned spaceflight. But this proposal, along with MISS and Project Adam, died a-borning because of events that were taking place at the White House. In retrospect, 1958 appeared to be the "year of the committees" to study what was going to be studied, by whom, and who had the responsibility for getting the job done.

In the month after the Sputnik launching, President Dwight D. Eisenhower established the President's Scientific Advisory Committee, headed by Dr. James A. Killian, president of MIT. The following March, the President's Committee on Government Organization, which included his scientific advisor, recommended that a new civilian agency be created to pursue an aggressive space program. The result was the National Aeronautics and Space Act of 1958 which created the National Air and Space Administration (NASA). Dr. J. Keith Glennon, President of the Case Institute of Technology, was named first Administrator of NASA and Dr. Hugh L. Dryden was named Deputy Administrator.

The organizational nucleus of the new space agency was the National Advisory Committee for Aeronautics (NACA) of which Dr. Dryden had been director. NACA had been involved in basic aeronautical research for 43 years, and most recently had focused on applying rocket propulsion research to manned flight which led to the development of the X-series aircraft. NACA also set up a special committee on space technology under the chairmanship of Dr. G. Guyford Stever of MIT. The Stever Committee met for the first time on 13 February 1958 and established seven working groups. The group named to study human factors and training was headed by Dr. W. Randolph Lovelace II. Serving with Dr. Lovelace on the ad hoc committee was a mixture of specialists, indicative of the interaction that would be necessary to determine man's capability in space: A. Scott Crossfield, test pilot; Hubert M. Drake, High-speed Flight Station, NACA: General Flickinger; Colonel Edward B. Giller; Dr. James D. Hardy, U.S. Naval Air Development Center; Dr. Wright Haskell Langham, Los Alamos Scientific Laboratory; Dr. Ulrich C. Luft, Lovelace Foundation for Medical Education and Research; and Boyd C. Myers II (Secretary) NACA.

The Committee's final report outlined means by which NASA should develop resources in life-sciences research. Thirteen technical areas were discussed: program administration; acceleration; high-intensity radiation in space; cosmic radiation; nuclear propulsion; ionization effects; human information processing and communication; displays; closed-cycle living; balloon simulators; space capsules; crew selection and training; and research centers and launching sites.

From the report: "The ultimate and unique objective in the conquest of space is the early successful flight of man, with all his capabilities, into space and his safe return to earth. Just as man has achieved an increasing control over his dynamic environment on earth and in the atmosphere, he must now achieve the ability to live, to observe, and to work in the environment of space."

130

The Working Group on Human Factors and Training urged that crew selection, survival, safety, and efficiency be considered in all experiments, and indeed, experiments with man could parallel those with animals. The success of the program would require a cooperative effort of life scientists and physical scientists representing diverse professional backgrounds. Accumulated experience would be applied to research on vital activities at the whole-body, organ, tissue, cellular, molecular, and atomic levels. The program should include the Army, the Navy, the Air Force, the Atomic Energy Commission, the National Bureau of Standards, the Public Health Service, and the National Academy of Sciences—with NASA having primary responsibility.

The critical goal of developing a manned satellite program would require a life sciences committee to study the immediate problems associated with manned spaceflight and to recommend specific research investigations to be undertaken by NASA. Membership of this committee should include not only representatives from the Department of Defense, U.S. Public Health Service, National Academy of Sciences, and Atomic Energy Commission, but also universities and foundations.

The National Academy of Sciences-National Research Council (NAS-NRC) president, Dr. Detlev Bronk responded by forming a 16-man Space Science Board in August to study scientific problems, opportunities and implications of man's advance into space. The next month, General Flickinger gathered his planning group together. The medical doctors included Lieutenant Colonel Robert H. Homes from the Army, Captain W. L. Jones of the Navy, and Dr. R. Keith Cannan from NAS-NRC, along with others. In October Dr. W. Randolph Lovelace, II, chaired a NASA Special Life Sciences Committee, consisting of military doctors, as well as government civilian scientists and engineers.

All told, by the fall of 1958, both the civilian and military scientific communities were fairly well organized for solving the biomedical problems of manned spaceflight.

The one serious ambiguity was NASA's role in the bioscience program. At the time of Project Mercury, there were four military medical doctors and one military psychologist, all on detached service with NASA. In addition, there were 28 engineers and three technicians concerned with life-support systems, instrumentation for physiological and environmental monitoring, animal programs for experiments in flight, and protective equipment and devices.

Yet another committee composed of leading scientists and chaired by Dr. Seymour S. Kety, Director of the Clinical Science Laboratory of the National Institutes of Health (NIH), submitted its report to NASA on 25 January 1960, then dissolved itself.

In essence, that report called for the integration of personnel and facilities in the military and other governmental agencies that related to space-oriented life sciences. NASA's mission was to put and maintain men in space thus leaving the military to concentrate on weapons systems and national defense. Consequently NASA established an office of Life Sciences and appointed Clark T. Randt, M.D., a member of the Bioscience Advisory Committee, as Director. Dr. Randt was replaced by General Roadman at NASA Headquarters. The Office of Life Sciences was not geared to the immediate problems of Mercury, but to the long-range space exploration program and left the management of Project Mercury to the Space Task Group (STG), headed by Colonel Stanley C. White. The STG had the overall responsibilities for the selection of astronauts, the development of life support equipment (environmental control, pressure suits, waste management, food and water systems, etc.), the animal test program and the operational medical support.

Meanwhile, the STG working at Langley, Virginia, to make that first primitive effort with existing technology and off-the-shelf equipment, depended almost entirely on the resources of the Air Force , Navy, industry, academic and private research institutions to develop workable life-support systems. Much of the work was done by C. F. Gell, H. N. Hunter, P. W. Garland and others at the Naval Research Laboratory (NRL), and by John Paul Stapp, S. Bondurant, N. P. Clarke, W. G. Blanchard, H. Miller, R. R. Hessberg, E. P. Hiatt, Eli Beeding and others in the military services.

It went without saying that teamwork would have to be of the highest order. Each scientist would have a piece of the responsibility regardless of what kind of hat he wore and the pieces would make a whole—namely a successful flight. Dr. C. P. Laughlin would record, process and analyze the physiological

132

stress information about the astronauts, including pre- and post-training physical examination; monitoring and tabulation of pulse, respiratory rate, body temperature and electrocardiogram; pre- and post-training vital capacity; pre- and post-training nude weight; and pre- and post-training volume and specific gravity of urine.

The major part of the physiological and stress information would be gathered by personnel of NIH and Dr. J. P. Henry of STG.

Fluid loss and vital capacity measurements would be under the direction of Dr. William Augerson. Insertion of the astronauts into the spacecraft would be done by one of two teams; Dr. William K. Douglas and Joe W. Schmitt, or Dr. C. B. Jackson and Harry D. Stewart. Drs. Douglas and Jackson would also evaluate the effectiveness of the biosensor performance.

The pressure suit and urine bag would be evaluated by Lee N. McMillion. William H. Bush would take over the electronic part of the biomedical recording, and Morton Schler would procure, install and monitor the environment control system. Gerald J. Pesman would evaluate the couch and restraint harness.

Dr. White noted as early as October 1959 that additional medical support in monitoring recovery and post-flight research was absolutely essential.

Dr. G. E. Ruff of the University of Pennsylvania, who during his tour of duty with the Air Force had participated in the astronaut-selection stress tests at Wright Air Development Center (WADC), concentrated on gathering basic psychiatric data. Simultaneous measurements were made of the emotional state, metabolism of adrenal medullary and cortical hormones, and control performance during their training. Blood and urine samples were taken before and after repeated exposure to acceleration. Urine samples were analyzed at the NIH, and blood samples examined by Dr. Kristen Eik-Nes of the University of Utah. Dr. Ruff also interviewed all of the original seven astronauts at least once during the training period, and tested them for their emotional state.

There were consultants for what one might call contingency plans. In April 1960, Dr. George Knauf, who commanded the hospital at Patrick Air Force Base, near Cape Canaveral, asked

133

each Surgeon General to provide a specialist in general surgery, orthopedic surgery, pathology, neurosurgery, plastic surgery, internal medicine and anesthesiology. The hospital would be integrated into the Mercury Medical Support System, and there would also be a forward medical facility at Cape Canaveral for emergency care in case of astronaut injury. Another facility would be on Grand Turk Island, and Navy destroyers would carry a technician who could perform laboratory duties. All selected physicians would be board-certified; the oral surgeon and the consultants would be on hand the day of the launch.

It would seem that the program was moving forward at a cautious though steady pace until it hit a political snag about six months before the planned suborbital flight. Events prompted by the 1959-60 recession, along with President Eisenhower's lack of enthusiasm for extended spaceflight plunged NASA to its lowest point to date. Programs beyond Project Mercury hung in precarious balance as the President presented his Federal Budget for Fiscal Year 1962. Eisenhower said he hoped the United States would have a manned orbital flight in 1961, but further testing and experimentation would be necessary to establish if there were any valid scientific reasons for extending manned spaceflights beyond the Mercury program.

This was the gloomy atmosphere confronting President-elect Kennedy in the weeks prior to his inauguration. Something was obviously wrong with America's space program and it all tumbled out in a report which he released on 12 January 1961. The report, prepared by an advisory committee headed by Dr. Jerome Wiesner set off a chain reaction profoundly affecting the biomedical aspects of Project Mercury.

The report strongly criticized NASA's organization and management and recommended a sweeping reorganization. NASA should make more effective use of the National Aeronautics and Space Council, develop a single direction within the Department of Defense in space efforts, and work out a more efficient tie with industry. The report criticized the Atlas launch vehicle, stating that it was "marginal," and that Russia had larger launch vehicles and would thus be the first to orbit a man in space.

134

Kennedy had asked Vice President Lyndon Johnson to recommend a NASA administrator and his choice of businessman-lawyer James Webb was an excellent one. It was he who grappled with the bickering forces of influential scientists who wanted to curtail manned space exploration and the military-industrial complex who favored turning over the major role to the Air Force.

During the transition from the Eisenhower administration to the Kennedy administration, the operations staff of Project Mercury continued its work and as yet, no known orbital manned flight had been made by any country. A U.S. suborbital animal flight was scheduled for late January 1961 with a manned suborbital flight soon after.

But in-house conflicts continued as the laboratory scientists pushed for more animal experimentation before exposing a human being to spaceflight, and the operations engineers insisted that

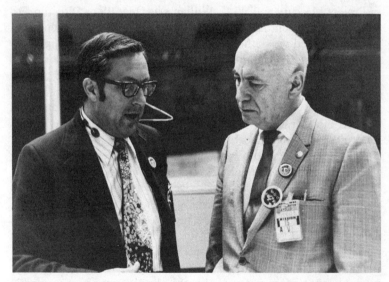

Dr. Charles A. Berry, Director of Medical Operations and Dr. Robert Gilruth, Center Director, Johnson Spaceflight Center, discussed inflight medical problem during Apollo 15 mission, July 1971./*NASA*

the X-15 experience had already provided the necessary biomedical background. The assessment of the Mercury biomedical program was to take place in March 1961 but by that time, Ham the chimpanzee had made a successful suborbital flight, thus demonstrating the validity of the Mercury spacecraft. This was a help, but there was still opposition to using man.

At this critical junction before the suborbital Mercury flight, the Aeromedical Research Laboratory at Holloman Air Force Base took responsibility for training the chimpanzees, preparing them for flight and handling them after recovery. Two Air Force physicians, Lieutenant Colonel James P. Henry and Lieutenant Colonel Rufus Hessberg, directed the animal program at Holloman. An Air Force veterinarian, Lieutenant Colonel Walter E. Brewer, headed the program at Cape Canaveral.

Events moved swiftly, following Ham's suborbital flight, and although there was still much trepidation, the STG aeromedical team was now convinced it was ready to sustain a human for a short space mission.

And it was a seasoned team at that, with Dr. Gilruth as Director of Project Mercury and W. C. Williams as Operations Director. Dr. Stanley White continued to direct Medical Operations while Dr. Douglas stayed on as the personal physician to the astronauts.

But the Russians did it again! By orbiting Cosmonaut Yuri Gagarin on 12 April 1961, they once more beat the U.S. in the space race and won the headlines.

During the next three weeks, the teams at Cape Canaveral worked more frantically than ever, checking last minute details before the step-one suborbital flight of astronaut Alan B. Shepard. True, there was yet to be an instrument perfected for measuring blood pressure during the flight, but this would come later. For the time being, there was an air of tenseness as the best aeromedical team that it was possible to put together, focused on one lone man, and two vital questions: were the technology, biomedical research and life-support systems adequate; and were all the millions of details adequately anticipated and dealt with?

There was no question in the minds of the thousands of people working in the space program that they had covered every possible aspect of the operation. The launch vehicle, the space capsule, the hardware, communications, telemetry, life support system—

136

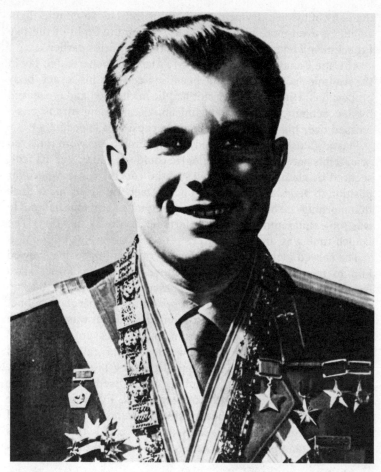

First man in space, Russian cosmonaut Yuri A. Gagarin, whose flight around the earth on 12 April 1961, won world-wide acclaim. His single orbit had a duration of 108 minutes. Seven years later, Gagarin was killed in a plane crash./*Novesti Photo*

everything was go. Aeromedical and biomedical research, concentrated and refined, had finally put the spotlight on one man who would initiate the actual flight operations of the U.S. space program. His short venture into space would consist of a full-dress enactment of what had been done dozens of times in simulation— suiting up, ignition, liftoff, flight, re-entry, splashdown, and recovery. The first American astronaut would fly higher and faster than any of his countrymen ever had before. His 15-minute flight would be even more historic than the 25-minute flight of the two Frenchmen who started it all, nearly two centuries earlier.

At Cape Canaveral on 5 May 1961, Alan B. Shepard, Jr., lay in the contour couch that had been molded to his exact body proportions. His shiny silver suit had been checked and rechecked by Joe Schmitt, space-suit technician. Restraining straps criss-crossed over his shoulders, across his chest and knees.

Plastic galoshes over his laced and zippered boots were removed prior to his entry into the capsule. He could see the tips of his feet, secured by clamps in the grooves of the couch. It was a peculiar position to be in, a most unique one, in fact. Up since one o'clock that morning, he had been in the capsule for nearly four hours. He was too exhilarated to be uncomfortable, too busy to worry. The launch time was drawing nearer.

The curved gloves with dots of rubber at the finger tips allowed him to manipulate the numerous switches and controls. Two earphones and two microphones assured Shepard of backup protection on his communications system. The fiberglass helmet with its plastic visor and thick-cushioning headliner was fitted onto his suit and locked in a manner similar to a pressure-cooker top.

As the countdown time grew closer, he talked into his microphone with Flight Operations Director Walter C. Williams, and heard the reassurring, routine words used many times in altitude chambers and in mock-up capsules. Every phase of the actual shot into space had been tested and retested. Every hazard the technicians, scientists and doctors could think of was anticipated, and precautions were set up to guard the astronaut's life.

A huge crane capable of plucking the astronaut out of his capsule in case of pre-flight trouble, stood by, as did an Army personnel carrier with its crew. Four miles from Pad 5, an abort rescue team waited anxiously. Six helicopters, carrying doctors, frogmen, and skilled technicians stood ready to liftoff to the rescue if necessary.

At sea were some 65-foot Navy crashboats; other craft were on the alert in case the capsule veered from its programmed track. In the splashdown area, the aircraft carrier *Lake Champlain* with helicopters and six destroyers stood by, monitoring the operation.

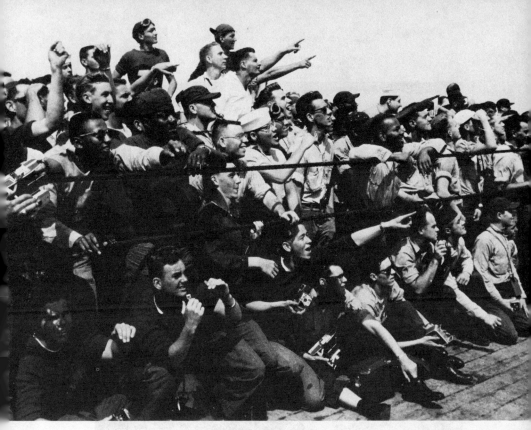

A crowd of cheering sailors aboard the *Lake Champlain* greet astronaut Alan B. Shepard, Jr., as helicopter recovery teams touch down on the flight deck with Shepard and his Mercury spacecraft./*NASA*

Thousands of electronic eyes viewed the capsule and the man inside. The world waited breathlessly as preparations were completed for launching the first American into suborbital flight.

After the 10-second countdown to ignition, the giant Redstone rocket roared with power. Inside the capsule, Commander Shepard felt the vibration of the liquid fuel engine as the brilliant tower of flame built up. Inside the blockhouse, technicians and doctors monitored the telemetering equipment.

"Liftoff!"

"Roger, liftoff, and the clock has started," Shepard reported.

So began the 15-minute spaceflight which propelled Alan Shepard into space, reaching an altitude of 116 statute miles for a downrange distance of 302 statute miles. Two months later, Virgil Grissom flew to an altitude of 118 miles and a downrange distance

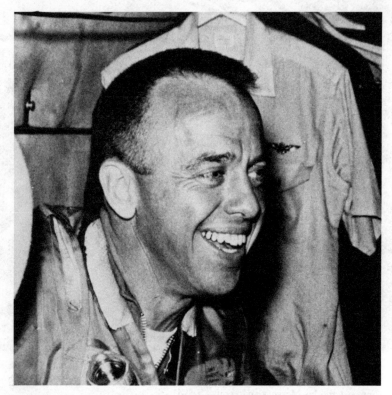

Beaming with elation after his first sub-orbital flight, Commander Alan B. Shepard, Jr., talks it up with Mercury project doctors while in flight from the recovery carrier, *Lake Champlain,* to the Grand Bahama Islands./*NASA*

of 303 miles. The subsequent orbital flight of chimpanzee Enos demonstrated the feasibility of the announcement by President Kennedy on 25 May 1961 that the national objective was a moon landing in the 1969-70 period.

Meanwhile, there would be more ambitious flights such as John Glenn's three earth orbits, the two-man Gemini series and finally the Apollo flights.

The bugs had been worked out of the administrative machinery as well the hardware itself—at least for starters. What worked were the countdown precedures, range monitoring and recovery techniques, bioinstrumentation and the control of environmental systems. In the Mercury-Atlas 2 and Mercury-Atlas 5 flights,

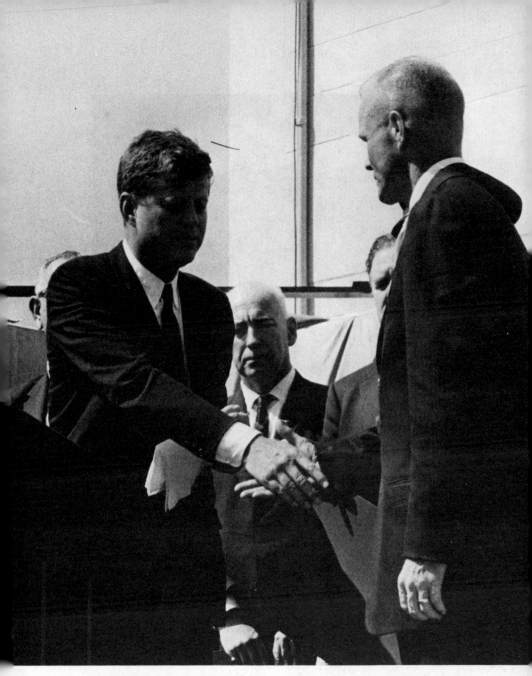

President John F. Kennedy flew to Cape Canaveral to award the NASA Distinguished Service Award Medal to John Glenn, following his three earth orbit in Friendship 7./*NASA*

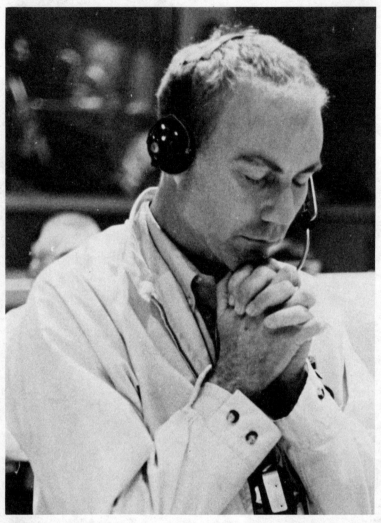

Come in, Friendship 7! The communications blackout during re-entry always provided a few minutes of almost unbearable suspense. As John Glenn went through that stage of his flight, Dr. W. K. Douglas, the astronaut's physician, did the best he could for a safe splashdown./*NASA*

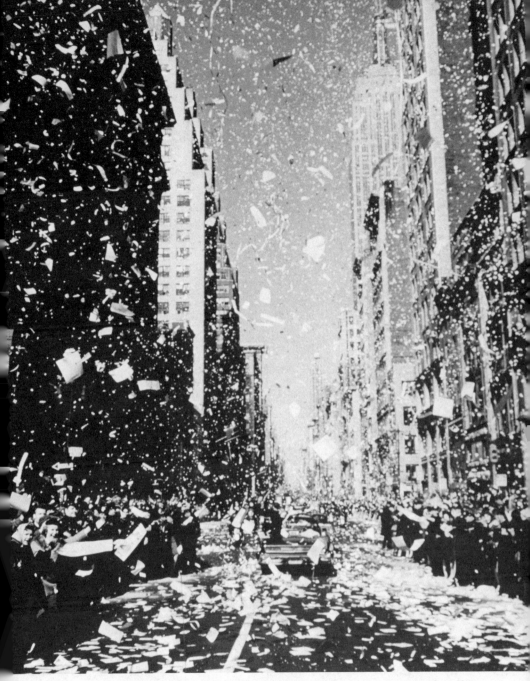

John Glenn, the first American to orbit the earth, gets a heroes' welcome from New York—a ride down Broadway in a blizzard of paper. The flight around the world and the ride down Broadway both took about the same amount of time./*NASA*

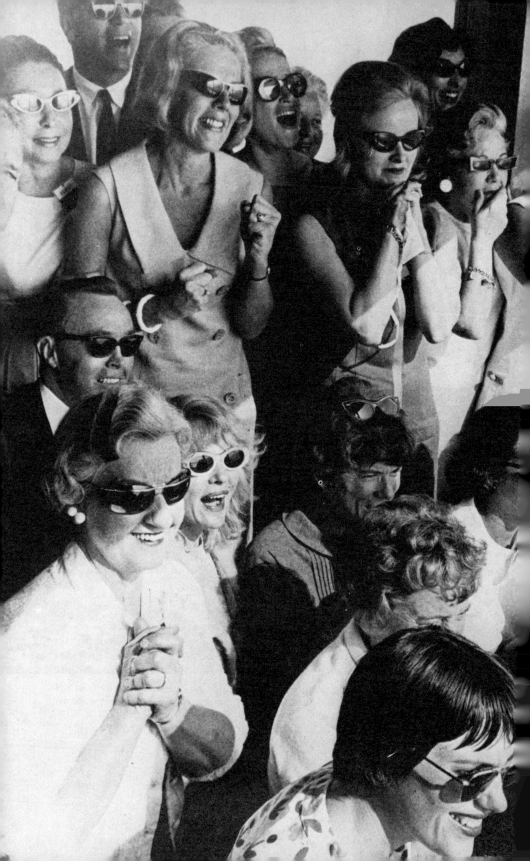

doctors learned that pulse and respiration were within tolerable limits during weightlessness; so was blood pressure in the peripheral arterial systems. Performing assigned tasks during weightlessness was also shown to be no big problem.

Following the Project Mercury series, Dr. Berry took over as Director of Medical Operation at Houston for the Gemini and Apollo series (he left the Air Force to do so) and Dr. Howard Minners took over for Dr. Douglas as personal physician to the astronauts and their families. Dr. Robert Gilruth stayed on and had the satisfaction of seeing the culmination of all the early anxieties—the first moon walk.

In June 1963, D. Brainerd Holmes, Director of the Office of Manned Space Flight resigned to return to private industry and Brigadier General Charles Roadman U.S. Air Force, Director of Space Medicine under Holmes, returned to duty with the Air Force.

The biomedical community still faced many unsolved problems of spaceflight. And in 1961 the orbital flight of Cosmonaut Titov in Vostok 2 produced another problem—Titov suffered from motion sickness. Was his condition induced by a first exposure to weightlessness, or was it the result of combined stresses of space-flight not encountered in atmospheric flight? Such questions, along with others concerning conditions or effects that could not be reproduced or simulated on earth, would continue to harass researchers. In effect, they needed to know the answers before they could send a man into space, but they had to send a man into space to get the answers.

The laws of Kepler and Newton were irrefutable, and the quality control of Lockhead and McDonnell-Douglas were of high degree, but some photographs of people witnessing early launchings, or waiting out re-entry and splashdown, showed that a few earthlings also believed in the magic of crossed fingers and the power of silent prayer.

They're off! As Gemini 3, with astronauts Grissom and Young aboard, lifted off from Cape Kennedy on a 3-orbit flight, their wives and friends displayed a wide range of emotions./*NASA*

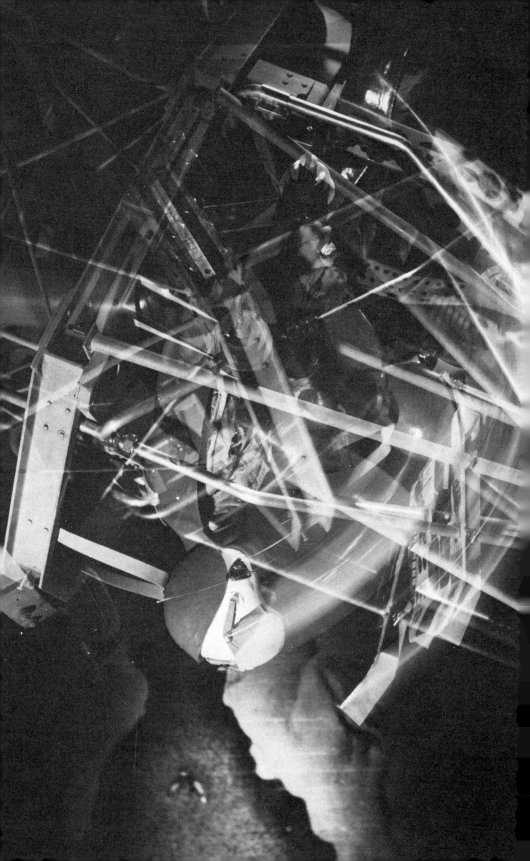

5

The Men Who Went to the Moon

For centuries man has watched the moon's mysterious wandering among the stars, marveled as it constantly changes shape in the night time skies, and dreamed of crossing space to explore the earth's nearest celestial neighbor. The centuries of dreaming ended on 20 July 1969 when Neil Armstrong descended from Eagle's ladder to the surface of the moon and said, "That's one small step for man, one giant leap for mankind." One might almost expect to hear cheers echoing down the halls of time, all the way from Galileo to Goddard—man had finally reached the moon.

Right behind Armstrong on the ladder was Edwin Aldrin, the second man to reach the moon. But circling around in Columbia, 64 miles above the moon's surface, was Michael Collins, who had come along for the ride, as it were, but would never set foot on the moon. Back at Canaveral and Houston were some two dozen astronauts who had flown in space—and some around the moon—but who would never get the chance for that memorable "one small step." And watching that first moon landing were several hundred more men who had volunteered for spaceflight but somewhere along the line had been selected out.

The Air Lubricated Free Attitude Trainer (ALFA) was in ingenious device which taught astronauts how to maintain attitude control and practice navigation in earth orbit. By using the Mercury hand-controller which actuated compressed-air jets, the trainer could be stabilized and controlled about all three axes./*NASA*

147

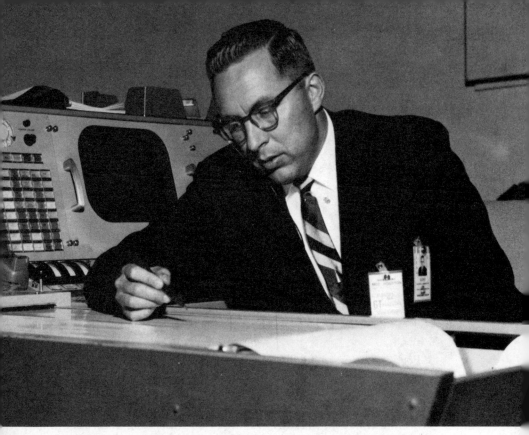

Dr. Charles Berry, Chief, Center Medical Programs, was generally known as the astronauts' chief physician during the Gemini and Apollo series. He is shown at the flight surgeon's console in Mission Control Center./*NASA*

At the Johnson Space Flight Center at Houston, Dr. Charles Berry, the man generally known as the astronaut's chief physician, during the Gemini and Apollo series, mulled over his part in the decision-making process. Even in his own elation at the success of the mission thus far, he hoped that his judgement, "Yes, these particular men are ready to fly to the moon," had been sound. One never knew. Flight surgeons don't always win popularity contests. Nevertheless, he considered that all the astronauts were his close personal friends. Their families socialized...he knew them all pretty well, on and off duty.

He was also aware that there had been resentments and hard feelings sometimes. No one likes to be told, "It's for your own good," least of all pilots and astronauts who are grounded temporarily or permanently. They wonder about the power of that one person, the flight surgeon, who can take that certificate off the wall and say, "Sorry, it's all over," or, "If we can get you fixed up, you're back in business." In fact, it was flight surgeons who determined who was fit to fly in the first place. In the case of spaceflight, it was the same old tug-of-war that pilots and doctors knew so well.

According to Dr. Berry, "Pilots and astronauts really feel they are invincible. All they need is a jock strap, a white scarf, and let's go. So the minute you start dealing with them, the question is, are they ever being truthful (about how they feel or what they really think)? In my situation, I was responsible for getting man to the moon safely, and back, and at the same time I have these guys saying, 'Well now, we think we can get onto the moon safely and back anyway.' And here I am having to make decisions with every single bit of data I collected being a fight. On the one hand, the scientific community, the conservatives accuse me of risking astronauts' lives, while the astronauts thought I was overly conservative..."

The problem of selecting and training astronauts was critical, particularly in the beginning of the space program because there was so little hard information to go on. Project Mercury was the first operational American flight laboratory in which man was able to test his physiological capabilities to withstand the hostile forces of the extraterrestrial environment for longer than a few seconds. Weightlessness, combined stresses, radiation, potential disorientations, and toxic hazards in spacecraft were among the problems about which earthbound research had been able to supply only limited information. Indeed, from the viewpoint of environmental medicine as an applied science, Project Mercury marked the swift transition from what had come to be known as aviation medicine to what is now recognized as space medicine. The task of setting up the criteria and conducting the selection program, for the first group of astronauts fell to NASA medical personnel, Doctors Stanley White, William Augerson, Robert Voas and George Ruff (the latter serving as psychiatric consultant).

At the time there were no textbooks specifically dealing with astronaut selection although the February 1957 issue of *The Journal of Aviation Medicine* published an article on "Selection and Training of Personnel for Space Flight." The article concluded that "spaceflight is not drastically different from most aspects of aviation which are now familiar." As matters turned out, it was a good deal more complicated than that but certainly historical precedents were leaned on for guidance.

At the beginning of powered flight, of course, there was no such person as a flight surgeon. The Wright brothers were the only two airplane pilots in the United States and they selected themselves to make their 1903 flight at Kitty Hawk. From then on, until 1914 the machine was developed faster than the techniques of examining the man who was supposed to fly it. In 1907, when the Army got its first airplane, the pilot's physical standards were the same for everybody entering the military service. He was to have no detectable disease, be physically strong and able to endure the discomfort and hardship associated with flying the fragile open-cockpit aircraft. The first obvious flaw in the system showed up in the fatal crash of the California glider pilot John Montgomery in 1911. He had suffered an epileptic seizure during the flight.

In 1910, the Germans became the first to set up physical standards and establish an Air Force Medical Service with special examinations, periodic re-examinations and psychological tests for their pilot candidates. Men were tested for "attentiveness, memory, quickness and sureness of movement, capacity to withstand fatigue, timidity, orientation and discrimination."

In America, a 1912 memo from the Army Surgeon General to the Army Chief of Staff called for preliminary examinations of candidates for flight training at the Signal Corps Aviation Field. It called for such standards as normal vision and hearing and the ability to judge distances. There were a number of logical impairments that would disqualify the candidate including poor equilibrium. These standards were probably never applied because in 1914 the Surgeon General came up with an official version, taken arbitrarily from a physiology textbook. They were so tough nobody could pass them during the first eight months of trial so they were lowered, again arbitrarily.

It took World War I to establish the flight surgeon as a new kind of medical specialist—a physician who combined medical skills with a knowledge of aviation. It was a period when men had to learn a lot fast, or pay a high price for ignorance. Many men flew in combat who shouldn't have, and others were unwisely

150

disqualified. Selection of flying personnel was in its infancy; American doctors looked to other nations for advice and instruction in all the aeronautical sciences. Often it was a case of the blind leading the blind.

Early in the war, aviator selection was haphazard though well meaning. For example it was reasoned that a daring cavalryman, used to reckless exhibitionist behavior and wild charges with sabre and lance, would be an ideal pilot. As it happened, they were right about at least one man who switched from horses to airplanes. Rittmeister Manfred Von Richthofen, the famed "Red Baron," became Germany's top scoring ace with 80 victories.

Some aces, however, under current selection would not have been in service at all, let alone flying. Britian's greatest ace, Edward Mannock, with 74 victories, had severe astigmatism in the left eye and was nearly blind. He had been working for the telephone company in Turkey and had been sent home because of his age, apparent bad health and defective vision. He bluffed his way through the medical examination for the Flying Corps by memorizing the eye charts and reading them with his good right eye. Leech, a Canadian pilot, flew successfully in combat with a wooden leg. When he finally crashed, and broke his wooden leg, he had to pay for its repair.

Guynemer, the French ace with 53 victories, had pulmonary tuberculosis and Oswald Boelcke, German ace with 40 victories, was periodically grounded because of asthma. William Thaw, known as the "Soul of the Escadrille Lafayette" had normal vision in only one eye, while Frank Luke, America's second ranking ace with 21 victories, would not have gotten past today's psychiatric examinations because of his moodiness and inability to get along with his squadron mates.

But for these few who flew successfully there were many others who were killed in action or in training because they were "flown out" or became stale from too much continuous duty. The British found that of every 100 aviation deaths, two were by enemy action, eight by defective airplanes and 90 for individual defects, 60 of which were a combination of physical defects and improper training. The latter was understandable, since many men in the Royal Flying Corps were there because they had been disabled by combat in France or Flanders. To counter criticism, the British finally set up a small medical research advisory committee and six stations for medical examinations of pilots. The emphasis was on cardiovascular performance after exercise and the breathing in and out of the so-called "flack bag" which was supposed to show how high a candidate could fly without oxygen.

In 1918, the French aeromedical service was reorganized for what it was hoped would be the better. The French, too, had been interested in the cardiovascular system, the middle ear and vestibular apparatus as well as the problems of insufficient oxygen. Under the new system, Doctors Nepper and Camus worked out a test for "nervous shock" whereby they measured changes in respiration, heart rate and vasomotor response when a revolver was fired close to the candidate's ear.

The Italians emphasized reaction time. Their laboratory had a *carlinga* "simulator," an airplane seat and nacelle with a control stick and rudder pedals connected to a light that measured the reaction time of the pilot candidate.

Although European air forces were having difficulty finding enough candidates to choose from, America had no such problems. In May 1917, Lieutenant Colonel Theodore C. Lyster, on duty in the Army Surgeon General's office, became the first Chief Surgeon, Aviation Section, Signal Corps, and established new standards for American flyers. Congress appropriated $640 million for aircraft and support for an increase from 131 officers (78 pilots) and 1,120 enlisted personnel to 20,000 officers, 611 cadets and 164,000 enlisted men.

He immediately set up 67 indoctrination centers where specially trained physicians examined would-be aviators. Standards were high; 20/20 visual acuity in both eyes, normal red/green color vision and 40/40 hearing in both ears were absolute requirements. Over 100,000 applicants were examined.

Rumors and gossip about the tough physicals flew thick and fast. There was the so-called "needle test" during which the blindfolded applicant held a needle between thumb and forefinger and a pistol was fired unexpectedly behind him. If the man pushed the needle through his finger it proved he didn't have much nerve. Another rumored test involved hitting the applicant over the head with a mallet when he least expected it. If he regained consciousness within 15 seconds he was assumed to be tough enough to make a good aviator.

The psychological make-up of applicants was given short shrift and there were many contradictions. Major William F. Patten, sent a study group to France, then summarized his confusion with an aviator profile: "He is a tall, short, stout, slim, blond, brunette, quiet, nervous, languid, alert, reckless, conservative individual."

Captain Floyd C. Dockeray, a psychologist who was sent to an overseas aeromedical unit in 1918 wrote: "As to the personality of the aviator, quiet methodical men were among the best flyers."

There were some early attempts to select candidates who were psychologically well equipped to be attentive and well coordinated at high altitudes. Cadets were also tested for various manual abilities and visual reactions.

Late in the war Edward L. Thorndike developed a "mental alertness" test to determine those most likely to succeed in ground school. He also studied the records of over 2,000 aviators to see if there was a relationship between actual success as a military flyer and such factors as age, social status, intelligence, business achievement and athletic ability. His test would have been adopted had the war not ended when it did.

During this period, doctors both in America and abroad were particularly concerned with the condition of candidates' vestibular apparatus. This structure, located in the temporal bone of the skull close to the ear (but not part of the hearing apparatus) consists of two types of specialized sensory receptors in the inner ear. The semicircular canals, filled with fluid respond primarily to angular motions of the head and its position in relation to the downward pull of gravity. The otolith organs, closely related to the canals are highly sensitive to linear accelerations and changes in the direction of gravity acting on the head. These two receptors acting together provide sensory information necessary to the perception of body position and movement.

A number of medical men felt that the vestibular apparatus could orient pilots in the air as well as on the ground. (It is now known that the semicircular canals can give misleading or false information in the air.) Isaac Jones, an otologist who became a flight surgeon wrote in his paper, "Equilibrium and Vertigo," that the vestibular canals were essential for orientation in the air and that "perhaps the ear would be able to tell us whether we were upside down or right side up." Jones later retracted this idea when experience showed that vision was the dominant factor.

Meanwhile, candidates were spun on piano stools and if they moved their heads and responded normally by vomiting they were rejected. In addition to measuring the response of the semicircular canals, the turning chairs established the important test for nystagmus—the jerky motion of the eyes to right and left, indicating sensitivity to rotary motion.

After the Armistice, the air forces of the victorious Allies dwindled to almost nothing, and there was time for serious reflection on the business of who should fly and who should not. In the United States, between 1919 and 1939 there were far more men who wanted to fly then there were airplanes; initial entrance standards were high and the training rigorous.

Because doctors found that 80 per cent of the groundings during the war were due to "nervous breakdowns," a number of personality studies and tests were devised. One such test developed in the mid-1920s by Major Raymond T. Longacre was the so-called ARMA (Adaptability Ratings for Military Aeronautics), which remained a part of flying physicals for over 30 years despite its questionable validity and considerable criticism. Another test, developed in the early 1920s was the Schneider Index to measure vasomotor stability and physical condition. Dr. E. C. Schneider's work was excellent in many areas, but the index through which he correlated the pulse rate with the blood pressure grounded many potential aces, and nearly grounded Charles Lindbergh. According to Dr. Stanley Mohler of the Federal Aviation Administration (FAA), "It was used religiously for years to select out unfit candidates for military flight training. And there were so many things the candidate had to do. They took his blood pressure in between his pulse rate, then added this and subtracted that. It all looked very scientific but some people, by virtue of the way they're made up—their emotional investment in their desire to fly came out beyond the zone of numbers that the test said made you fit to fly..." The Schneider Index was accepted until 1943 when a study by the School of Aviation Medicine shed so much doubt on its value that it was dropped.

154

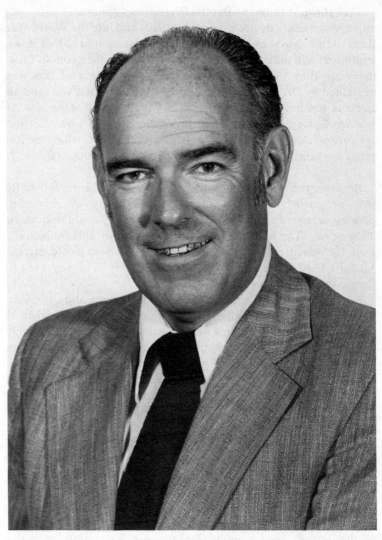

Dr. Stanley Mohler of the Federal Aviation Administration (FAA) feels that formerly many aviation candidates were unwisely grounded by the tests that did not accurately predict physiological or psychological problems that might occur. The author of *Wiley Post, His Winnie Mae,* and the *World's First Pressure Suit,* Dr. Mohler is currently Program Director of Aerospace Medicine; Professor and Vice Chairman of the Department of Community Medicine at Wright State University in Dayton Ohio./*Department of Transportation*

155

The Howard-Dolman Depth Perception apparatus was yet another screening device used in the 1920s and into the World War II era. Army, Navy, even civilian pilots were required to look down a tube and pull little wires to line up two rods. If they couldn't line them up, they were out of the picture. The fallacy of this was explained by Dr. Mohler: "The theory was that when you land an airplane you have to see both sides of a rock or both sides of what you are looking at so you get a three dimensional view. But the eyes are so close together that beyond about 30 feet, whatever you see is the same anyway. Lots of one-eyed pilots do superb flying.."

Between the wars, many military pilots who still wanted to fly took up barnstorming as stunt aerobats and gypsy birdmen, piloting surplus Jennies or Wacos wherever they could find an air show or fair. The question of who was physically and emotionally fit to fly was often of little more concern than who would drive a Model T Ford down the boulevard. If pilots felt sick, they went to their own private physicians.

Airplanes were flying higher and faster and carrying passengers; it appeared that civil aviation was the travel boom of the future and something had better be done to regulate it. In 1926 the Department of Air Commerce was established under the Department of Commerce. From then on, civil pilots had to be examined and their airplanes inspected and licensed. Furthermore they were required to follow established safety rules. Airlines formed their own standards for physical examinations and "recklessness in pilots" was cause for immediate discharge from the job. Dr. Louis H. Bauer, former Commandant of the School of Aviation Medicine at Mitchell Field and at that time the most distinguished specialist in aviation medicine in the U.S. became the first medical director of the Aeronautics Branch of the Department of Commerce.

It was Dr. Bauer who drew up the first standards based on those of the International Commission for Air Navigation, and the military standards of the British and Americans. Three classes of airmen were established, with physical exams to be administered only by designated examiners.

On paper, this was fine, but in practice not everyone wanted to be bothered with it. Early aviation medical pioneers were constantly pressured to lower their standards and a number of people didn't want doctors involved at all. Edward P. Warner, editor of *Aviation* magazine, wrote in the January 1934 issue that "...Exams for student and private pilots should be conducted by a flight inspector at a flying field instead of by a physician..." In 1945, T. P. Wright, the Civil Aeronautics Administrator, ruled that any registered physician could give an airman an examination which meant that chiropractors and osteopaths were acceptable. Even podiatrists got into the business of signing forms that allowed people to fly. The Aero Medical Association, organized in 1929 (later the Aerospace Medical Association) bitterly opposed such bureaucratic decisions, but changing federal policy on the grounds of aviation safety was not easy to do. In this case it took years.

During World War II there was never a clear-cut agreement on the role of the medical elements of the Army Air Forces. Military leaders argued among themselves as to what constituted the combat mission of the air arm. Meanwhile doctors did their best to hurriedly select those who were best qualified to fly. Probably the most memorable contribution was a classification test battery, consisting of six apparatus tests of coordination and speed of reaction, along with 14 printed tests, including mechanical comprehension, perception and visualization. Weighted scores were derived from these tests and each candidate received a series of score ratings. The term "stanine," a contraction of the words "standard nine," was coined to simplify interpretation. Three aptitude stanines for pilot, navigator and bombardier were developed, using different combinations of tests in the battery.

Pilot selection took a new turn with the coming of high speed, high altitude military jet aircraft. Now, in order for a pilot to fit into the cockpit of the new jet fighters, seated height could be no more than 41 or less then 32 inches. Anyone who did not fit within those limitations would experience visual distortion through the canopy and would have difficulty in making an emergency ejection.

With the creation of the Federal Aviation Administration (FAA) on 28 August 1958, its Bureau of Aviation Medicine finally got enough money and recognition to move forward in civil aviation medicine. There was a return to the system of using only

157

designated medical examiners, and existing physical standards were reviewed and revised. Diabetes mellitus requiring insulin or a hypoglycemic drug for control was ruled disqualifying for all classes. A history or diagnosis of a psychotic disorder or evidence of coronary heart disease grounded pilot applicants. Visual standards were generally liberalized.

The new agency approached the problem of age limit for airline pilots and by March 1960 had ruled that pilots reaching the age of 60 had to retire from air carrier operations. Although large European airlines had forced pilots to retire at 55 or 60, this was the first time the American government set a maximum limit for any group in private industry. Research to detect and measure physiologic aging and the prediction of incapacitation could mean that future airline pilots will be retained on an individual basis rather than by an arbitrary age cut-off. Until then, the cut-off is age 60.

Selecting and training astronauts for space flight was in some ways a grand finale to all the efforts to date in trying to match man with machine. On 8 October 1958, the Space Task Group was unofficially established at Langley Field, Virginia where the NACA Langley Laboratory had been located since 1917. Robert R. Gilruth, who had headed the former NACA Pilotless Aircraft Research Laboratory at Wallops Island, Virginia, was named Project Manager, and Charles J. Donlan, Technical Assistant to the Director of the Langley Laboratory, was made Assistant Project Manager. Thirty-five key staff members of the Langley Laboratory, who had worked closely with the Wright-Patterson Laboratory personnel on the Man-in-Space plan, were transferred to the new Space Task Group, as were 10 other persons from Lewis Research Center, Ohio. These 45 people formed the nucleus of the work force for the spaceflight program with headquarters at Langley. On 14 November the highest national priority procurement rating was requested for the manned spacecraft project (although it was not granted until 27 April 1959). On 26 November, the program was officially designated as Project Mercury.

Now that man was definitely scheduled to fly in space, several big questions were posed. Who? What type of individual would function most effectively as an astronaut? What sort of professional qualifications, training and experience would be the most valuable? By what physical and mental criteria should he be judged, and for that matter, who should do the judging?

The aeromedical team composed of Drs. Stanley White, William Augerson and Robert Voas, together with other representatives from the Space Task Group, NASA Headquarters, and the Special Committee on Life Sciences, worked almost around the clock for several weeks. They finally came up with a beginning, a "duties analysis" of what the astronaut was expected to do. The astronaut was to fly in space and survive, thus proving man could do it. He was to demonstrate that he could perform useful tasks in space. He was to serve as backup for the automatic controls and instrumentation, thus adding reliability to the system. He was to act as a scientific observer beyond what the instruments and satellites had done, and report on these observations. And finally, he was to serve as an engineering observer and, acting as a true test pilot, to improve the flight system and its components.

Once the experts had decided on what was expected, the next step was to determine qualifications. These included environmental stress capacity, toughness and resilience, motor skill, perceptual skill, maximum age of 35 (later changed to 39), an engineering or scientific degree and a height no taller then 71 inches in order to fit into the capsule.

The next question was, what professions ought these super-achievers to come from? And there were a number of strong opinions and valid arguments, along with bizarre suggestions. Some thought mountain climbers would be ideal because they were used to high altitudes. Others felt that doctors, racing drivers, astronomers or midgets would be suitable candidates because of their specialized skills and configuration. The *Journal of Science,* published by the American Association for the Advancement of Science, proposed that Eskimos would be good astronauts because "...these people are not concerned with the passage of time." Buddhist monks were recommended because they could put themselves in a state of suspended animation and would not be concerned with sensory deprivation. One researcher asked NASA to give him two weeks on the moon. It wouldn't matter if he didn't get back. Fortunately, the idea was rejected. Balloonists, submariners, deep sea divers (particularly those with

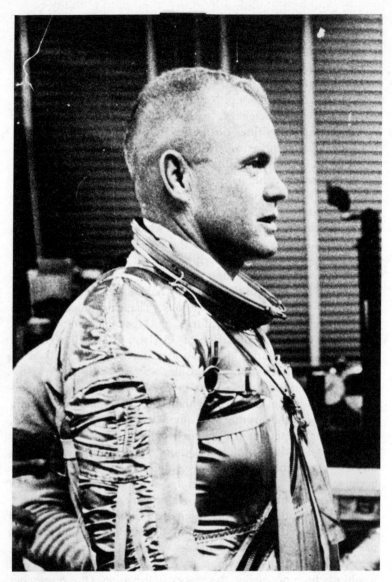

John Glenn, a lieutenant colonel in the U.S. Marine Corps, was selected to be the first American to orbit the earth. He is wearing the full pressure Mercury suit, developed by the U.S. Navy./*NASA*

experience), Arctic and Antarctic explorers, and metorologists were all considered as candidates during the summer and fall of 1958.

It was finally decided that test pilots were the most appropriate group from which to choose. An important factor was their demonstrated capability of meeting threatening situations in the air with accurate judgement, quick decisions and motor skills.

In late December 1958, the White House issued verbal orders that only active military test pilots were to be used as astronauts in Project Mercury. This was a sound decision, because here was a solid group, largely preselected and preexperienced, whose records were available for preliminary screening (which was not true of commercial or civilian test pilots). Most of them had graduated from military test pilot schools where entrance and graduation requirements were stringent; furthermore they were familiar with full-pressure suits and complex cockpits.

Once the decision to use only military test pilots was made, the selection committee added two requirements. The candidates must have been graduated from a test pilot school and have had at least 1,500 flying hours and be fully qualified in top-performance jet aircraft.

More then 450 names were selected for further consideration including 200 Air Force, 200 Navy, 23 Marine and 40 Army pilots. Of these, 58 Air Force, 47 Navy and five Marine test pilots met the preestablished criteria. These 110 were divided into three groups for interviews according to general qualifications obtained from the records.

There were a number of practical considerations. Would younger men in their mid-twenties with less experience, training, education and maturity be better choices than those who were 10 years older, who were highly seasoned, whose past performances were well-known, but who had fewer useful operational years left? The choice went to the older group.

Timing was another factor in the Mercury Program. In order to keep on schedule, the selection process, begun in January 1959 had to be completed by the end of March 1959. That allowed only three months to cull through the nation's top military pilots and come up with those few men destined for future stardom.

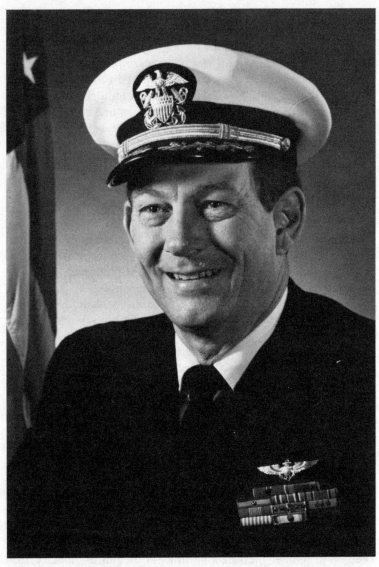

Captain Frank Austin (MC), U.S. Navy, was, at the time of the Mercury astronaut selection, the only jet qualified flight surgeon in the services, and Lieutenant Commander. He was disqualified because he was too tall. Next time around he was found to be too old. According to Captain Austin, it's easier to take off a few inches than a few years/*U.S. Navy*

At that time there was only one jet qualified flight surgeon in the military services—Lieutenant Commander Frank Austin, (MC) U.S. Navy. He was disqualified because he was too tall. Next time around he was disqualified because he was too old. Said Austin, "I could have gotten shorter before I could have gotten younger."

The first group of 69 pilots reported to NASA in Washington for briefings and individual interviews which eliminated those who did not want to volunteer for the spaceflight program. Those remaining took a battery of written tests to measure general intelligence and aptitude for engineering and mathematics, which included Miller's Analogy Test at the graduate level, the Minnesota Engineering Analogy Test and the Doppelt Mathematical Analogy Test. Finally the volunteer completed a biographical inventory developed by NASA for selecting scientific research personnel. Each applicant had four interviews by senior management people. They were also interviewed by each of two Air Force psychiatrists to determine their relationships with their families and associates.

In the final interview, flight surgeons reviewed their medical records, filled in any possible blank spaces in their histories and by the end of the second week, 32 candidates were still in the running.

The next two phases of the medical evaluation were carried out at the Lovelace Foundation for Medical Research and Education, the Lovelace Clinic in Albuquerque, New Mexico, and at the Aerospace Medical Research Laboratories (AMRL), Wright-Patterson Air Force Base, Ohio. The 32 volunteers were divided into five groups of six men each and one group of two. One group at a time reported for an exhaustive series of examinations while the other men remained at their home stations. At the Lovelace Foundation, under the direction of Dr. A. H. Schwichtenberg who headed the Department of Aerospace Medicine, candidates had their medical and aviation history taken and were given extensive physical examinations. There were laboratory tests, radiographic examinations, physical competence and ventilatory efficiency tests and finally an overall evaluation.

At the AMRL, a testing program had been going on for several years. The people there had extensive physiological and biochemical tests integrated into their stress program. There was a

163

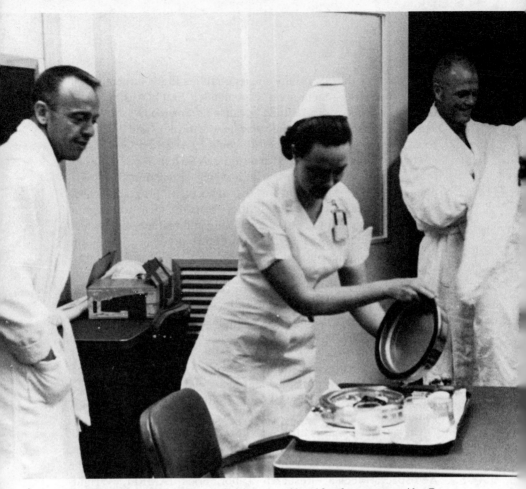

Air Force Captain Jean McKay, a dietician, served breakfast for astronauts Alan B. Shepard, Jr., (left) and John H. Glenn, Jr., prior to physical examinations for Shepard's sub-orbital flight. This was one of the pleasanter aspects of being selected for the Mercury program./*NASA*

human centrifuge, low-pressure chambers, thermal exposure chambers, C-131 and KC-135 aircraft modified to fly Keplerian trajectories for weightlessness studies, tumbling turntables and an anechoic chamber for sensory deprivation observations. Men experienced every stress anticipated during an actual Mercury flight, except for extended weightlessness.

The tests were extremely uncomfortable at their worst, annoying at best, but little by little, valuable data accumulated for each individual—data that would go into the swelling bank of information so necessary for man's first flight into space. In spite of the heavy research that had been going on for years, there was still so much to learn in a hurry that no detail could be considered insignificant.

Finally, on 2 April 1959, the seven astronauts for Project Mercury were chosen. There were three Air Force officers; Captains Leroy G. Cooper, Jr., Virgil I. Grissom, and Donald K. Slayton; three Navy officers, Lieutenant Malcolm S. Carpenter, and Lieutenant Commanders Walter M. Schirra and Alan B. Shepard, Jr.; and one Marine, Lieutenant Colonel John H. Glenn. Within 24 months these names were to become household words throughout the world—names that symbolized the dreams and hopes of everyone, that space would at last be explored by humans.

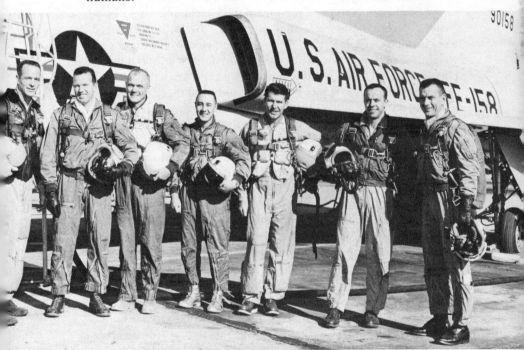

On 2 April 1959, the Original Seven astronauts for Project Mercury were chosen. They were Malcolm Scott Carpenter, Leroy Gordon Cooper, Jr., John Herschel Glenn, Jr., Virgil I. Grissom, Walter M. Schirra, Alan Bartlett Shepard, Jr., and Donald Kent Slayton./NASA

165

These men, the "Original Seven," did indeed earn and deserve the adulation they received, not only for their accomplishments but for what they endured during the pioneering selection process. By the time of the Apollo Program, the system had been improved: the stress tests at AMRL (with the exception of the exercise tolerance) had been eliminated and biological and blood sampling tests had been made more efficient. Psychological evaluations were streamlined and conducted by carefully selected interviewers.

Although most astronauts accepted what the doctors did to them with stoic good humor, a few had some black thoughts in retrospect. Michael Collins, the Apollo 11 astronaut who later wrote *Carrying the Fire*, mentioned the "...pleasant lab technician, part Dracula and part leech..." who took blood samples. He complained of the uncertainty and indignity of being "poked, prodded, pummeled and pierced..." No orifice, he stated, was inviolate. Flying the Keplerian trajectory to experience weightlessness was no picnic either, although a few thought it pleasant at first. They nearly always wore pressure suits which in Collins' opinion were rarely well-ventilated. And there was always a lot to do during the 25 seconds of the parabola; drinking, swallowing, voiding and whatever else the doctors could cram into the time limit. Repeating these 40 to 50 parabolas in a day, with the body alternating between 2gs and zero g, induced a lot of wear and tear. Cameramen, engineers and supporting personnel assigned to the flights invariably threw up.

While all of this was going on, the astronauts were being exposed to the greatest public scrutiny in recorded history. As Collins wrote: "All of them were Gordon Goodguys, steely resolve mixed with robust muscular good humor, waiting crinkly-eyed for whatever ghastly hazards might be in store for them 'up there'." There were background investigations on morals; one later astronaut left the program because of an impending divorce—in those days astronauts did not get divorced. There was what Collins calls the "charm school" where the men learned to make impromptu speeches, talk, dress, stand and sit. They were told to wear knee length socks so their hairy legs wouldn't show when they sat down. For drinking at parties, they were told to take a long one, and make it last. They were even instructed on how to hold their hands on their hips (thumbs forward for ladies, thumbs back for men).

But the Mercury astronauts weren't the only ones undergoing the super-strenuous physiologic and stress testing. Along with them was Lieutenant Colonel William Douglas, who was assigned as their family physician. "General Flickinger wanted me to go through the selection process myself and personally experience all the things the astronauts would have to go through. I went at once to the Lovelace Clinic in Albuquerque and inserted myself into the physical examination procedure. Roughly six or seven candidates came in each week. Some of the things they were subjected to at the AMRL, I was not. For example, I did not spend several hours in the anechoic sensory deprivation chamber because I was more useful elsewhere."

One unusual test that Dr. Douglas did participate in with the first astronauts was conducted in the human gradient calorimeter, a huge facility in the bio-energetics department of the Naval Medical Research Institute in Bethesda, Maryland. The program itself, under the direction of Dr. Theodor Benzinger, represented the latest state of the art in the physiology of body temperature and heat stress and it was important at that time to acquaint the astronauts with what they might expect to encounter.

According to Dr. Benzinger, the world's first human gradient calorimeter had a response time of 50 seconds; its temperatures were controlled to 0.01°C. and errors in complex heatflow measurements were within 1 percent of human heat loss. "Even so, it would not have been possible to discover the mechanisms of human temperature regulation with this instrument, had not the method of tympanic thermometering been invented for precision measurement of the temperature patterns in the brain, close to the site of measurement, near the stem of the internal carotid artery..."*

The Mercury astronauts and Dr. Douglas spent two weeks in June 1959 undergoing the tests. During the preceding months, the Department had discovered that sweating and widening of the

*This method of clinical thermometry was not applied to the later astronauts because it might have produced tickling sensations in the ear and interfered with voice communication. The method has been used elsewhere in clinical surgery.

blood vessels of the skin are not elicited, as previously believed, by the sense of temperature in the skin. Instead, they are elicited by a second, a central sense of temperature, a small organ in the depth of the brain stem in the anterior hypothalamus. The location of a center indispensable for temperature regulation in animals and man had been known since 1885; at last its function as a "human thermostat," had been found.

The Mercury astronauts were, except for the investigators, the first group on which the "setpoints" of their human thermostats were determined, when sweating first occurs with rising brain temperature.

Each man spent several hours, often with strenuous exercise, in the calorimeter at 45°C. where all heat flows by radiation, conduction, convection and evaporation of sweat and all relevant temperatures of the body were measured at high precision and without inertial distortion. (One record obtained on Alan Shepard later became a textbook figure.)

After the experiment, the body fluid lost by the astronaut measured by calorimeter, was collected. Dr. Benzinger recalls, "When I held up the glass flask with the crystal clear liquid, the astronauts all contended it was the gin of the night before..."

The pay-off on the many tests came on 5 May 1961 when Alan B. Shepard made his 15-minute suborbital flight in Freedom 7, and proved that the doctors had made a good choice in selecting him. Shepard, with the other "Originals," became the first skilled astronauts in the U.S. and the nucleus for successive manned space flights.

During the first decade of the U.S. manned spaceflight program, there were six selection programs. In the 1960s, two scientist-astronaut groups were included. The plan from the beginning had been to have foresight and flexibility so that as spacecraft and missions became longer and more complex, the human requirements could be adjusted.

In the beginning, the pioneering one-man missions of the Mercury astronauts called for a spacecraft operator, an experimenter, a brains-behind-the-machinery type and a keen scientific observer. They were generalists, rather than specialists. Each man was on his own in flight.

During Gemini flights, test-pilot astronauts coordinated their activities, performed extravehicular activities (EVA) and got along with each other for up to two weeks in confined quarters. The two Gemini astronauts had increased scientific observations to make which were of academic value.

In the Apollo project, a third member chosen for scientific background had to be fully qualified to manage the operation of either the spacecraft or the Lunar Module (LM).

Meanwhile, the medical evaluation process was streamlined by turning the whole job over to the USAF Aerospace Medical Center at Brooks Air Force Base, San Antonio. At nearby Houston, the new NASA Manned Spacecraft Center (MSC), later renamed Lyndon B. Johnson Space Center, Space Task Group members transferred from Langley Research Center, Hampton, Virginia and veterans of the Mercury flight began serving on the selection board for the new astronauts.

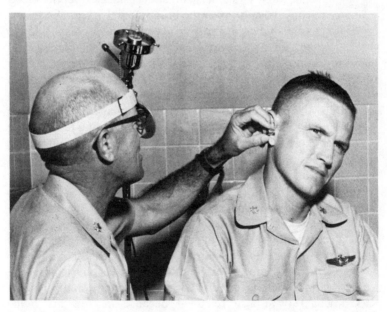

Before a pilot was selected for duty in the space program, he was examined, checked, and tested to the point of near non-endurance. Frank Borman, who flew in Gemini 7, is shown here having his ears checked./*NASA*

169

Astronaut Donald K. Slayton, Director of Flight Crew Operations, held the key position in astronaut selection and training, while Dr. Berry left the Air Force to become the first permanent civilian Director of Medical Operations at the Manned Spacecraft Center. It was Berry's responsibility to shape the future course of medical and related qualifications of pilot-astronauts and later scientist-astronaut candidates. By early 1962, methods for selecting the next five sets of astronauts, combining medical factors and team evaluations, were established.

The medical evaluation, as explained by Dr. Lawrence E. Lamb at the School of Aerospace Medicine,* was divided into four parts. The first concerned the detection of significant diseases or abnormalities—those not apparent in regular histories and physical exams. Candidates were checked for abnormalities that, under normal circumstances on earth would be relatively unimportant but could cause problems on prolonged space voyages; renal stones, silent gallbladder stones, peptic ulcer, evidence of convulsive focus in the brain, dental apical abscesses, rectal polyps and diabetes. The second concerned predisposition to disease or limited performance capability, for example, obesity and borderline glucose tolerance. The third category was a complex evaluation of mental and character dynamics such as motivation, intellectual ability, learning aptitude, emotional adaptability and maturity. The fourth emphasized physiologic capacity under different loads and stresses, including tests during maximum exertion, use of the tilt table for evaluating autonomic control of the cardiovascular system, and physiologic stresses such as hyperventilation and breath-holding combined with orthostatic influences.

The two scientist-astronaut selection programs, 1965 and 1967, found Dr. Berry and his staff screening 84 men with average ages of 32, all of whom were from the scientific community. Among the first group was geologist Harrison "Jack" Schmitt who later become a U.S. Senator from New Mexico, two physicians, Joe Kerwin and Duane Graveline (who later resigned), and physicist Kirk Michael (who also resigned because he felt his field,

*Aeromedical evaluation for space pilots, *"Lectures in Aerospace Medicine,"* Brooks AFB, Tex., SAM 1964

theoretical physics was impractical for an astronaut). The 1967 group included two more physicians, Bill Thornton, who held an electrical engineering degree prior to his M.D., and F. Story Musgrave, physiologist, M.D., glider pilot, parachutist and surgeon.

The selecting and testing of the scientists was similar to that of the pilots; the difficulties lay in the lack of ready-made medical history and screening that the pilots had. Some of the candidates had medical problems that disqualified them; almost none had had psychiatric and psychological evaluations, and unlike the pilots, they were unused to the physical stresses and hazards of flying high performance aircraft.

Following the 1976-77 Skylab missions where true weightlessness in a relatively "roomy" house in space was experienced for 85 days, there was a new look at future selections of space travelers. Legs, it was seen, were not of much use; in fact, they hindered mobility. These nuisances caused cardiovascular and muscular problems in the absence of gravity. Dr. Robert P. Heaney of Creighton University in Omaha, Nebraska, seriously proposed that amputees be considered for future space missions. "Their tissue requires food and consumes oxygen, and if we exercise them, they consume even more. The ultimate fuel cost of legs on long missions must be really staggering."

Another doctor felt that the strong, athletic types of astronauts had to spend too much time exercising to keep their muscles in shape. "Now if we were to send a skinny older person (like myself) who didn't care about keeping in shape, maybe all the energies could be directed toward the jobs at hand..."

These views were not generally accepted, even though they indicated that visionaries were still very much a live breed.

Scientist-astronauts will play an ever increasing role in the space shuttle missions; so will women and minorities. Of the 35 new candidates selected in July 1978 for the space shuttle program, six were women, three were blacks and one was an Oriental-- American.

Among the six women chosen from 8,079 applicants, Dr. Shannon W. Lucia, a 35-year-old biochemist of Oklahoma City is the mother of three young children. Dr. Anna Fisher is a physician, Dr. Judith Resnik, an electrical engineer, Sally Ride, a

171

researcher in physics, Dr. Margaret Seddon, a resident in surgery, and Kathryn Sullivan is working for her doctorate in geology. Women in space, of course are nothing new; Soviet cosmonaut Valentina Tereshkova made 48 orbits aboard the Vostok 6 spacecraft in 1963. Of the minorities selected, one is an engineering specialist, another a physicist in optic physics, and the third a pilot. Captain Ellison S. Onizuka, an Air Force engineer from Kealakekua, Hawaii, is of Japanese descent.

There is one male physician, Dr. Norman E. Thagard. The others are astrophysicists, aeronautical engineers, astronomers and military pilots.

The longest tests, according to the 21 women and 187 men who made it to the finals in November 1977, were interviews with two separate psychiatrists—"Psy one," and "Psy two."

Women were asked how they'd react to "running around in their underwear," with men in space. Men were asked how they'd respond to seeing women in their underwear. Suppose a disabled spacecraft had only one space suit for six people. What should the senior astronaut do about the others who were his responsibility?

Politics were probed (the Panama Canal question and Northern Ireland were then news-worthy) and so was the race issue. What would the black candidates do about South Africa if they were President? Jews were asked about their feelings on the Middle East; whites were quizzed on their willingness to fly with blacks and everyone was asked if they would fly with Russians.

"I'd fly with little green men if it meant getting into space," one woman replied.

By space shuttle time, no one had to ride the centrifuge and nobody had to take a Rorschach Test to see what the ink blots meant. All candidates, however, enjoyed physical exercise and exposure to physical risk—mountain climbing, scuba diving, sport parachuting and the like. One new astronaut is a judo champion; one of the women is a former tennis pro.

The selection and training of astronauts continues to be a highly sensitive and personal relationship between the would-be space voyager and physician. Once selected, what then for the astronauts and their families? And what about their support, their trackers and telemetry personnel working in remote areas of the world?

Historically, aerospace medical specialists were spread all over—from the launch pad where industrial accidents could occur to the far corners of the earth where they functioned as medical monitors. Navy flight surgeon Frank Austin recalls: "I was one of six or eight Navy surgeons who joined in with the Air Force, Army and civilian surgeons to go on loan to NASA as Mercury and Gemini medical monitors. After indoctrination at Langley, Virginia, we went out on assignments to some 16 different stations. I always had a suspicion they chose us Navy guys because they had two ships they had to man; one in the Atlantic, one in the Indian Ocean. They were 325-footers, run by civilian crews, all of whom were ancient mariners subject to kidney stones, heart attacks and so on. So when we went out to work with these ships we carried our medical bags. On the ships, we set up equipment so as to read medical measurements on the astronauts. We got the EKG, respiration, heart rate, environment (oxygen, CO_2) temperature and so forth. The best indication of alertness was the voice..."

While Austin was on board ship in the Indian Ocean a crewman became critically ill with appendicitis. There was no way to get him back to civilization and a hospital in time to save his life. Dr. Austin rigged a galley table for the operation, and using sterilized soup spoons as retractors, performed the appendectomy on the spot. Ten day later, the man walked off the ship in good health. "Just routine surgery at sea," said Austin.

During the John Glenn orbital flight one of the crewmen had a heart attack. "Ironically we could get an EKG from a man in space or on the way to the moon, but we had no way of getting one of a man on board a ship." Fortunately, he was able to treat the patient successfully. "By having a doctor on the ship, we were able to keep the ship on station. Otherwise we'd have had to sail 600 miles back to Mauritius and there would be no tracking ship for that portion of the space flight..."

Physicians who became involved with the space program generally fell into two groups; the biomedical scientists who were involved in life support systems, and the astronauts' doctors and personal physicians.

In the beginning, Colonel William Douglas, on loan to NASA was identified as *the* astronauts' flight surgeon. He was on hand

173

when they were selected and it was his job to take care of them and their families. Dr. Howard Minners was at that time at Langley Field for a year of training in aerospace medicine. He recalls: "That year of training was broken into segments and one of those segments was called the Space Task Group. So I sort of split my time between Bill Douglas' personal doctoring work and Stan White's biomedical sciences group." When Dr. Douglas returned to the Air Force, his place was taken by Dr. Minners.

"At that time the organization was growing very rapidly. The name was changed from Space Task Group to Manned Spacecraft Center (MSC) and was moved from Langley to Houston...Dr. Charles Berry came aboard then and we formed an office called the Flight Crew Effectiveness Branch; the original two people in that office were Dr. Berry and myself." Soon, several more doctors were assigned.

Dr. Berry's group grew into a medical operations office, totally responsible for the medical care to the astronauts and their families. "In addition, we participated in the preflight preparation of the astronauts, their medical examinations and in some cases, control of their diet and postflight examinations. In fact, in the early days they made an extraordinary effort to have the same doctor or doctors examine before and after the flight."

An example of this was Scott Carpenter's flight in the Mercury-Atlas 7. "I woke him up in the morning so I saw him when he opened his sleepy eyes and said, "Now we're going someplace today." And Dr. Minners was one of the last to see him get into the capsule. "I examined him that morning...then I went down to the launch pad and watched him get into the capsule. I was one of the last to see him, and one of the first ones to see him after the flight. We picked him up in the ocean and in this case flew him to Grand Turk Island and examined him down there..."

As testimony to the success of the medical care given the selected astronauts and cosmonauts and the caution that was exercised by the coordinated efforts with the systems engineers, there were only two fatal accidents in actual space operations. Even though the Russians gave their cosmonauts excellent medical care, Colonel Vladimir Komarov was killed on reentry of the Soyuz 1 in April of 1967, when his parachute failed. He had made a previous orbital flight in Voskhod 1, with a total of 24.3

hours in October in 1964. The other was the Soyuz 11 tragedy in June, 1971, in which cosmonauts Dobrovolskiy, Volkov and Patsayev died of anoxia and dysbarism due to hatch seal failure, resulting in rapid decompression of spacecraft prior to reentry.

Some astronauts were killed in routine flight operations. Ted Freeman, flying a T-38, hit a snow goose on a landing approach at Ellington Air Force Base, and crashed. Charles Bassett and Elliot See were making a low visibility landing at St. Louis when they hit the McDonnell building. Yuri Gagarin, the first man in space, was killed during a routine training flight near Moscow, 27 March 1968. He had spent one hour and 48 minutes in space. C. C. Williams, returning to Houston from Cape Kennedy, crashed when his T-38 went out of control. Gus Grissom, Edward White and Roger Chaffee died in the tragic fire in the spacecraft on the launch pad at Cape Kennedy on 27 March 1967.

The shock of losing these men was profound, and felt all over the world. For the physicians who selected them, helped train them, and cared for them and their families, the personal loss was impossible to measure. Years later, they still find it difficult to discuss objectively.

Who will fly? The selection process has come a long way from the days of giving a send-off to derring-do aviators in goggles and fluttering white scarves. Biomedical experts carefully built a base from which they could decide who would most likely succeed in the epic space voyages. If the doctors hadn't known what they were doing, and staked their professional reputations on their choices, Armstrong, Aldrin and Collins might still be waiting for their flight orders.

175

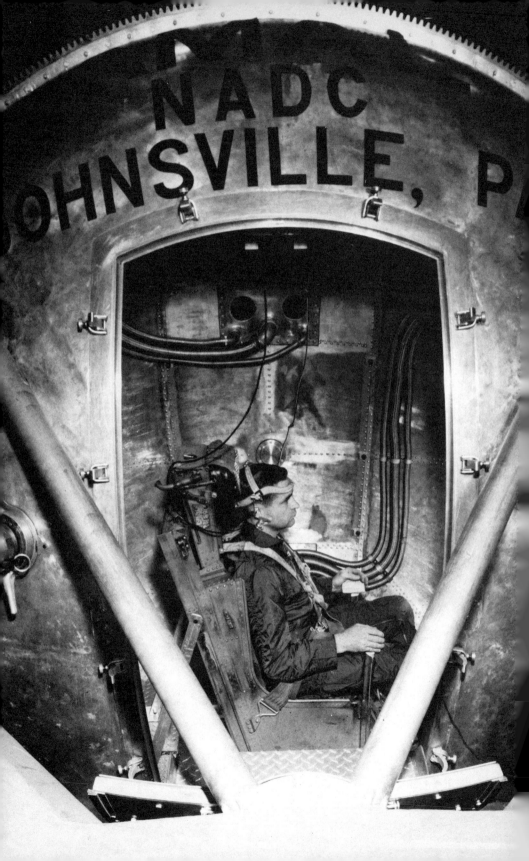

6

Space Medics Have Long Ears

On the afternoon of 20 July 1969, half the world listened as the Apollo 11 mission moved into highly critical moments—man's first landing on the moon. The lunar module was in powered descent, about 4 miles from the surface of the moon when Mission Control Center at Houston told the Eagle "You're go for landing." Neil Armstrong talked his craft down as if he was shooting a practice landing back at Houston: "Hang tight. We're go, 2000 feet...750, coming down...400 feet...contact light. Okay, engine stop... Houston, Tranquility Base here. The Eagle has landed."

Possibly the only person who knew how excited Armstrong was in those moments was flight surgeon Berry at the Control Center in Houston, monitoring physiological aspects of the flight through biotelemetry. Armstrong's usually normal heart rate of 90 a minute had gone up to 156 at touchdown.

It's simple enough to check temperature, pulse, and respiration if the patient is where the doctor can lay hands on him, but quite another matter if the subject is flashing through space at 17,000

An early example of biotelemetry is this hook-up designed to record physiological conditions of a man riding a 50-foot centrifuge at Johnsville, Pa., in 1952./*U.S. Navy* miles an hour, or walking around on the moon 243,000 miles away. At the end of World War II the whole idea of monitoring the physiological conditions of a man by long distance communications seemed close to impossible. One man who had much to do with making biotelemetry a fine art was Doctor Norman Lee Barr, who in 1947 was involved in setting up a human centrifuge for the Navy at Johnsville, Pennsylvania, about 17 miles north of Philadelphia. One purpose of the centrifuge was to determine tolerance to acceleration, and this had to be done while a man was under a heavy g-force, not after the machine stopped spinning and he climbed out.

By 1948, working with the Army, Air Force, and Navy, there had been organized a program for the gathering of information needed to put a man into an orbiting satellite. But what was urgently needed was a physiological data transmission system that would collect data on a subject in flight and make it available for recording by ground bases. At that time, Dr. Barr set up a project, Research Aerospace Medicine (RAM) which picked up the physiological information communication work being performed at the Naval Medical Research Institute. RAM soon had a 4-engine Douglas aircraft which was equipped as a flying electronics laboratory, manned by 17 mechanics and technicians.

Dr. Barr, who had started out as a physicist, then became a naval aviator, and then a medical doctor, not only managed the laboratory—he flew it. He also assembled the logistic support one learns how to acquire after a few years in military and government circles: "...I secured people (paid for by the Bureau of Aeronautics)...the development in the laboratory of the communications apparatus was done largely at the Naval Medical Research Institute in Bethesda, and that was paid for by BuMed...When there was a need for additional personnel, I got them through BuMed and assigned them to the Naval Medical Research Institute. I also got additional personnel from the Chief of Naval Operations, officer types, all scientists, the kind that could use tools and help build the equipment—electronics technicians. They were all paid for out of various budgets, but all assigned to Project RAM. There were no other doctors in the project."

178

The flying laboratory was equipped to transmit measurements of subjects aboard the craft to a ground base several hundred miles away. This included pulse rate, respiratory rate, respiratory volume, and electrocardiograms. The airborne transmissions, after being picked up by a ground station were first fed into a telephone and could then be sent anywhere the phone system serviced.

A first full dress rehearsal of the system came in February 1949 when the Chief of Naval Operations authorized Barr to use his flying laboratory in cooperation with an aircraft carrier to check out long distance data transmission. Selected heart patients in a hospital in Athens, Greece, were examined and the results transmitted to the aircraft, then relayed to the carrier off Port Lyautey in Africa, then meshed into the naval communications system, picked up in Washington and sent by telephone to Bethesda. The system was set up to work both ways—information on patients in Bethesda was sent back to Greece at the same time. Doctors at Bethesda, plus the chief of the cardiac service of Georgetown University, actually read the transmissions from Greece and were able to diagnose for the Greek patients.

In a striking demonstration of airborne biotelemetry at the 1953 meeting of the Aero Medical Association in Los Angeles, Dr. Barr set up a laboratory as one of the displays. He also had a flying laboratory at 8,000 feet and a jet fighter flying at 52,000 feet, and from both aircraft physiological data measurements—electrocardiograms, pulse rate, respiratory rate, respiratory volume, electroencephalograms, and myograms were transmitted to the ground laboratory for the amazement of the medical people, and the press. At that demonstration, a reporter, perhaps less amazed than the others, asked Dr. Barr: "Would it be possible to put a man on the moon?" Barr believed it was possible, even then, and replied "Yes, if someone wants us to do it and wants to pay for it, we can do it." It would be five more years before Sputnik encouraged others to agree with Dr. Barr.

Here it is worthwhile to enumerate the various physiological data and response measurements of a man in space which biotelemetry makes available to ground observers: body and skin temperature, conditions of spoken voice; cardiovascular functions (heart rate, electrocardiograms, blood pressure, pulse pressure, oxygen content of the blood, brain tissue and muscle tissue, and heart sounds); measurements of respiratory functions, such as rate, volume, and breath sounds; measures of gastrointestinal functions, such as swallowing, regurgitation, water and food intake, evacuation; measures of nutritional state—substitutes for body weight are required—to include girth, biceps, and leg measurements; measures of urinary frequency and volume; measures of muscle activity with myograms of selected muscle groups; measures of central nervous system activity—electro-encephalogram; galvanic skin responses; problem solving ability, orientation, auditory perception and response, visual perception

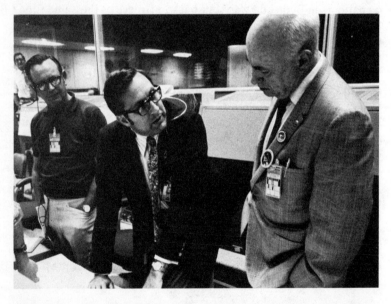

By the time of the Apollo 15 flight in July, 1971, biomedical telemetry had been greatly perfected. Here, at the Johnson Space Center, an EKG trace of arrhythmia (irregular heart beat) of one of the astronauts is checked by the Center Director, Dr. Robert R. Gilruth, Dr. Charles A. Berry, and Director of Flight Operations, Christopher C. Kraft./*NASA*

and response, and touch, smell and taste perception; performance measurements—experiments to be based on graduated task difficulty and performance adequacy.

It can readily be seen that an astronaut occupied with the multitudinous tasks of handling astronavigation, engine control, photography, communications, and on-board control of power systems, has no time to check his own blood pressure or EKG and must leave such details up to the sensors and telemetry.

The instrumentation required for making physiological measurements in space consists of electrodes and transducers for gathering information and converting it into electrical equivalents ready for radio transmission; the necessary transmission system; and receiving, relaying, recording and presentation equipment on the ground.

Telemetric information from spacecraft in orbit or on a lunar mission is transmitted on a "real time" basis—as it is collected or happens—or taped and then transmitted when the spacecraft is in range of a particular ground station, or ship. There were 18 stations in the original network, on three continents and islands in two oceans and several specially equipped ships could be stationed wherever needed during a mission. This arrangement permits direct communication between a spacecraft and a ground station for five minutes out of every fifteen during earth orbit; on a lunar mission the spacecraft is out of communication only when it goes "around the corner" behind the moon—for about 30 minutes each lunar orbit. The global system called Manned Space Flight Network (MSFN), was first used for the Mercury flights. Set up by Western Electric, Bell Telephone Laboratories, Bendix Corporation, Burns and Roe, Incorporated, and IBM, the original system cost about sixty million dollars. All stations are connected by 102,000 miles of teletype lines, 60,000 miles of telephone lines, and 15,000 miles of high speed data circuits. At the Goddard Space Flight Center, near Greenbelt, Maryland, where all U.S. orbital satellites and space flight missions are tracked through that enormously complicated electronic system, teleprinters and computers handle the incoming data. Goddard records as much as 75 miles of magnetic tape weekly.

Ground-based monitoring of men in actual high-altitude flight

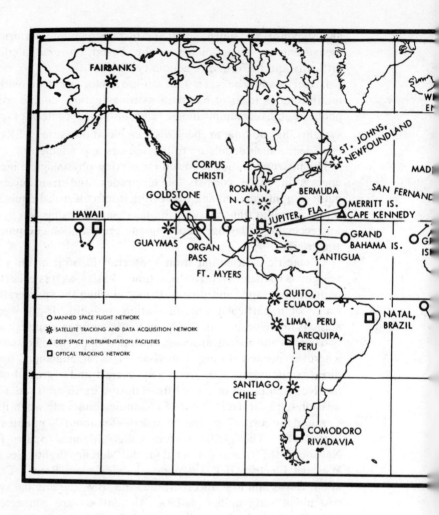

The Manned Space Flight Network, with stations positioned all the way around the world, keeps a spacecrew in constant communication with the control center./NASA

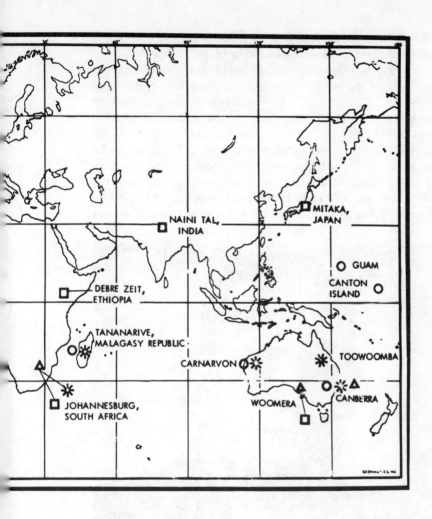

NAINI TAL, INDIA

MITAKA, JAPAN

O GUAM

DEBRE ZEIT, ETHIOPIA

CANTON ISLAND O

TANANARIVE, MALAGASY REPUBLIC

CARNARVON

TOOWOOMBA

WOOMERA

CANBERRA

JOHANNESBURG, SOUTH AFRICA

conditions was a part of all Explorer, Stratolab, and Man-High flights. During one of these, when Barr was monitoring the flight from the laboratory in Bethesda, Maryland, and the balloon was over Minneapolis, one of the pilots suddenly showed a deviation from normal heart trace known as the WPW syndrome, (so called for Wolff, Parkinson, and White, who discovered it). Barr

183

immediately detected the unusual heart condition, the first time a medical condition was diagnosed at long range.

And in 1961 biotelemetry actually went into space with the orbital flight of Enos, the chimpanzee, launched from Cape Canaveral on 29 November. The worldwide system of tracking stations had been established by then, and Enos had been fitted in accepted astronaut style with the usual array of sensors and catheters. At the monitoring station in Bermuda, Dr. Berry, as he recalled later, "...danced all around the console. I absolutely went wild. I could hardly believe that we were really seeing this, the first EKG from space." Then Enos began showing ectopic beats, which worried the doctors until he was recovered and it was

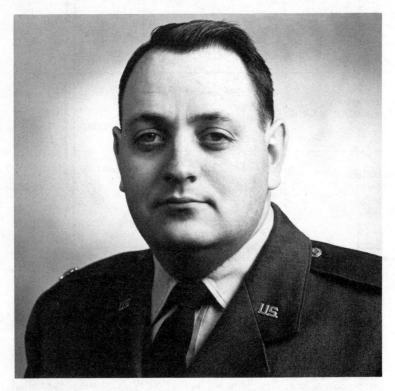

During the sub-orbital flight by Virgil I. Grissom, Air Force medical officer, Colonel Stanley White, kept a close watch on incoming physiological measurements provided by telemetry./*NASA*

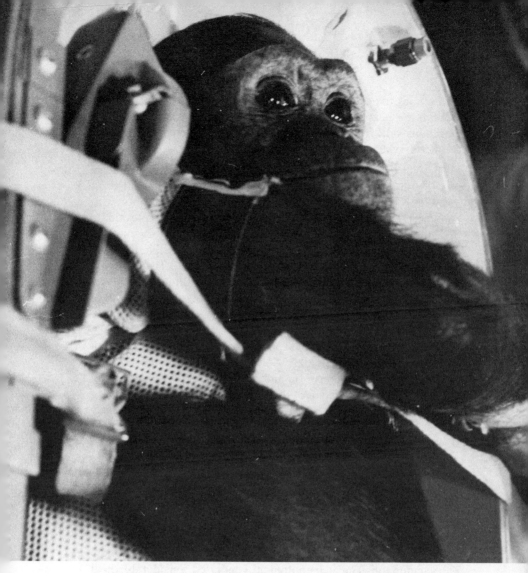

Space-chimp Enos, on his historic flight, had reason to look worried. The cardiac catheter, transmitting his heart beat back to earth, had been improperly inserted and was tickling one wall of his heart./*NASA*

discovered that the cardiac catheter had been inserted just a little too far and it was tickling the wall of the ventricle.

Astronauts still do not like the tickling—a mild word for it—that goes along with being prepared for a space flight. An astronaut suiting up for a mission must have several sensors taped to his body—in a few early flight missions, the locations were marked with tattoos to ensure that the sensors would be fixed in the same location the next time they were needed—and all these lead to a unit in his suit, from which a harness of wires connects him to the telemetry system of the space craft.

The fact that improper insertion of the catheter in Enos' heart was noted from a ground station pointed out the inherent advantage of biomedical telemetry. The Mercury flights with chimpanzees aboard offered the first U.S. opportunity to evaluate the physiological and behavorial aspects of a living organism in space. Subsequent manned orbital flights made possible full time monitoring of humans in the space environment. These flights proved that it was possible to exercise medical flight control of a man in space, and set a pattern followed in all subsequent space missions—the medical flight controller became a full-time member of the flight control team.

All this technique and sophisticated equipment was not developed overnight. Telemetry—derived from the Greek *tele* (far off) and *meter* (to measure), and now understood as meaning measurement at a distance—had its first primitive beginning almost a century ago. A patent for an electrical telemetry system was issued in 1885. Biotelemetry began two years later, when A. D. Walker first did an electrocardiogram on a human heart.

William Einthoven in 1906 sent an electrocardiogram by wire to a laboratory a mile away from the hospital. In 1925 the Russian scientist Pyotr A. Molchanoff first used a radio in a balloon to obtain measurements of temperature and air pressure during experiments in atmospheric research. The first airborne telemetering equipment used in high-altitude balloon flights was juryrigged together out of whatever radio equipment was handy. The vacuum tubes in such equipment generated considerable heat and the batteries added excessive weight to the capsule.

After World War II, the development of transistors, printed circuits, and the resulting miniaturization of all components made possible great savings in space required by electronic equipment. Now, as many as five thousand transistors and resistors can be integrated in a hundred printed circuits, all about the size of a postage stamp. Electronic miniaturization, it is estimated, has in the past twenty years reduced the weight and bulk of electronic equipment in the ratio of 20,000 to 1.

Telemetry involves the simultaneous transmission of many kinds of information; this can be done over a single transmission link by multiplexing—the use of many subcarrier frequencies, each modulated by a source of information. Transmissions are either in the analog system in which signal strength varies continuously, or the digital system involving binary numbers. Signals received by a ground station are taped, then processed through computers which produce a printout of the information received. This allows repeated review of all data collected, whenever desired, by playing the tapes back through suitable equipment, such as oscilloscopes, audio systems, or teleprinters. Of course, all real time data can also be presented for immediate analysis on appropriate equipment at the same time it is being tape recorded.

Many of the measurements, such as heart action, respiratory action, brain activity and skeletal muscle action, involve the development and release of electrical activity which is proportional to and characteristic of the phenomena of interest. Electrocardiograms and electroencephalograms are based on this principle. The acts of swallowing, hiccoughing, regurgitation and defecation are subject to electronic surveillance. Measures of mental alertness are obtained from myograms of the muscles on the forehead. The electrical currents originating in these physiological processes must be amplified by transducers before they can be transmitted. Even emotional activity can be monitored by detecting changes in the electrical resistance of the skin as they take place.

Transducers are required for all physiological measurements, as well as for the measurement of environmental factors and performance. These tranducers convert physical and chemical changes into electrical equivalents, proportional to the measure of interest, which activate the transmission system. Ultra-high frequency gives the advantage of wide band widths on which numerous and varied items of information can be carried. The low frequency of the various items of physiological information makes it possible to use narrow band widths on the subcarriers and place these frequencies close together to provide a large number of channels. Furthermore, much of the data changes at a very low rate and permits commutation—one band can carry several types of information, with each being transmitted for a fraction of a second, and all being recorded in sequence.

The suborbital flight of 15 minutes, made by Alan Shepard, on 5 May 1961, marked the first time that physiological and behavioral techniques were combined in evaluating the functional efficiency of a human subject in space (The Russian cosmonaut Yuri Gagarin had orbited the earth on 12 April of that year, but Russian releases of information on the flight were noted for their lack of detail.) For the first time, ground observers monitored body temperature, chest movement, heart action, and electrocardiogram of a man moving at high speed, out of sight, in a space environment.

In the early Mercury flight, body temperatures were measured by a rectal probe. The Mercury astronauts, understandably, found a few hours of this more than enough, and later an oral thermometer was used. Respiration rates, first measured by a thermistor on the helmet microphone, were later taken by an impedance pneumograph. Blood pressure recordings began with the third Mercury flight.

It was soon realized that biotelemetry gave the flight surgeon a much better link with the astronaut than the direct voice communication system considered necessary in the Man-High and Skyhook operations with balloons. Voice transmissions, of course, are maintained with astronauts on all missions, and they enable ground control to check on their conditions through normal flight reports and answers to queries. In fact, voice transmissions are so effective in indicating an astronaut's condition that in later missions, tapes of the voices of each man involved were sent to tracking stations around the world, so that everyone in direct communication with the astronauts would be acquainted with their normal voices and recognize any variations indicating change in their condition.

As it is now developed, biotelemetry, magnetic tape recordings, and computer techniques make it possible, long after a mission is completed, to "fly" it again by running the tapes. With voice recordings and television also on tapes, the actions and reactions of astronauts can be examined at great length and in detail not possible during the stress of an actual operation, making possible a more thorough understanding of their physical and psychological processes than ever before.

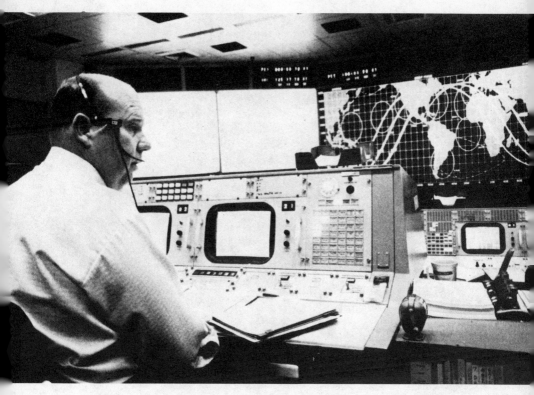

Mission Control Center during the launch of Skylab 2, with Flight Director Philip C. Shaffer at the console. A display of the Manned Space Flight Network appears on the far wall. Note that space-age pencil sharpeners are still hand powered./*NASA*

Through telemetry, the flight surgeon, who may never go into space, has become a medical flight controller, and a valuable member of the flight control team. Wherever an astronaut goes, through the magic of radio telemetry, a trained and devoted member of the medical profession goes with him.

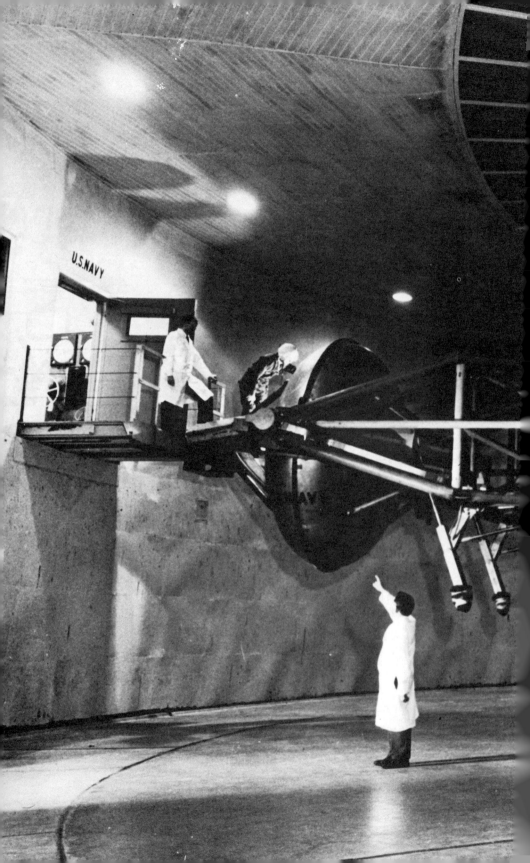

7

Fast Starts and Crashing Stops

Acceleration and deceleration are the invisible, but very noticeable, effects of a fast start, or rather sudden stop in any sort of vehicle. A jack-rabbit take-off from a green light pushes one back into the seat—the effect of acceleration. A panic stop in highway traffic results in deceleration that throws one into the dashboard or against the seat belt.

In an airplane on the takeoff run, acceleration pushes passengers back into their seats as the pilot runs the engines up to full power. And on landing, as reverse thrust of the engines brings the plane to a quick stop, deceleration throws the passengers against their seat belts. The same thing happens in an express elevator coming down in a tall building—acceleration as the car commences its drop lifts passengers off their toes, and deceleration as it slows for the ground floor makes their knees sag.

Scientists became concerned with the problem of acceleration and deceleration as an aspect of flight operations almost from the

For many astronauts, the voyage into space began in the human centrifuge at the Naval Air Development Center, Johnsville, Pennsylvania. The effects of acceleration and deceleration, and all the aspects of space flight, can be simulated here./*U.S. Navy*

191

beginning of aviation. Restraint gear was developed for those fast stops in the old biplanes and eventually, as high performance military aircraft were developed, pilots learned what their bodies' physiological behavior was during acceleration. Colonel Rufus Hessberg explained the early acceleration investigation this way: "An early concern was to avoid spinning in and crashing in an airplane when you are making, say, a turn on a final approach and you have to turn your head to change radio channels. It's the combination of moving your head in the force field of an acceleration environment. If you hold your head still, you and the system move at the same time—that is, if you're making a nice slow turn at the airport. But if you're making a fighter approach and then the tower says, 'okay, now change from an air traffic frequency to tower frequency,' and you turn your head (down) to switch to the other frequency, then you can get pretty disoriented. These are the practical aspects to it, and this is why it was important to aviation. This is why Dr. Graybiel and others studied this and began to explain it. Then we, the practitioners, explained it to the pilots so that they could avoid it...disregard their feelings and believe in their instruments..."

The studies involved the use of a centrifuge, a means of producing slow onset, and steady, continuous acceleration loads. "That's how we determine black-out thresholds by having the acceleration force drain the blood from the head. That's why you gray-out and you go a little further and you black-out..." And it all has to do with the basic laws of physics.

Here it is necessary to flash back to a remote past, long before the laws of physics were discovered, or even suspected, to a time when man led a simple primitive life. The terrestrial environment in which he evolved offered near laboratory conditions. He lived in the temperate zones, in clean unpolluted atmosphere, in normal gravity, and moved about over the surface no faster than his legs or a good horse could carry him. The unseen forces delineated by the laws of physics discovered over the centuries had little effect until steam engines, internal combustion engines, and then aircraft and rockets translated the laws into the bonecrushing reality of acceleration and deceleration. Certain high-speed flight operations also exposed pilots to the hazards of "centrifugal

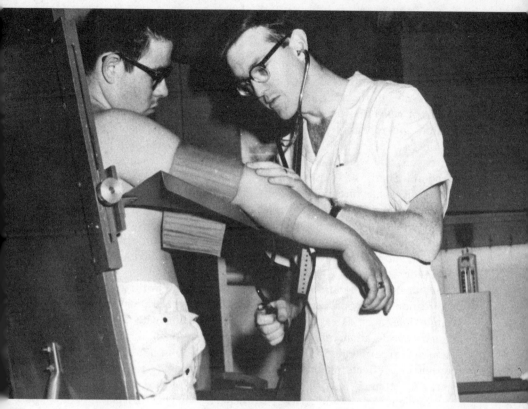

A long, simulated ride into space, in a study of the functions of the inner ear and its relation to motion sickness, was made in "slow rotation room" at Pensacola in 1965. This sailor, 19-year old Terrence L. Duverney, rode the SRR for 28 days, constantly spinning at ten revolutions per minute./*NASA*

force," a term that until World War II, pilots felt belonged exclusively to scientists in their labs. But in World War II bomber crews found they simply could not make emergency escapes from damaged aircraft spinning down out of control. They were pinned inside by suddenly developed centrifugal force.

Centrifugal force is a natural phenomenon. The earth itself, rotating on its axis, is a huge centrifuge. This rotation, which, with the Coriolis* effect it produces in the earth's atmosphere and oceans, is responsible for the ocean currents; the Japan Current, Gulf Stream, Humboldt Current and Brazil Current. These, in turn, create the temperate climates around much of the earth. The same force and effect set up typhoons and hurricanes. Coriolis effect is due to the varying rotational speeds of the earth, the surface of which moves eastward at a speed of 1,000 mph at the equator, and appears to be standing still at the poles. This effect must be considered in firing long-range ballistic missiles, and it is the reason why water going down a drain spins in a clockwise direction. South of the equator, of course, it goes in a counter-clockwise direction. Coriolis effect is beyond any normal frame of reference. It is imperceptible unless one were to "ride" the slow-rotating device at the Navy's laboratory in Pensacola. In this darkened circular roon, the eyes play tricks, the equilibrium is distorted, and it is impossible for a novice to toss a sponge ball into a receptor.

Technically, acceleration refers to a rate of change in the speed or direction of motion. *Linear* acceleration is acceleration in a straight line, such as experienced in a taxi starting with a jerk. *Angular* acceleration refers to rotation or change of direction. Scientists experimented on both, determined to pinpoint the physiological effects on the human body. According to Colonel George C. Mohr, U.S. Air Force, who is Director of Research and Development at Headquarters Aerospace Medical Division, Brooks Air Force Base, Texas, they worked on four categories; the magnitude as stated in g units (gravity), the duration as expressed in seconds of time, the rate of onset, which is the increase in g units per second, and the direction in which the acceleration acts on the subject.

An acceleration of lg is the normal gravitational acceleration of the earth, equal to 9.81 meters per second squared. The action of the earth's gravitational force is to give all objects weight. All evolution from amoeba to astronauts, developed under the influence of a standard gravitational lg acceleration. A body falling toward the earth, because of the pull of gravity, accelerates at the

*Named for the French mathematician Gaspard Gustave de Coriolis who studied it in 1835. Coriolis acceleration is twice the product of the angular velocity and the relative velocity of the affected particle, perpendicular to the axis of rotation.

rate of 32.2 feet per second squared (9.81 m/sec^2). If an object is accelerated at the rate of 64.4 feet per second squared, the force required is twice the earth's gravitational force, and the object's weight is twice its normal weight. An acceleration of 10g is associated with a weight ten times as great; 20g, 20 times, etc. A 200-pound man accelerated at 10g has an apparent weight of 2,000 pounds.

In measuring the acceleration, impact acceleration is considered to be less than 2/10 seconds; abrupt acceleration is from 2/10 seconds to 2 seconds; brief acceleration is set at from 2 to 10 seconds.

This kind of finite measurement is based on theories and research tools established a long time back. Centrifuges, now in use by many nations for physiological investigation, were first constructed for treatment of patients. The idea was suggested by the English physicist, Erasmus Darwin in 1794; the first operational centrifuge was used in the psychiatric clinic of the Charité Hospital in Berlin in 1818 for spinning mentally ill patients. By today's standards, it was quite small, with a radius of just over 12 feet, turning at 50 rpm, and producing a G-load (force) of 5G. By contrast, an "ultracentrifuge" developed by the Swedish scientist Theodor Svedberg, a Nobel prize winner in 1926, had an incredible top speed of 10,000 revolutions per second which resulted in a G-load (force) 900,000 times as intense as the force of gravity. It must be remembered that this was a small, table-top model, certainly not intended for use in testing a human being.

Very little work was done with centrifuges until pilots, subjected to the increasingly high speeds of aircraft in World War I and the decade following, began reporting symptoms such as temporary blindness during steeply banked turns. Gray-outs and black-outs worried researchers and in France, in 1917, the Ministry of War authorized experimentation with dogs. These canines were subjected to the heavy, and fatal force of 98G. The American Interplanetary Society in 1932 determined that a mere 30G for two minutes was fatal to guinea pigs. A year earlier in Berlin, Wernher von Braun found that a force of 200G had a fatal effect on mice.

The first centrifuge capable of handling human subjects was designed for the Luftwaffe by two Germans, Heinz von Diringshofen, a medical doctor and pioneer in airborne

195

acceleration research, and his brother Bernd, an engineer, who helped design the centrifuge and develop airborne flight instrumentation. Located in the Military Medical Academy, which also housed the Aeromedical Research Institute of the Luftwaffe in Berlin, it began operation about 1934. With a 10-foot radius, it could develop 20G. Monkeys, as well as volunteer scientists were subjected to high G forces, and X-rays of their visceral organs showed displacement that could be duplicated by forces encountered under actual flight conditions.

The Germans planned on replacing their old 1934 model centrifuge during World War II, with a highly sophisticated model designed by F. Ranke and Otto Gauer, but Allied bombing raids forced them to stop work on it. Hydraulically driven, it was capable of producing high G forces very quickly.

Serious experimental work on centrifuges began in the United States in 1936 when the U.S. Army Air Corps commenced operating a human centrifuge at Wright Field in Ohio. As was common in much of the aeromedical research in the pre-World War II period, funds for such work were limited. Captain Harry Armstrong, who in 1936 founded the Air Corps Laboratory, U.S. Army Physiologic Research Unit (later to become the USAF 6570th Aerospace Medical Research Laboratory) got $100 a year for supplies and had no model to work from in building a centrifuge. He salvaged the electric drive motor from a power plant, and got all the aluminum tubing he needed from wrecked aircraft. At that time, Armstrong would have had difficulty getting official sanction for any project because he had publicly stated that he expected aircraft would eventually fly as fast or faster than a 45-caliber bullet. Design engineers considered the idea as pure fantasy and suggested that a mere medical officer had no business making such predictions.

Right behind the Americans and their research on the effects of high speed flight came the Canadians. In 1938, after the German-Italian-British-French discussions at the Munich Conference produced headlines of "Peace in our Time," the general jubilance was tempered with doubt in some quarters. At the University of Toronto, in Canada, Sir Frederick Banting called his staff of research scientists together to commence work in the field of war aviation medicine.

With the outbreak of World War II, Dr. W. R. Franks, a Canadian medical researcher, began investigating the problems of acceleration in flight. A design for a human centrifuge was worked out, and the completed installation was operational in the summer of 1941. The centrifuge was extremely advanced for its day because it satisfactorily duplicated conditions of flight—the chair in the rotating cab could be inverted for negative G studies, and an automatic cam mechanism made it possible to stage standard reproducible runs. Electrically driven, it could accelerate the cab from dead stop to 20g and slow it to dead stop in five seconds. During the war years alone the centrifuge made over 17,000 practice runs without a mishap.

Although developed by the University of Toronto, the centrifuge was under operational control of the Royal Canadian Air Force. An important result of RCAF research was the development of the first operationally practical anti-g suit which was worn by pilots during combat. And the problems of gray-out and black-out, earlier explored by von Diringshofen were clarified.

Colonel Hessberg explained it this way: "What you're really saying is that you have a column of blood that goes from the heart to the brain and it's so many centimeters high and at atmospheric pressure in our 1G environment you measure a person's blood pressure and that's what it takes to drive it from the heart up to the brain."

"If you double that force which would be like 2Gs, because fortunately the cardiovascular system has the capability to respond to a 2G stimulus, the heart rate will increase and the blood pressure will increase to compensate. The capacity of the heart chamber when it fills with the venous return of 50cc and a heartbeat of 80, moves 80 times a minute, or 4,000cc of blood per minute. When you add resistance by acceleration from head to foot, you decrease the flow, and the venous return goes from 40cc to 35, but if the heart rate goes from 80 to 120 beats per minute, you are going to move approximately the same amount of blood around. You've compensated for the increased pressure or acceleration force. It gets more difficult to move that column of blood up from the heart or compensate when you get to 3½ to 4G. Then you do get gray-out, which is fuzzy vision, because you're reducing the circulation. Then, if you go a little further, 4½ to 5G, then the blood can't get there even enough to maintain the gray-out, and you get black-out..."

NOMENCLATURES OF ACCELERATIONS REFERRING TO THE DIRECTION IN WHICH THEY ACT

Direction of Acceleration	Direction of Inertial Force (Reaction)	Three Axis Nomenclature	Other Nomenclatures	
Back-chest	Chest-back	+Gx	Supine position	Transverse
Chest-back	Back-chest	—Gx	Prone position	g loads
Left-right	Right-left	+Gy	Leftwards	Lateral
Right-left	Left-right	—Gy	Rightwards	g loads
Seat-head	Head-seat	+Gz	Positive	Spinal
Head-seat	Seat-head	—Gz	Negative	g loads

Soon after the RCAF centrifuge in Toronto went into operation, the Mayo Foundation in Rochester, Minnesota, established an Aero Medical Unit and set up an Acceleration Laboratory in which a centrifuge with a 15-foot radius was built. By 1942, research was underway on linear acceleration, deceleration, and rotary (angular) acceleration. Experiments were backed up by actual flights in a Douglas Dauntless aircraft furnished by the Navy. From October 1942 to October 1945, 400 volunteers—three physiologists and a technician—made nearly 3,000 runs on the centrifuge, sometimes with anti-black-out suit protection and sometimes without. As reported in the *Journal of Aviation Medicine*, October 1947*, runs of 15 seconds or more in duration were made 92 per cent of the time. One subject experienced 1198 runs at more than 2.5g with totals of 226.3 minutes at 4g and above, and 43.6 minutes at 6g and above.

*An article titled "Do permanent effects result from repeated blackouts caused by positive acceleration?" The volunteers were Dr. C. F. Code, Dr. E. H. Lambert, Dr. E. H. Wood, and Mr. Roy Engstrom.

The experiments demonstrated that if blood circulating to the brain was interrupted for from five to seven seconds, unconsciousness would result but that most people would make a complete recovery in from five to 60 seconds after circulation was restored. Experiments with dogs showed that complete interruption of blood circulation in the brain for more than six minutes would produce neurologic damage. The experimenters concluded that a human subjected to complete anoxia of the brain would not last quite as long as a dog.

The U.S. Navy, too, commenced research in the forces that would be encountered by space-age pilots, with installations at Pensacola, Florida, and Johnsville, Pennsylvania, among others.

The Pensacola centrifuge, the first one completed for the Navy, began operation in 1945. With a 20-foot radius and angular velocity of up to 60 rpm, it could produce 9g. The central feature of the centrifuge (outdated by the Johnsville installation in 1950) was a 56-ton flywheel, friction-driven by a rubber tire coupled to a natural gas-powered engine; maximum onset rate to reach 9g was 1.48 g/sec.

The Johnsville centrifuge, with the awesome title of Dynamic Flight Simulator (Human Centrifuge Computer Complex)* of the Aerospace Medical Research Department, U.S. Naval Air Development Center, is the giant among U.S. installations. (The Royal Air Force centrifuge at Farnborough, built in 1965 surpasses it in one aspect—it has a radius of 62.5 feet, whereas the Johnsville centrifuge has a radius of 50 feet.)

Development of the Johnsville centrifuge began in 1945, with Commander Ralph L. Christy (MC) U.S. Navy, acting as liaison officer between the various naval activities and commercial contractors. There was at first considerable rivalry between the Air Corps and the Navy over the project, but the Bureau of Medicine and Surgery, the Office of Chief of Naval Operations, and the Bureau of Aeronautics finally convinced the Medical Sciences Committee of the Department of Defense Research and Development Board that the Navy had solid, well-conceived requirements for the centrifuge.

*Reorganization over the years has changed that title to the even weightier Life Sciences Division, Aircraft and Crew Systems Technology Directorate, U.S. Naval Air Development Center, and mail no longer goes to Johnsville, but Warminster, although the centrifuge is right where it always was.

It is difficult to describe the Johnsville centrifuge, and its capabilities, without resorting to superlatives. The main building, 124 feet in diameter, houses a 180-ton, 4,000-horsepower motor that drives a 50-foot long, 45-ton steel arm at speeds up to 48.5 rpm; it can be driven from a dead stop to 180mph, the equivalent of 40g, in less than seven seconds. A spherical steel gondola at the end of the centrifuge arm is mounted on power gimbals so it can be oriented in the resultant of normal gravity, centrifugal G and tangential G-force, or tumbled in order to simulate an aircraft out of control for work on high-speed escape problems. The gondola can also be used as a low-pressure chamber to simulate pressure altitudes of up to 100,000 feet, or the extremely high heat generated by a spacecraft on entering the earth's atmosphere from space.

The centrifuge can be controlled manually by an operator "on the ground," through a system of cams, or by a pilot operating controls from within the gondola, or by a computer. A pilot riding the centrifuge "flies," in one of two modes. In closed-loop simulation, the pilot handles the centrifuge by means of cockpit controls and so receives the appropriate linear acceleration components. In open-loop simulations, a computer programs the operation of the centrifuge, and the pilot "flies," as a passenger.

The modification that allowed computer control, and closed-loop simulation, was accomplished by Dr. John L. Brown, Dr. Randall M. Chambers, James D. Hardy of the Laboratory, and Captain Walton L. Jones (MC) U.S. Navy, of the Bureau of Aeronautics. The computer installed at that time was one of the largest in the United States.

The subject riding the gondola can be monitored by closed circuit TV, and telemetry furnishes constant readouts on pulse rate, blood pressure, ear opacity, respiration, electrocardiograms, electroencephalograms, and other physiological parameters.

The sophisticated design of this centrifuge makes it especially valuable for simulating and testing flight performance, pilot tolerance to G forces, pilot restraint, cockpit instrumentation, control system design, and emergency procedures such as escape from a damaged high-performance aircraft. At Johnsville, as research in problems of space flight assumed high priority, the centrifuge was also used to imitate the acceleration a man might experience riding a rocket-driven spacecraft, or the sudden deceleration such a craft would meet on reentry into the earth's atmosphere.

The Johnsville centrifuge played an important part in acceleration training for U.S. astronauts, in Projects Mercury, Dynasoar, Gemini, and Apollo. The first attempt to simulate the reentry performance of a specific aircraft began in January and February of 1959, with a group of 23 pilots from NASA, the Navy, Air Force, and the Marine Corps, and the use of some flight simulation procedures developed earlier in preparing pilots for the X-15 flights. Two closed-loop systems were used; one connected the pilot's control responses with the driving system of the centrifuge, and the other connected his control responses with the driving mechanisms of the indicators on his instrument panel. A total of 231 runs were made, during which pilot performance and physiological responses were recorded.

In the summer of 1959, the Mercury astronauts received acceleration training, including familiarization runs using predicted Atlas launch and reentry, and abort profiles ranging up to 18g. In addition, engineers and scientists made a large number of runs in order to experience the anticipated conditions of acceleration.

A second acceleration training program for Mercury astronauts, commencing in the spring of 1960, represented a major step forward in providing total simulation; it included full-pressure suits, realistic breathing conditions, depressurization of the gondola, and a more realistic pilot restraint system and contour couch, display panel, control devices, communications network and physiological instrumentation. A computer-controlled program put the centrifuge through a two-stage Atlas launch at 8g, booster burnout, retro-fire, and re-entry, including opening of drogue and main parachutes.

Just before the first manned Mercury flight, three of the seven Mercury astronauts were put through a simulated suborbital flight designed to collect additional physiological data on the effects of acceleration on blood pressure, EKG, respiration and pulse rates, to refresh their memories about anticipated accelerations, and to determine how these accelerations might affect their ability to perform control tasks. Later, each astronaut made a complete, real-time simulation run of 4½ hours, the equivalent of a three-orbit mission, in a complete cockpit instrumentation of the Mercury display panel.

In all, between January of 1959 and May of 1963, seven centrifuge programs were run for Mercury astronaut training. "Complete mission training" included all the events of a regular space shot—early morning suiting-up, psychiatric testing, waiting in the gondola for the countdown, launch, orbit, reentry, recovery, escape training, post-flight testing, and debriefing, on a real-time basis.

A centrifuge simulation and astronaut training program for Project Gemini was conducted in June and July of 1963, during which a number of "flights" were made. Launch profiles were prepared on a magnetic tape which the computer used to drive the centrifuge in open-loop system. The astronauts selected for the Gemini mission were put through normal launch and reentry problems, fuel failure aborts, premature ignition, engine failure, and guidance systems failure.

Finally, there was full-scale centrifuge simulation of the Apollo space vehicles in October and November of 1963, with an Apollo cockpit installation provided by the North American Aviation Company. Tests provided information on pressure suits, the g-couch, the Apollo instrument panel, the pilot's control stick, and miscellaneous cockpit instrumentation. Six Apollo pilots and other selected pilots made 284 runs. As in all centrifuge runs at Johnsville, biomedical telemetry monitored all physiological responses; closed circuit TV was also used.

Beginning in 1970, under the direction of Dr. Harald J. von Beckh, a research program aimed at protecting pilots and flight crews was developed which took advantage of the fact that pressure within the gondola could be controlled during a run. Volunteers were exposed simultaneously to increased G loads *and* pressure changes, as might be expected during accidental decompression and subsequent emergency descent of high altitude multi-mach transport aircraft. That was the first time that the gondola of a turning centrifuge was used as a controlled decompression-recompression chamber.

Some astronauts, and many people on the ground, considered that in their efforts to anticipate and train for every possibility encountered during space flight, they over-trained. One such step encountered by all astronauts on their way into space was a training session in the most horrifying of all simulation devices, the Multiple Axis Space Test Inertia Facility called MASTIF for short. A ride in MASTIF subjected a man to the forces he would encounter if a capsule began to tumble in space—it spun him at 30rpm in three planes at once, and forced him to use stick and rudder to counter all forces and bring his couch to a position of zero motion.

The training paid off though. During the Gemini 8 mission in March, 1966, after Neil Armstrong completed the first docking maneuver in space, the capsule and the Agena rocket began tumbling. Gemini backed away, but even so, tumbled faster—one complete revolution every second—until Armstrong triggered auxiliary rockets to break the spin. The mission then had to be aborted.

To date, most astronauts have been subjected to strong accelerative forces for only a limited time. The effects of prolonged acceleration on speed are like compounded interest—the end result is amazing. A long ride on the Johnsville centrifuge was made by Carl C. Clark, who spent *24 hours* under a force of +2G, in general performing routine duties such as an astronaut might carry out during a planetary mission. In that time, had he been in a spacecraft under that acceleration of 2g, he would have traveled 45,000,000 miles and reached a top speed of 3,800,000 miles an hour.

The next best thing to riding a spacecraft is to make a simulated flight on the centrifuge at the Manned Spacecraft Center in Houston. All Apollo astronauts trained there. The centrifuge is (or rather *was*, since it is no longer operable) capable of simulating all the effects of an actual launch-lift off, first stage separation, second-stage ignition and separation, and third-stage ignition. The peaks of acceleration during a rocket launching, as recorded by NASA during the first orbital flight of the Mercury series (John

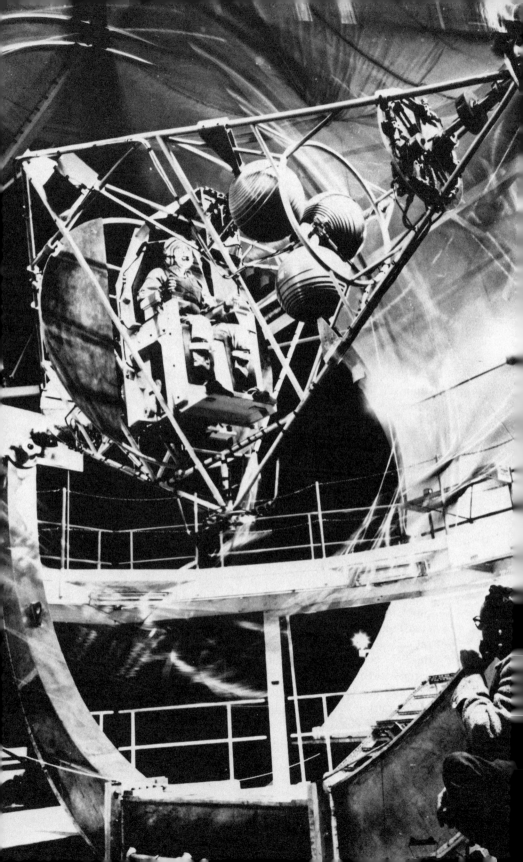

Glenn, 20 February 1962), were just prior to burnout of the second stage engine—6.4g for 54 seconds.

In any summary of who had what, and where in the way of centrifuges, it should be pointed out that in 1969, the U.S. Air Force began operating the Dynamic Environmental Simulator at the 6570th Aerospace Medical Research Laboratory at Wright-Patterson Air Force Base. This centrifuge has a 19-foot main arm,

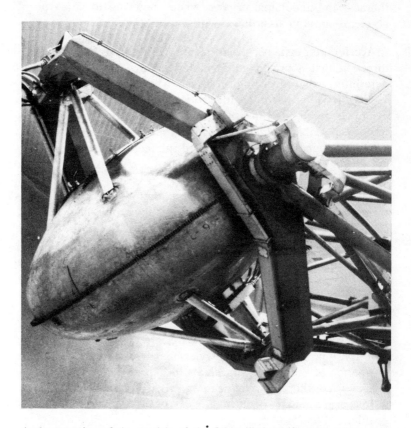

A close-up view of the gondola of the Johnsville centrifuge resembles some futuristic spacecraft. It can subject a man to 40g in less than seven seconds./*U.S. Navy*

The Multiple Axis Space Test Inertia Facility (MASTIF) can, in effect, turn a man every way but loose. It spins him in three planes at once until he uses conventional controls to stop all motion../*NASA* and in closed loop operation is capable of simulating vehicle dynamics, target dynamics, and cockpit display read-outs.

In order to understand the effects of acceleration on the human body, the types of acceleration mentioned earlier must be better defined. It is also necessary to understand that because the human body is essentially a fluid system, the reaction of the vascular system and to a certain extent the entire body, including the thoracic and abdominal organs, when subjected to any type of acceleration, is in accordance with Pascal's law.*

Acceleration instantly produces an effect on the body, and the direction that a prolonged accelerative force acts on the body determines what physiological effects will occur.

+Gz (Positive G or Headward Acceleration) means that the aviator is accelerated in a headward direction by the centripetal force. The *centrifugal force*, the force that the aviator is aware of, acts in the opposite direction toward the feet. Common examples are during a pullout from a dive or when a pilot executes a high speed bank and turn.

-Gz (Negative G or Footward Acceleration) occurs when the accelerative force acts on the body in a footward direction. In this case, the centrifugal (inertial) force is toward the head. Typical examples are during a nose-over and an outside loop.

+Gx (Backward G, Forward Transverse Acceleration) occurs when the accelerative force acts across the body at right angles to the long axis in a back-to-chest direction. The centrifugal force would also be across the body, but in the opposite direction or in a chest-to-back direction. An astronaut lying semi-supine in a special couch is exposed to +Gx during exit and also during re-entry. It occurs during re-entry causing a shift in the couch due to rotation of the entire spacecraft to expose the heat shield to denser atmosphere. A pilot seated upright in aircraft such as the X-15 is exposed to +Gx during the exit or firing phase of the flight profile.

---

*Named for Blaise Pascal (1623-62), a French mathematician and philosopher who discovered the effect of pressure on fluids and stated it thus: an external pressure applied to a fluid exerts an equal pressure in all directions.

-Gx (Forward G, Backward Transverse Acceleration) occurs when the accelerative force acts across the body at right angles to the long axis in a chest-to-back direction. The centrifugal force would also be across the body in a perpendicular direction but in a back-to-chest direction. Piloting aircraft such as the X-15 or space shuttle in the re-entry phase of the flight would expose the astronaut to -Gx. He is forced forward against his straps and has a tendency to be pitched out of his seat unless tightly restrained.

±Gy (Right or Left Lateral Transverse G, Left or Right Lateral Acceleration, respectively) Accelerations of this type are encountered only briefly in normal flight and never in space flight unless an emergency situation arose in which the space craft was exiting or re-entering in a non-stable manner.

Tolerances to a positive vertical G force can be greatly diminished by various factors. Associated hypoxia will reduce the tolerance level, and during what might be considered a normal G force, circulatory collapse might also result. Recent illnesses may cause decreased g tolerance for as long as three weeks after all symptoms have subsided. Tolerance to G forces can also be decreased by sunburn, or exposure to warm, humid environments. On the other hand, g tolerance can be increased by exposure to cold. In general, the greater the magnitude of acceleration, the more severe the effects. The effects of acceleration are also related to duration—5g (positive G-force) for 2-3 seconds is harmless, but 5g (positive G-force) for 5-6 seconds causes blackout and possibly unconsciousness.

When research into acceleration first began, investigators sometimes failed to discriminate between acceleration and inertia, and referred to head-to-seat acceleration, when what they really meant was the head-to-seat *inertial load* produced by seat-to-head acceleration. Eventually a standard system of nomenclature was established which enables researchers to exchange information more accurately.

There is another system, termed "Investigator's jargon," which follows Pascal's law in expressing acceleration effects. In that system, the inertial reaction force is described by the effect it has on the eyeballs. Back-to-chest acceleration produces an eyeballs-in reaction, or EBI. Seat to head acceleration produces an

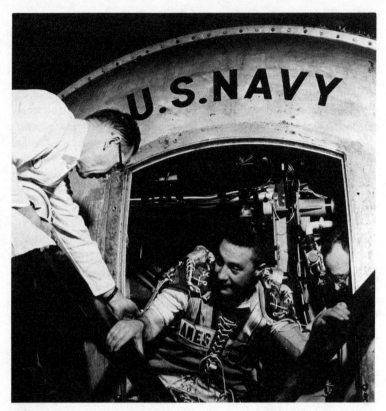

Before he made a sub-orbital flight in 1961, astronaut Virgil I. Grissom went through all the stages of simulated space flight in the Johnsville centrifuge./*NASA*

eyeballs-down reaction, or EBD. It sounds colorful but it is still somewhat confusing.

Prolonged acceleration, which is usually radial, seldom builds up to more than 10-15g, and lasts for only a few seconds. The skeleton and semi-solid body tissues can withstand such Gz forces. but the cardiovascular system will be affected, as will the cerebral spinal fluid.

Under headward acceleration, the physiologically important inertial reaction force acts in a footward direction, with tremendous stress on body organs and an apparent increase in their weight. The cardiovascular system fails to supply the head and brain with an adequate blood flow, and there will be some heaviness of limbs and head at +2Gz, extreme heaviness at +3Gz, dimming or "graying" of vision at +3-4Gz, loss of peripheral vision at +3.5Gz and +4.5Gz and complete loss of vision at +5.5Gz. Facial tissues sag, producing an aged look, but after cessation of acceleration, consciousness returns in about six seconds.

The concern over blood pooling in the lower extremities of a man in space had some basis in fact, but only after the Apollo flights were completed was there solid confirmation that the remarkable human body could handle the stresses after all. So far, over 100 Americans and Russians have been in space—some of them for as much as 140 days, and while some were a little heavy on their feet at first, they soon returned to normal.

What all this boils down to is the fact that researchers frantically sought parameters on which they could base man's ability to withstand the G forces that were predicted in order to launch him and get him to orbital altitude and speed. Said Hessberg: "Actually, we found out that the only way you could do it was taking it across the body—from chest to back—rather than from head to foot. We did find that out during the early work at Wright-Pat. And the same thing with landing in the Pacific under the parachutes. You could take those landing loads safely..."

Specifically, pilots in a supine position with their bed or couch inclined to an angle of approximately 20 to 25 degrees with the vertical can increase their threshold for g tolerance up to a level of 9 or 10g. As a spacecraft attains 26,400 feet per second in reaching orbital velocity, staging through three peak G-loads with the second at about 8G, men were well able to tolerate the forces. In fact, an individual leaning forward approximately 25 degrees can take 4.5G for as long as 15 minutes. A much heavier G-load was tolerated by volunteers in 1975 centrifuge experiments at the Naval Air Development Center, when they were placed in a supine position—seat back angle of 75 degrees from the vertical. They withstood 14G for 45 seconds without visual impairment or other undesirable symptoms.

But what of deceleration forces, the crashing stops? What would happen to space travelers who had withstood all the other hazards "up there" only to be crushed during the triumphal reentry into earth's atmosphere?

Work on "impact" probably received more press attention than any of the other fields of pre-spaceflight investigation because of the drama, and certainly the fright, that surrounded the sled rides. Impact! That means stopping at one-tenth of a second from a very high speed without slowing down at all. It's like hitting a brick wall or experiencing a head-on collision on a freeway.

Hessberg explained it this way: "I've done many different things in my life, like jumping out of airplanes 97 times and I rode the centrifuge until heck wouldn't have it, but I will tell you, sitting in that damn seat, knowing that gun's going to go off, is the scariest thing you can imagine."

A number of doctors, scientists and test subjects, including animals rode the sleds down the track to learn what could be endured when there was a sudden impact—stop! One of these, Hessberg, recalled: "We had the old Daisy sled, 120 feet of track, and we operated it with ejection seat catapults. We'd fire those and drive the sled down the track. We had a large plunger on the front of the sled that went into the water brake. It was a hydraulic stopping system which had a lot of plugs in it which we could unscrew. The way we patterned the deceleration was by figuring out how many holes we would make in it so that the water could get out. But what would happen, occasionally...we'd have a delay in our ride and you'd sit there in the desert sun and those catapults would get super-hot, and, boy, they would fire hot. And you'd get a super-hot firing...!"

Air Force Captain Eli Beeding took one of those super-hot firings in 1961. It was the most severe shock observed in human testing. While seated facing to the rear, he suffered an impact of 82.6g at 382g/sec. He showed no blood pressure for 30 seconds, complained of lower back pain, and lost consciousness. He was hospitalized for three days, and fortunately made a complete recovery.

The most famous "sled-rider" is Colonel John Paul Stapp, Air Force physician, who at the time of his experiments was called, "the fastest man on earth," and also, "the bravest man in the world." Both terms were right—Stapp's rides were on a sled using rocket propulsion. A Stapp sled ride went like this...

Inside a small sunbaked cement building at Holloman Air Force Base in New Mexico's Tularosa Valley, an engineer stood beside a remote-control panel. In the corner, a loudspeaker droned the final

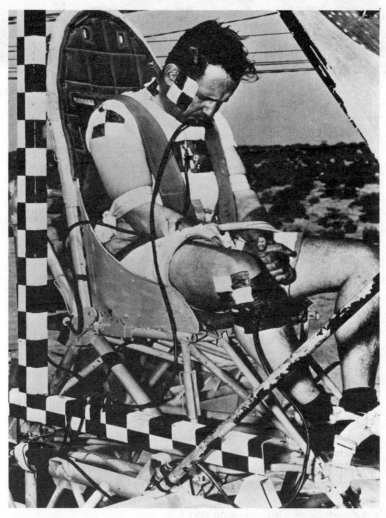

A ride in the rocket-powered Sonic Wind was considered to be not habit forming. Colonel John Paul Stapp, an Air Force physician, rode the sled 29 times. At 46G, his body withstood a force of five tons for a quarter of a second./*NASA*

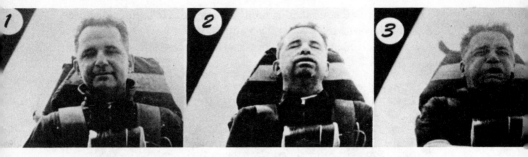

Incredible physical stress is shown in these photographs, as Colonel Stapp went from a standing start to 632mph in 5 seconds, and then made a smashing stop. He endured a peak of 40g, and had two black eyes./*NASA*

seconds of the countdown, as Air Force and Northrop technicians watched tensely through the periscope window.

Ten... nine... eight...

Outside, a squat steel sled, painted in red and white stripes so that it resembled a robot spider, sat quite still on its 3,500-foot long tracks that ran all the way to nowhere. Strapped to the sled was Colonel Stapp who had made the ride 26 times before. Twice he had broken an arm, fractured a rib, and had suffered a hemorrhage of the eye retina, various degrees of concussions, headaches and stiff muscles. Sled-riding was not apt to be habit forming *except* when one had questions that required answers. And when the questions concerned high altitude, high-speed bailouts, crashes and the return of space vehicles to earth's atmosphere, Sonic Wind No. 2 was the ideal vehicle to provide the answers. Close behind Sonic Wind No. 2 was another similar vehicle powered by nine great rockets which, on ignition, would release 40,000 pounds' thrust and send the Air Force doctor down the tracks at 200mph faster than last year's 421mph. Beneath each sled was a scoop which would hit the pool of water at the end of the track and stop the vehicle with bone-jarring finality. The jolt would be equivalent to driving an auto at 120mph into a brick wall and the subject would experience the same gravity pressures and wind blast of a man who ejected from a jet moving at a speed of 1,000mph at an altitude of 40,000 feet.

Near the red and white sled a blue Air Force ambulance stood ready, just in case. Overhead, a T-33, piloted by Captain Joe

212

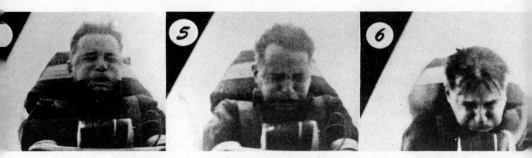

Kittinger, lined itself up for the race. Stapp, in the sled, concentrated on the cord in his hand which would trigger a movie camera aimed at his face. He breathed with his diaphragm, a procedure necessary because chest straps held him so tightly to his seat. Across his lap was a large safety belt; shoulder straps were snapped to this and then to the seat to keep his limbs from flailing. His elbows were locked to his sides by a strap running across his back. Above and below his knees, powerful straps held his legs in place; his wrists were lashed to the strap above his knees. His teeth were clamped on a rubber bite block; equipped with an accelerometer, this bite block would reveal valuable data on the test.

Hours before the test, Stapp had been given a thorough physical examination which included X-rays and an electrocardiogram. He had slipped into his blue wool flight suit, put on his thin leather flying gloves, and lowered the fiberglass helmet over his head. Stapp was ready; but he told his friends, "I assure you I'm not looking forward to this." Even so, he was determined that these tests on which they had all worked so hard would provide aviation and space scientists with an accurate graph showing human tolerance limitations.

Said Dr. Charles Lombard, who knows Stapp well, "His determination was almost a hate in his life. He hated the fact that not enough was known about acceleration to save the lives of jet pilots in bailouts, so he went to great extremes to learn more, then to educate the world..." This hate accounted for the fact that nobody ever "told" Stapp to go through this kind of punishment for the cause, or for that matter ever "asked" him to. In fact, much of his earlier work at Edwards Air Force Base was accomplished furtively with "moonlight requisitioning" for needed help, parts and materials in exchange for medical care at his "curbstone clinic." Eventually he would be "ordered" to stop participating as a subject in the experiments because he had become too valuable an authority to run such risks.

But before that happened, he and his assistants had a lot of work to do. Of his new helmet for this particular sled ride he said, "Now I have a helmet that will stay on my head, whether or not my head stays on my body." And on that morning of December 1954, he had called everybody to admire the beautiful sunrise because even he wondered if he would ever see another. At such proposed speed, his eyes could well be torn from their sockets.

Seven... six... five...

The countdown continued, while Stapp thought over details. As a doctor, he must report every symptom he, the subject, experienced. The words formed in his brain as he stared down the track. "Subject experienced considerable apprehension and uneasiness, with cold sweat of axillae (armpits) and palms..."

The engineer closed the ten-second time relay switch. The circuit to the igniters was activated.

Four... three... two... one... FIRE!

Nine rockets exploded with the force of a freight train ramming Stapp's sled from the rear, shooting it forward with a speed that paralyzed observers. Behind him, an enormous mountain of smoke leaped into the air as orange-red flames seared the sky. Overhead, Captain Joe Kittinger in his T-33 had dropped down to pace the test. Shoving the throttle all the way forward to more than 500mph, he nosed ahead of the rocket sled below. As he looked down, he found it impossible to believe that a human being rode—voluntarily—aboard that monster.

"...I will never forget, as long as I live, the incredulous awe I felt at that moment as Colonel Stapp accelerated like a bullet away from my own speeding airplane," wrote Kittinger in his book, *The Long Lonely Leap*.

Incredible but true, Colonel Stapp reached a speed of 632mph within five seconds from a standing start. Then suddenly spray shot up in a fountain as the sled's metal scoops slammed into the water at a speed of 927 feet per *second*. The rate of onset of deceleration for the doctor was 600g per second, reaching a plateau of 25g for longer than a second, with peaks of 35 to 40g's.

The ride was over. The fire crew moved in, swiftly but carefully, to spray the burning-hot rocket chambers with a layer of foam. Eager though concerned workers gathered around Stapp and began unfastening his harness. "I can't see," Stapp said, trying to force his eyelids open with his fingers. Someone tried to give him oxygen but he refused it. Part of the test involved recovery without such aids. A stretcher was brought alongside and he was gently lifted onto it.

For a full two minutes Stapp was blind, his only vision being that of shimmering salmon. Later, he described the effects of tremendous deceleration as he hit the water brakes. "It went from black to yellow. I saw the water splash when I hit the brakes. Then came the red-out. After that I didn't see a cockeyed thing." As for the pain in his eyes, "It felt as though my eyeballs were being pulled out of my head...somewhat like the extraction of a molar without an anesthetic."

When the shimmering salmon turned to blue and he could actually see the world around him, Stapp remarked quietly, "That was one of the pleasantest moments I've ever gone through."

His injuries? Numerous bruises, where the harness and straps had dug into his body, and a pair of the most beautiful shiners anybody ever had. After five days in the hospital Stapp was anxious to go again. Now he was more convinced than ever that scientists had been underrating man's physiological limits. Given proper restraints and protective clothing, man could take an awful walloping in an emergency and still come out all right.

During his 29 rides between the years 1947 and 1954, he took as high as 46g and had proved the fact that the body could withstand a force of 10,000 pounds for a quarter of a second. It was something no astronaut would ever have to do.

From the time Alan B. Shepard made his sub-orbital flight on 5 May 1961, 43 Americans have flown in space for a total of 95 million miles. The men who rode the centrifuges and rocket sleds may never have been rewarded with the thrill of actual spaceflight, but they saw 12 others land on the moon and return to earth safely, proving that their long and sometimes painful hours were well spent.

215

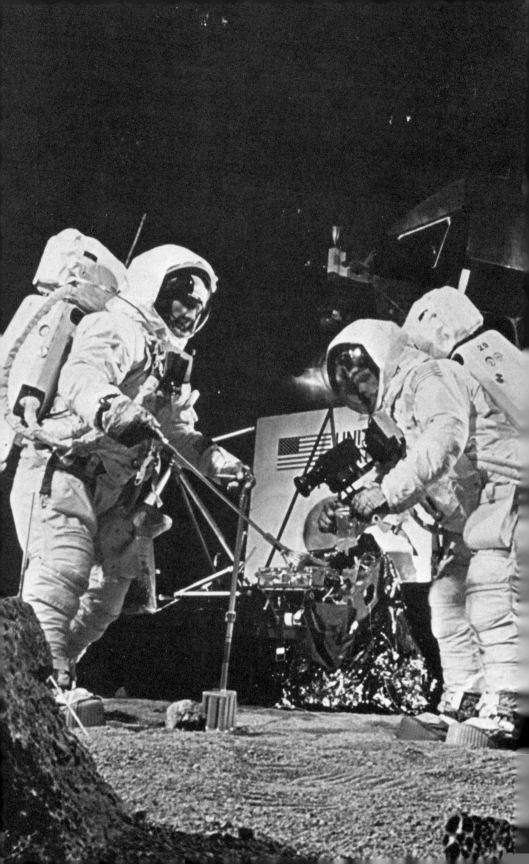

8
Pressure Suits and Shirt Sleeves

Just less than a century after men first ventured into the sky in a primitive balloon, they had so improved the state of the art that balloons were capable of reaching miles above the earth into the "critical zone," where normal breathing was impossible. In 1875, three balloonists topped that deadly level, to an extreme 28,000 feet, but only one of them came back alive. Balloons had not yet reached their maximum ceiling, but man had exceeded his physical limits—beyond and above the temperature range and oxygen content of a normal environment, there was an impassable barrier to further exploration in the sky.

Yet less than another century had passed when the world looked up to see men walking on the moon. There they were, 245,000 miles from their home planet, facing temperatures ranging from 250°F. down to -280°F. in a complete vacuum. Their bulky life-support backpacks provided them with pressure, oxygen, and air conditioning—a micro-environment similar to that of the earth they had left far behind them.

Before men walked on the moon, they practiced for it. In a simulated moon landing (note beams and lights overhead at upper right), Apollo 11 module pilot Edwin E. Aldrin worked at picking up "moon rocks" while the spacecraft commander, Neil Armstrong, held the camera./*NASA*

217

It was clear even before powered flight became possible that the higher man went, the more protection his body needed. As early as 1838, an armored suit for warding off hyperbaric pressures in undersea operations was designed by Taylor. Jules Verne, in 1872, wrote about pressure suits that would protect space travelers from the reduced barometric pressure of higher altitudes. In 1875, Soviet chemist Dmitri I. Mendeleev designed a gas-type gondola for use in stratospheric balloon flights. These were strange and curious ideas for their day, but all three of them were expanded upon by later developers.

Meanwhile, early balloonists fought the cold and hypoxia. In World War I, aviators suffered and sometimes died for lack of refined oxygen supply systems, impact restraints or suitable protective clothing. Parachutes were regarded as fit only for crowd-thrilling stunts; the bulky contraptions got in the way in cramped cockpits and were untrustworthy at best. Besides, pilots flew with a romantic creed of gallantry; a pilot whose plane was hit in combat expected to go down in flames. Only after a German aviator made a successful bail-out late in World War I did Allied pilots begin carrying parachutes.

Civilian aviators in the early 1900s had no flight suits—they wore ordinary street clothes with caps turned backwards in the fashion of the Wright brothers. Army daredevils turned up in cavalry uniforms, riding boots and white silk scarves. Some adopted high-crowned reinforced leather headgear which was supposed to protect the skull from injury if the wearer were thrown out on his head. But as one authority remarked, "Its chief virtue was to keep the brains from splattering." Some pilots wore goggles to protect their eyes from wind and insects, a fairly adequate precaution for low level flying.

In 1918, the so-called "Big War" ended and flying men who managed to stay in uniform wound up with a few surplus warplanes, mostly old Jennies and DH-4s. There was little money for gas and operating costs but a large need for justifying their passion for flying. It was in this atmosphere that the Army seized every opportunity to get into the limelight; Army pilots engaged in aerobatics, races, endurance hops, parachute drops, inflight refueling, altitude attempts, forest fire patrols and border guarding. Pilots used their own judgement as to what pieces of available gear they might wear. Pilots, motorcycle riders and drivers of Stutz Bearcats sometimes all looked very much alike.

By May of 1923, Army Lieutenant John A. Macready, with his companion pilot, Lieutenant Oakley G. Kelly had set a world flying-endurance record and made the first nonstop flight across the United States in the Air Service's new single-engine Fokker T-2. With Captain Albert W. Stevens operating the camera, they set a world altitude record in aerial photography. But it was Macready flying alone into the stratosphere that proved how seriously hostile the elements were; the machines were ready but man wasn't.

Macready flew to 30,000 feet no less than 50 times in his LePere biplane which was equipped with oxygen flasks and supercharger. Flying in an open cockpit, he faced temperatures as cold as -83°F. and struggled with lack of oxygen and insufficient air pressure while coaxing the Liberty engine to perform at unprecedented heights. Macready truly earned his "icicle crown." To withstand the intense cold, he wore two or three suits of wollen underwear and over that, a heavy knitted garment of wool, with a thick, heavily padded leather-covered suit of down and feathers over it all; fur-lined gloves; fleece-lined moccasins over his boots; and a leather head mask lined with fur which, with the oxygen mask, covered his face completely.

To prevent formation of ice inside his goggles, he coated them with anti-freeze gelatin. Some warmth was brought into the cockpit from the engine by an asbestos-covered tube. This was fine until he started a downward glide with his body exposed to the frigid blast of a 200mph wind.

At times his fingers became so cold they were useless, and he had to manage the control stick with the base of his hands or his wrists. Other times, fire from the engine exhaust forced him to dive the plane to put out the flames. But throughout all these harrowing and sometimes painful experiences, Macready was gathering facts about temperatures at different altitudes and seasons of the year. He also investigated the problem of lack of sufficient oxygen, for he found that even harder to bear than the cold.

219

Getting enough oxygen into the lungs at high altitude, using bags, flasks and finally oxygen masks was the first major step in developing life support systems. Protective suits, helmets and other equipment were developed but not at a pace concurrent with the achievements of airplane engineers and designers.

Oxygen masks enabled pilots to fly to 40,000 feet, but beyond that point, positive pressure breathing systems had to be used to force oxygen into their lungs. Finally, at 50,000 feet, 10 miles above the earth where the air pressure is only 11 per cent of that at sea level, the lungs become completely filled with carbon dioxide and water vapor and there is no room for oxygen. In that unfriendly sky, a pilot will die in moments without an artificial environment. These facts, along with the temperature extremes, were well known; the solution involved an orderly progression from enclosing the cockpit, to pressurizing the cabin, to finally sealing it to provide a "shirt-sleeve" environment. Suits were developed as back-up systems in case of decompression.

But it was not always a smooth race between aircraft producers and the medical people who were trying to devise ways of keeping flyers alive under such rapidly changing conditions. Safety systems cost weight and weight costs speed and performance; in the middle were pilots who considered themselves invincible.

The first serious efforts to design and build a workable pressure suit was instigated in 1933 by Mark Ridge, an American balloonist. He prevailed upon physiologist John Scott Haldane (who had suggested such a suit in 1920) and Sir Robert H. Davis, a British diving suit specialist, to design and build him a protective suit. The team agreed; young Ridge wore the suit in a number of low-pressure chamber tests in London in the last of which he achieved an ambient pressure of 17mm Hg—a pressure altitude of about 90,000 feet for 30 minutes with no ill effects. These tests were the first in the world where a human was successfully protected in a pressure suit at low barometric pressure simulating an extremely high altitude. In spite of this success, Ridge was unable to raise the necessary financial backing to buy a balloon or aircraft; he died a disappointed man in 1962.

With aircraft breaking speed and altitude records in the 1930s, a number of countries were developing high-altitude pressure suits; the United States and the Soviet Union in 1934, Germany and

Spain in 1935 and Italy in 1936. It was said even then, however, that anybody could design a pressure suit; the problem was, making it wearable and workable at the same time.

Wiley Post, noted for his first round-the-world flight of eight days, 15 hours and 51 minutes in 1931 and the second in seven days, 19 hours in 1933, was the first to discuss biological rhythm disruption in transmeridional flight in his book, *Around the World in Eight Days,* 1931. He is credited with making the first aircraft flight wearing a pressure suit. After he won the 1930 Bendix race and made his global flight he then set out to break the New York-Los Angeles speed record, the world's altitude record of 47,572 feet held by the Italian, Donati, and to win the 10,000-pound prize in the 1934 London-Melbourne race. Success could well depend on his developing a pressure suit that would enable him to live and fly in "rarefied" atmosphere of 40,000 feet where the pressure was as low as 2.7 psi.

Post probably had read about the Haldane-Davis Stratosphere Flying Suit in a British aviation journal; at any rate, at the suggestion of Jimmy Doolittle, he approached the B.F. Goodrich Company in Los Angeles, a firm already successful in the production of aviation rubber products, and presented his idea. He wanted a suit, similar to those used by deep sea divers, and he wanted a metal helmet through which all connections would be made. The rubberized fabric would be joined to the helmet by a "vulcalock" sealing process.

The suit was made of six yards of double-ply rubberized parachute cloth glued together on a bias; pigskin gloves and rubber boots were joined to the suit. The 3½-pound aluminum helmet was equipped with a foam rubber pad in the crown, earphones, a double-layer xylonite plastic visor, a hinged door at the mouth level and front and back tie-down fasteners.*

The suit was static-tested in the Los Angeles plant on 18 June 1934 where it held a pressure of 5 pounds per square inch (psi) "with only a minimum of leakage...in between the two parts at the waist joint..." Post then had the suit shipped to Ohio for further

---

*The helmet, all that remains of the first pressure suit made in the U.S., is in the Smithsonian Institution's National Air and Space Museum. It was donated in 1963 by the B.F. Goodrich Company.

testing at Wright Field. A medical officer was on hand and for the first time, liquid oxygen (LOX) was used to pressurize the suit.*

Several tests were made at different altitude equivalents and temperatures but the suit failed because it leaked at the waist where top and bottom were joined.

With three months to go before the London-Melbourne race, Post persuaded the Goodrich people in Akron, Ohio, to modify and improve the first damaged suit. The project engineer was Russ E. Colley, who later directed the development of the full-pressure suits for Project Mercury astronauts, the U.S. Navy and the U.S. Air Force. He perfected a new upper and lower torso, a unique waist clamp, oxygen hose fittings below the helmet visor and metal rings at the elbow and knee joints to facilitate limb movement.

On a hot, humid July day in 1934, Post climbed into the suit and promptly got stuck. He simply could not get out of it because his arms, shoulders and neck were tightly bound by the suit. His attendants vainly tried to free him; finally they moved him to a refrigerated storage room for golf balls where they literally cut him out of the suit. Post probably suffered the world's first case of pressure-suit claustrophobia.

Post's third suit, built by Colley and his wife who sewed the outer fabric on her home sewing machine, had two layers instead of one. Each layer was designed to serve different functions; the inner rubber bag contained liquid gas under pressure and the outer cloth fabric maintained the desired suit shape. The new suit also had a large neck opening through which Post entered, rather than the troublesome waist entrance.

Wiley Post tested his third suit in low-pressure runs in August 1934, and later that month wore it when he flew the *Winnie Mae* out of Akron. He made at least 10 documented flights in the suit, all in the *Winnie Mae*, and tried unsuccessfully several times to break Donati's altitude record of 47,352 feet.

Post never competed in the London-Melbourne race; *Winnie Mae*'s supercharger had been severely damaged during a test in September and he was unable to get it repaired in time. Nevertheless, he demonstrated the feasibility of pressure suits in high-altitude aircraft and the use of liquid oxygen to provide

*The testing at Wright Field was so secret that Captain Harry Armstrong, who was in the building at the time, did not learn about it until 40 years later.

pressurization and breathing gas. According to Dr. Stanley R. Mohler, an avid historian on the subject, Post made several cross-country stratosphere flights wearing his pressure suit, early in 1935.* One was a record flight from Burbank to Cleveland in the jet stream, the weather phenomenon he first discovered in December 1934 while flying the *Winnie Mae* over Bartlesville, Oklahoma.

Considerable work was being done during this era that would not become general knowledge to the aviation medical community until years later. A German, Professor Heinz von Diringshofen, had been experimenting with humans in flight since 1931 to determine ways of reducing the symptoms produced by rapid changes in speed and direction of airplanes. Going back even further, Harald J. von Beckh, M.D. who is currently Director of Medical Research at the Naval Crew Development Center, pointed out that Jimmy Doolittle who won the Pulitzer Trophy in 1922, stated that he became unconscious when making turns. The winner in 1923 is said to have been in more or less of a daze...not being sure how many laps he had completed. The answer to why the blood was driven from the head, thus depriving the brain cells of the necessary oxygen, seemed to be centrifugal force.

In America, Lieutenant Commander J. R. Poppen (MC) U.S. Navy, who later headed the Naval Air Development Center's Aeromedical Laboratory, in 1933, exposed dogs in upright positions to pull-outs of 4.5g. Measuring by invasive techniques the pressure in the carotid artery, he showed a decrease of pressure at the level of the head. He also experimented with an abdominal belt which—when inflated prior to the onset of g loads—mitigated their effects. These early tests by Dr. Poppen, were actually the basis for the present anti-g garments. The Navy Surgeon General clamped a tight security classification on the tests and they were not published until 1950.

Elsewhere, between 1934 and 1943, and again in 1946 to 1955, Russia had an excellent high-altitude pressure suit program. According to Air Force Major Charles L. Wilson, ''From 1934 to

*Post died in a plane crash at Pt. Barrow, Alaska, in August of 1935; the famed humorist, Will Rogers, died in the same crash. His pressure suit, the third model, is in the Smithsonian Institution's National Air and Space Museum.

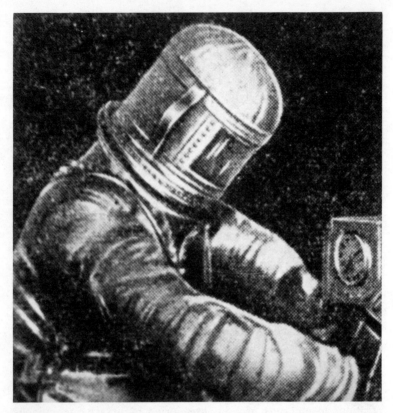

Long before World War II, Dr. Vladislav A. Spasskiy of the Soviet Institute of Aviation Medicine instituted a program for high altitude protective suits. This one, resembling a deep-sea diving outfit, was tested and used in the years 1935-1937./*Institute of Biomedical Problems, Moscow*

1940, the Soviet program at least equalled and probably exceeded in scope and excellence the combined efforts of all other nations in this technical area. Soviet aerospace life scientists in general have been serious and vigorous in their efforts to protect their aircrew members.''

The Soviet's programs began under the direction of Dr. Vladislav A. Spasskiy of the Soviet Institute of Aviation Medicine. They used the best talents available from many disciplines, their facilities were superior for their day and they were allowed to work uninterruptedly, with Ph.D. theses often serving as incentives.

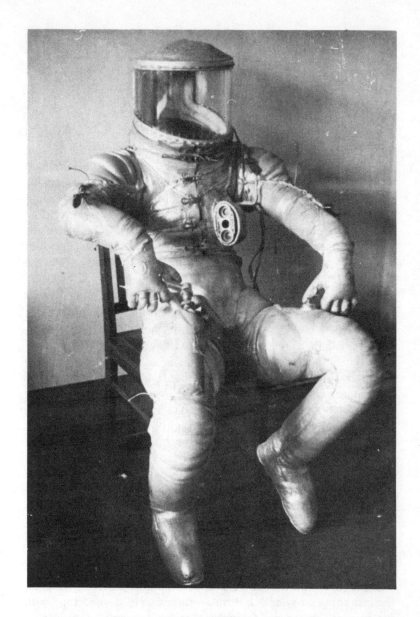

Russia had an excellent high altitude pressure suit program, commencing in 1934 and continuing through World War II. Further development took place from 1946 to 1955./*Institute of Biomedical Problems, Moscow*

Among the weaknesses of their program, according to Dr. Wilson, was their lack of appreciation of benefits of denitrogenation, their early lack of appreciation of benefits of pressure breathing, lack of accurate formulae to estimate alveolar gas tensions and their reliance on a closed circuit life support system. The Soviets did no original work on bladder and capstan suits.

Other pioneers of the period were the German meteorological flyer Klanke and British high-altitude record flyers Swain and Adam. Lieutenant M. J. Adam, on 30 June 1937, reached an altitude of 53,800 feet; he found that any movement beyond his suit's "neutral" position was exhausting and had a rebound effect. Klanke's suit, which he designed himself, was so rigid he could hardly move. Moreover, the entire suit had to be bandaged to prevent it from over-inflating under pressure. It was clear from these early studies that the suits would have to have joints if the pilot was going to be able to fly.

The Germans, although they considered pressure suits only as makeshifts for specific research projects or substitutes for pressure cabins, nonetheless did develop an operational outfit. The Dräger suit, made of strong, rubber-lined ticking, was the first to have pressure-independent universal ball joints at the shoulders, elbows and hips. Slightly bent gloves were attached to the suit by a closure lock and could be removed by pressing the two closing bolts together. The helmet had a sliding window which could be kept open during low-level flights. However, during such flight, the ventilation and regulation of the suit's temperature had to continue. As soon as actual pressurized flight began, the pilot put on his oxygen mask through the sliding window, then closed the window. The suit inflated until a pressure was reached which had previously been adjusted by the air relief valve. When this pressure limit was exceeded the compressed air entering continually escaped through the relief valve. The rapid increase of the air pressure within the suit could be compared to a nose dive which sometimes produced ear pain.

The Dräger suit was developed in one and two-piece garments, the last being a coverall, but the Germans were never happy with the suit, or the concept for many reasons. It seemed a necessary evil, but a half-baked approach to flight in high altitudes. As pressure suits for high altitude flying were being developed, so too

226

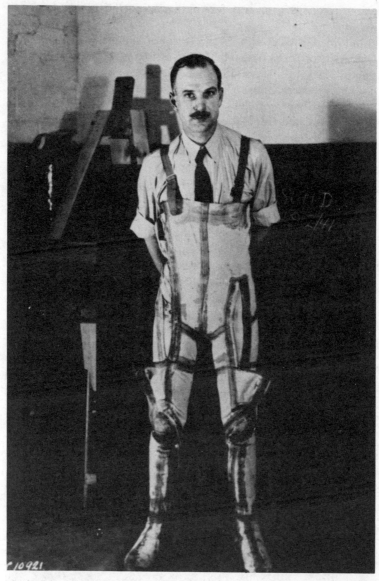

In Canada, Doctor W. R. Franks developed the first anti-g suit to be used in actual combat during World War II. At first, fluid pressure was used against the calves, thighs and abdomen to prevent pooling of blood in the veins and causing blackout; later, gas was used./*W. R. Franks*

were protective measures for counteracting the severe forces of gravity.

In 1939, Dr. W. R. Franks, Professor of Medical Research, at the University of Toronto, had begun investigating ways of preventing pilot "blackout"—loss of vision during aerial maneuvers. In earlier cancer research he had seen that glass tubes spun in a high speed centrifuge were less apt to break if they were supported in water. He tested this flotation-in-a-fluid hypothesis on mice in a small centrifuge and found their tolerance for centrifugal force increased up to 240g. The next step was to apply this principle to humans. A suit was made which he tested in the air in 1940 to find that he could withstand far more g-force than normal without blacking out.

But testing the g-suit in aircraft was troublesome, slow and dependent on the weather, so they decided to build a human centrifuge—the first of its kind on the Allied side. The Germans' most sophisticated centrifuge was at the Aeromedical Research Institute of the Luftwaffe. The one at Tempelhof was much smaller and less efficient. The Canadians had the only centrifuge entirely electrically motivated and controlled and having a rotating cab. Franks' Mark III flying suit became the first anti-g suit to be used in actual combat air operations anywhere in the world.

The principle of the anti-g suit is that a fluid pressure (later gas) is applied to the calves, thighs and abdomen and extremities, and also supports the increased pressure due to acceleration in the arterial blood of the same regions. If pooling is prevented, there is an adequate return of blood to the heart which being likewise supported on the arterial side, can then pump blood to the eyes and brain against the increased load, thus preventing blackouts and unconsciousness and delaying onset of fatigue.

The suit, first used by the Royal Navy's Fleet Air Arm in the Allied invasion of French North Africa in November 1942, consisted of a rubber bladder lining and a non-stretchable outer covering. Worn between flight clothing and underwear, the suit was filled with water as the pilot sat in his plane; after that, the action was entirely automatic. As the blood got heavier under g-loads, so too did the water in the suit which pressed against the body's tissues. The water suit's advantage was that it was entirely automatic—there were no connections to the plane to hinder emergency escape and no special fittings needed. The disadvantage was that it was uncomfortable to wear on the ground, hot in the tropics, and hampered getting out of the cabin in an emergency.

There were also controlled air-pressure suits which were lighter, cooler and more comfortable. Their disadvantage was that the pilot had to be connected to the plane, and since there was little pressure gradient they were suitable only for a g-force of short duration. In fact, the early British fighter planes *had* no readily available source of air pressure; later fighters and jet aircraft of course did.

The Mark VI F.F.S., a harness type or cutaway model air-activated anti-g suit could be worn either over or under the clothing. It lay in place and zipped up on the legs and abdomen. The lacings were then tightened so the suit fit snugly and comfortably. The knee and hip joints were not covered; otherwise there was a continuous air bladder to put pressure on five areas; the two calves, the thighs and abdomen.

The Mark VII F.F.S., also air-activated, was designed to be worn in place of ordinary trousers. When high g force was anticipated, the zipper which ran the full length of the leg was zipped up, thus snugging the trousers so that when air pressure was applied, there was sufficient pressure on the calves and thighs to prevent pooling of blood in them.

But regardless of the kind of protection offered, pilots and many high ranking military officers were opposed to anti-g suits of any kind. They said the added gadgetry hindered the pilot, complicated the aircraft and wasn't effective anyway. Nevertheless, the World War II "believers" at such centers as the Mayo Clinic, Wright Field, the Naval Air Crew Equipment Lab (NACEL) in Philadelphia and various industrial firms did develop suits and concepts that worked. For example, a small company owned by veteran suit designer Dave Clark, working with Mayo specifications, came up with 21 different models of g-suits; the accepted model passed the rigorous centrifuge tests at Wright Field and was finally approved.

As anti-g suits became an accepted fact, so too did body armor, or flak suits, which served to protect B-17 bomber crews during bombing missions over Germany. They were developed in 1942 by

Major General Malcolm Grow when he was surgeon of the Eighth Air Force in England; craftsmen of the Wilkinson Sword Company fashioned them with plates of 20-gauge manganese steel with a thickness of 1mm., secured in pockets to overlap 3/8 of an inch. It was later concluded that these flak suits prevented about 74 per cent of wounds in covered areas. Continual improvement of this type of equipment led to the development of strong, light-weight protective armor which was used extensively by fighting forces during the conflicts in Korea and Vietnam.

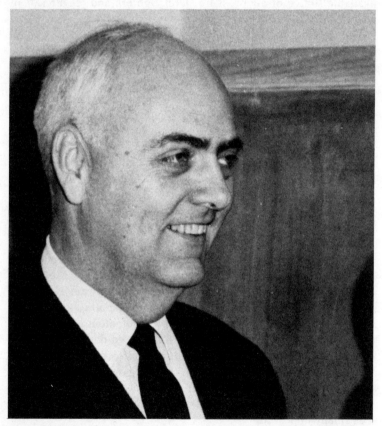

Captain Walton L. Jones (MC) U.S. Navy, assigned to the Bureau of Aeronautics, was among those responsible for developing the Mark IV full pressure suit which was used as an emergency back-up to Mercury's environmental control system./*U.S. Navy*

230

During the 1950s the U.S. Air Force began experiments with the rocket research plane, the X-15, which took a pilot in a full-pressure suit to an altitude of 354,000 feet, near the fringe of space. Meanwhile, NACEL came up with a combined compensated breathing regulator which separated the respiration system completely from the pressurizing gas; the simplified breathing mask required no check valves. The Navy's Mark IV full-pressure suit which ultimately became the first space suit worn by the Mercury astronauts, underwent a strenuous operation test in May 1961 with a world record balloon altitude of 113,700 feet, reached in the two-place open gondola Stratolab.

The Mark IV full-pressure suit, used as an emergency back-up to the Mercury's environmental control system, was developed under the management of Wayne Galloway of the Goodrich Company, Captain Roland Bosee, (MSC) U.S. Navy and James Coreale of ACEL—and Les Snyder and Captain Walton L. Jones, (MC) U.S. Navy, of the Bureau of Aeronautics. Mr. Coreale later left ACEL and headed NASA's space suit efforts.

As the cabin's interior was small, there was little need for mobility except for shoulder and hand movement and because the flights were short, body wastes could be controlled by pre-flight diet and a urine collection device installed in the suit. The tailormade suit itself had a variety of zippered openings for donning and doffing; vulcanization prevented leakage, and there were air-tight bearings and fluted joints which allowed the astronauts to move. It was made of four layers of loosely fitted material, the outer layer being a high-temperature-resistant metallic fabric. The second layer was a woven net to restrain the suit from ballooning when pumped up like an automobile tire to 2.7psi. The third layer, the gas bag or bladder was made of thin, neoprene rubber, contoured to fit the body, and the inner layer next to the astronaut's body was smooth, soft nylon. The bubble helmet, with its built-in communication system was attached to the suit by a special padded neck ring.

Oxygen was fed into the suit through a connector in the torso area, circulated to the extremities, and then to the helmet for breathing. The exhaled waste bled off through a headpiece connector into the environmental control system where it was disposed of. The temperature and oxygen control system assisted

231

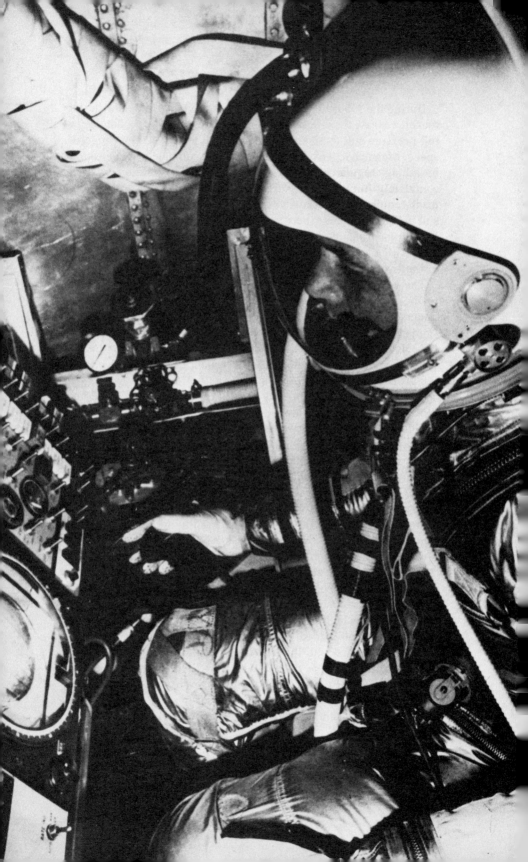

the astronauts in maneuvering at temperatures of plus or minus 100°F.

Among the many crucial decisions that had to be made, even as the suit was being readied for functioning as a component of the craft's environmental control system, was the selection of the gaseous environment. Ideally the atmosphere would most closely resemble sea level conditions. But the state of the art had not advanced sufficiently to handle the weight such a system entailed and there was not yet a reliable regulation system for controlling the gas mixture. Also, at that point, engineers dared not rule out the possibility of sudden decompression of the cabin. The system therefore called for minimum weight and volume, minimum power usage, simplicity in regulation of gases, reliability, ease in maintenance, and compatibility of cabin and suit systems with everything else.

For the engineers and physiologists, the single gas, 100 per cent oxygen at 5psi was the simplest, most reliable and lightest-weight type of atmosphere to deliver with the available technology. They also felt it gave greater protection against decompression. Physiologically, a mixed gas would have offered protection against atelectasis, or collapse of the air sacs of the lungs. No one yet knew what would happen under decompression if a mixed gas of 50 per cent oxygen and 50 per cent nitrogen at 7psi was used. Tests were made at NACEL to determine how long it was necessary to pre-breathe oxygen at sea level to protect the body from the bends, should an early mission decompression occur and whether a person would be protected after breathing 50 per cent oxygen, 50 per cent nitrogen at 7psi. It was shown that three hours of preoxygenation at sea level prevented the bends, following a decompression in 40 seconds from sea level to an altitude of 35,000 feet; without preoxygenation, 18 hours exposure to the 7psi, 50 per cent oxygen, 50 per cent nitrogen gives protection against bends to an altitude of 35,000 feet in one minute. The study also indicated that astronauts should be carefully screened for their susceptibility to the bends.

Environmental control for Project Mercury included the protective suit as well as the arrangement of knobs, switches and dials so that an astronaut could keep track of them all. Considering the close quarters in a Mercury capsule, the engineers and suit technicians were successful./*NASA*

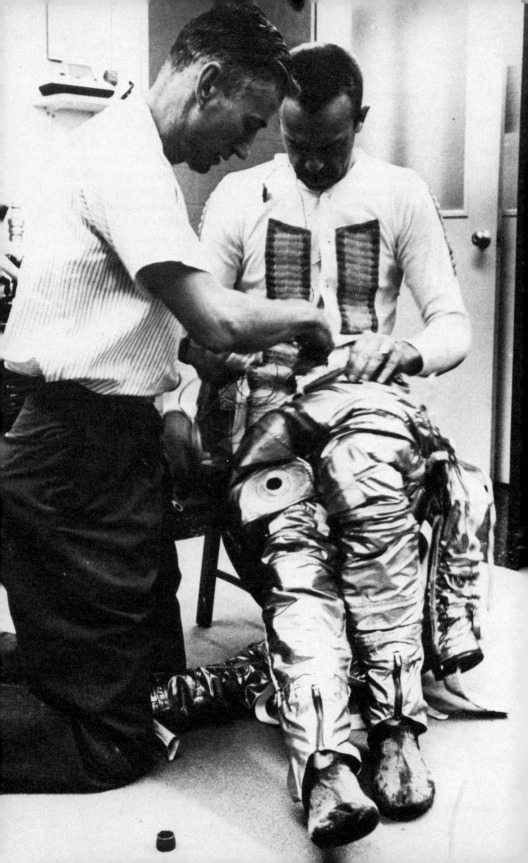

The greatest physiological unknown factors involved with the 100 per cent oxygen 5psi atmosphere were the hazards of atelectasis, and the postflight development of a vacuum in the middle ear, following absorption of the oxygen that would lead to the collecting of fluid and pain in the middle ear on return to normal atmosphere. It was generally known that pure oxygen at low pressures would present no pulmonary oxygen toxicity problem. However, investigations were required to determine the need of an inert gas in any artificial atmosphere. Both industrial and Department of Defense laboratories worked on the problem for NASA.

The 100 per cent oxygen atmosphere was used until the tragic fire on the launch pad at Cape Canaveral, 27 January 1967 in which astronauts Virgil Grissom, Edward White and Roger Chaffee were killed. Following that, along with removal of flammable materials in the cabin, there were engineering changes in the escape hatches; an emergency suit mix of 60 per cent oxygen, 40 per cent nitrogen was used until the mission was well underway and it was safe to gradually switch to 100 per cent oxygen.

Meanwhile during the many years of pressure-suit development, scientists and engineers worked towards making aircraft cockpits and cabins habitable. As early as 1928, the Germans at the Junkers plant developed a two-man removable altitude cabin for fighters and in the 1930s, Captain Harry Armstrong at Wright Field was involved with perfecting a sealed cockpit for the stratosphere flights of Anderson and Kefner. Using the X-C35 aircraft, systems were developed to maintain sea level pressure, oxygen supplies, disposal of carbon dioxide, ventilation and problems connected with explosive decompression. This led directly to pressurized cabins in passenger aircraft with nine Boeing 307 Stratoliners being placed in operation early in 1939 by Transworld and Pan American Airlines. Late in World War II, cockpit and crew stations of bomber and fighter aircraft were sealed off and air under pressure from the engine compressor was forced into the area, providing constant circulation which in turn drew off the carbon dioxide. It was soon learned, however, that

Alan B. Shepard was suited up by technician Joe Schmitt for the Freedom 7 Mercury sub-orbital flight of 5 May 1961. This was America's first space shot and it was highly publicized. That suit *had* to work./*NASA*

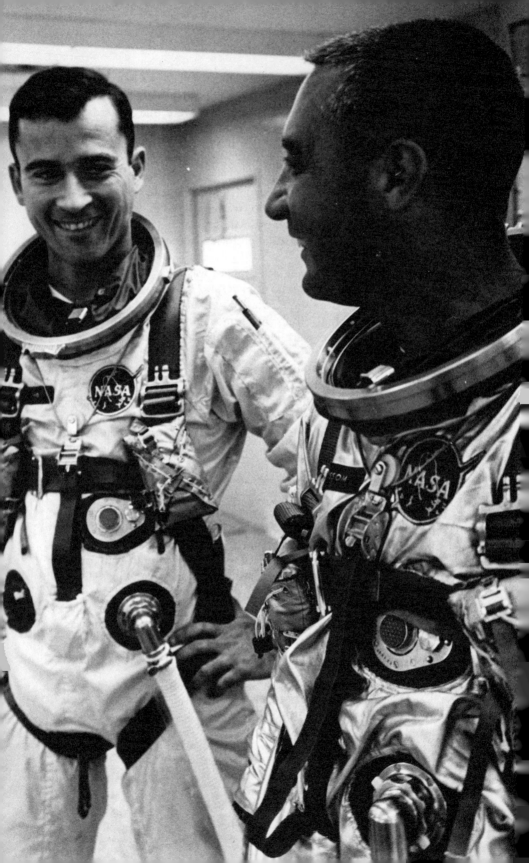

aircraft pierced by bullets decompressed so a compromise was reached whereby sealed cabins would be pressurized only enough to make the atmosphere tolerable; the crew wore oxygen masks or pressure suits that were at cabin operational altitude equivalence, inoperative in normal flight but capable of increasing pressurization in an emergency.

After the war, a great deal was learned about artificial environments during the biological tests with animals in nose cones of V-2 rockets. By 1950, Dr. Hubertus Strughold was publicly stating that the time had arrived for bold action: "We have today these pressurized cabins. They are in conventional planes and in military aircraft to protect against the low atmospheric pressure outside. But they would be ineffectual at certain altitudes. There would be no protection because of technical aerodynamic and toxicological reasons. Such altitudes begin at 80,000 feet. We have to resort to a new type of cabin—a sealed cabin, one I would prefer to call a hermetic cabin. You all know that our altitude chambers are not reproducing the effects of outside atmosphere. There is nothing now in the world where a man's relationship to a completely closed atmosphere can be tested. We will have to know this. We will have to know what happens to a man within a sealed atmosphere. This is a very important problem and project in spaceflight. It is equally important to the safety of our pilots who are already flying towards the fringes of space. We must build a prototype of a spaceship cabin to find out just to what extent the atmosphere in such a cabin is changed by the presence of a human occupant..."

Strughold's plan was businesslike, calling for the groundwork to be done in the laboratories. First there should be a one-man chamber, completely closed, for testing air regeneration devices. The first test which was made in 1954 at the Department of Space Medicine, School of Aviation Medicine at Randolph Air Force Base, was aimed at determining the best kind of artificial atmosphere (composition and pressure) that could be obtained with a minimum of volume and weight. In the program, too, was

The 100 per cent oxygen atmosphere was used until the tragic fire on the launch pad at Cape Canaveral, in which astronauts Virgil Grissom (right), Edward White and Roger Chaffee were killed. Shown here with Grissom is astronaut John W. Young./*NASA*

237

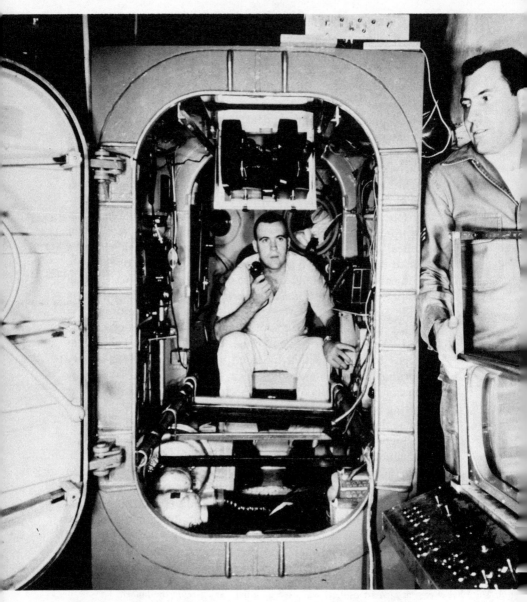

Airman Donald Ferrell made history with his seven-day simulated "moon" flight in 1957, under the direction of Dr. Hubertus Strughold and Colonel Paul Campbell, at the School of Aviation Medicine./*U.S. Air Force*

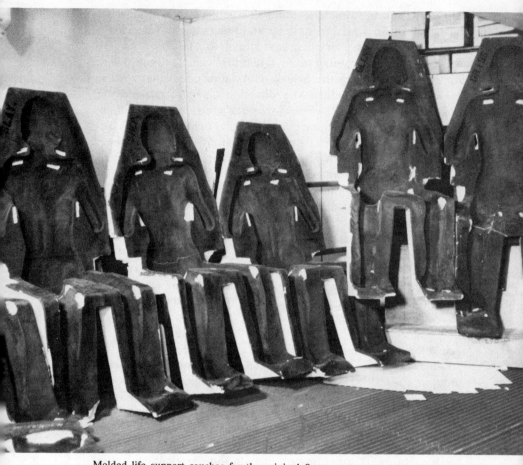

Molded life support couches for the original Seven astronauts at the U.S Navy Aviation Medical Acceleration Labortory in Johnsville, Pa., provided the basis for the couches installed in Mercury space capsules./*NASA*

the miniaturizing of bioinstrumentation such as recording equipment, oxygen sensors, carbon dioxide sensors etc., and physiological reactions as recorded by the electrocardiogram, electroencephalogram, respiratory movements and body temperature. It all had to include telemetry which had as its base the "biopacks" used in animal rocket experiments.

239

The space cabin simulator could also be used to determine the best pattern for work, rest, sleep and psychological reactions to confinement in a sensory deprived situation. The first such test was all set to go, according to Dr. Willard Hawkins, at that time an Air Force Major with the School of Aviation Medicine, "Major Julian Ward and I, under the direction of Dr. Strughold and Colonel Paul Campbell, wanted to send a man on a seven-day simulated flight, when along came Sputnik I in October 1957. The country was at a low ebb as a result of that. Well, we went ahead with our 'flight' shortly afterwards with Airman Donald Ferrell, and he got along very well. Senator Lyndon Johnson came down to welcome Ferrell when he returned from his 'flight'."

By September of 1958, a two-man space cabin was ready for human testing. The "guinea pigs" were Dr. Bruno Balke, and Senior Master Sergeant Samuel G. Karst, who spent 10 days in the cramped space cabin before they emerged to breathe some fresh air again. Dr. Robert T. Clark, in charge of the tests, reported the men in good physical condition and gave his opinion that, "...men could undergo the hardships of high altitude without harming their physical performance."

In 1963, scientists at the Krasnoyarsk Institute of Physics, the Siberian branch of the USSR Academy of Sciences, launched a program aimed at creating artifical ecological systems for extended space voyages. The main difference between the Soviet experiments and similar ones carried out in other countries, notably the United States, was that the researchers were placed in conditions that were as close as possible to terrestrial. They conducted various scientific experiments and observations, raised grain and made bread for themselves, cooked all sorts of meals on a usual electric range, did the laundry, watched TV programs and regularly cleaned their quarters, which were furnished with conventional furniture.

A major problem turned out to be food. Since it would be impossible to stock enough supplies to last four months—the distance equivalent to that between Earth and Mars—the Siberian scientists concentrated on controlled biosynthesis. This meant increasing yields of cereals and vegetables. Sixty per cent of the daily diet would be vegetable food.

The apparatus in which Gennady Asinyarov and Nikolai Bugreev "traveled," to Mars over a period of four months in 1978 is the hermetically sealed Biosatellite-3. It consists of four modules; living, technical (life-support system), and two modules containing "plantations." These served to raise potatoes, tomatoes, cucumbers, garden radishes, a wheat variety specially evolved for cultivation under intensive light conditions in a closed environment, and other crops. The rest of the food was of animal origin, taken into Bios-3 in vacuum-dried form without loss in nutritional value. All production processes were fully controlled by the crew members. The only external links were the supply of power and the removal of extra heat.

An old Russian tradition was broken on the day the experiment ended; instead of receiving the usual bread and salt of welcome, the terranauts themselves presented to those who met them a fresh-baked loaf of sweet cookies of their own making.

As the cabin environment for space travel was being refined through the years, so too were the suits being upgraded for comfort and maneuverability. When the Gemini program began in 1965, the whole suit philosophy changed from that of a back-up protective garment to a prime life-sustaining system. Wearing a fully pressurized suit, a Gemini crew member would leave the space craft for varying lengths of time to perform duties in the void of space. And because the two-man cabin was too small for donning and doffing a complete suit, the garment had to be comfortable enough for 14 days of continuous wear. Because of such varying requirements, two different suits were developed.

It was the most serious challenge to date, despite the tremendous amount of research and development that had produced the earlier suits. What was finally selected was a multilayered garment with an outer layer of high-temperature-resistant nylon able to withstand temperatures as high as 500°F. Beneath that was a link-net restraining layer under which was the neoprene-coated nylon gas retention layer. Next to the body was a nylon oxford suit which was worn for comfort. Quick disconnectors allowed the astronauts to remove their gloves and helmets when they were not needed, and a pressure-sealing zipper running from the small of the back through the crotch made dressing and

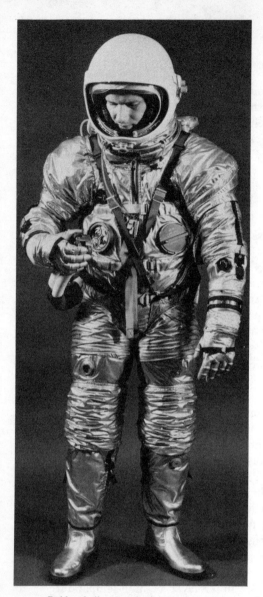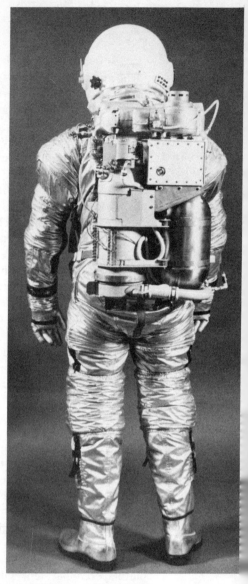

Rubber bellows at the joints of arms, legs and torso provided increased mobility when the Apollo suit was pressurized. The helmet had an airlock feeding device used for eating and drinking in conditions of weightlessness./NASA

The life support back pack developed for the Apollo Moon-landing program supplied oxygen and ventilation, controlled temperature and humidity, and removed respiratory and body contaminants from inside the suit./NASA undressing easier. A bioinstrumentation and communication connector was installed in the suit torso, as were connectors for the environmental control system (ECS). A built-in disposal system took care of urine.

Oxygen entered the helmet for breathing, then circulated to the extremities for thermal control. The suit also contained such everyday necessities as a handkerchief, pencils, survival knife, scissors and neck and wrist dams to prevent water from entering the suit during recovery from the sea. There was a parachute harness and pockets on arms and legs to hold charts and log books.

With the decision to have one of the crew members "walk in space" during the Gemini 4 mission in June 1965, the extra-vehicular activity (EVA) suit had to provide thermal, micrometeoroid and visual protection, as well as certain redundancies essential to crew safety. The outer cover of the GT-3 suit was replaced with a multilayered overgarment, the outer cover of which was fabricated from a high-temperature-resistant nylon. A layer of felt was used as a spacer layer; several layers of a high reflective Mylar provided superinsulation; and two additional layers of high-temperature-resistant nylon completed the multi-layered overgarment. The other layers remained as before.

The new EVA helmet was equipped with a removable visor assembly; the outer visor provided visible and infrared sun-ray protection and the inner lens, with its special coating to prevent fogging, gave protection from impact and attenuated ultraviolet rays. Thermal overgloves protected the hands from conductive heat transfer in exposed sunlight. In the Gemini 4 flight, astronaut White wore this suit with no difficulty; in fact it was decided the cover layer bulk and extra visor material could be dispensed with for astronaut McDivitt's EVA in a later flight.

The extravehicular life support system included a 25-foot umbilical assembly which allowed the astronaut to move back to the spacecraft adapter section. The assembly's electrical wires supplied continuous communication and bioinstrumentation during the EVA. The 1,000-pound-test tether line kept the astronaut attached to the spacecraft and the oxygen hose carried oxygen from the spacecraft to the suit. Emergency oxygen was available from a high-pressure oxygen bottle so if the umbilical system failed the astronaut could manually operate the emergency supply.

Space walks are a tricky business at best. The Soviets learned that in February 1978 when Cosmonaut Yuri Romanenko, aboard the 96-day orbital flight of the Salyut 6 space station, took an unauthorized space stroll. Only Georgi Grechko had been slated for such a walk and Romanenko was to remain behind at open hatch. Both were wearing a new type of space suit equipped with radio and an hour's supply of oxygen. Thus, when working outside the spacecraft they required no umbilical link to the mother ship except a simple tether to keep them from floating away. All was well until the Salyut passed over the western Pacific Ocean, out of range of Soviet ground stations. Suddenly Romanenko, who was not tethered, jumped out of the hatch.

There was no explanation for this daring plunge other than U.S. speculation that he might have gotten "space rapture." Grechko reacted quickly, made his way hand over hand along Salyut's rail and grabbed the end of Romanenko's safety line. By then, Romanenko was about 13 feet from the ship. A few seconds more and Romanenko would have been on a "2001 Space Odyssey."

For the Gemini 7 14-day mission in December 1965, there was another suit to be worn inside the cabin. Since the crews reported that some of their activities were hampered by the bulky versions of the old suits and because by this time the cabin pressurization system was sufficiently reliable, the astronauts were fitted with a lighter weight garment originally developed for the Air Force by the David Clark Company. This suit had a soft fabric hood instead of the hard preshaped helmet, and a polycarbonate visor and pressure-sealing zipper. The long zipper allowed the astronaut to remove the hood and stow it in the compartment behind his head. The suit itself weighed only 16 pounds as compared to the previous 23.5 pounds and could be completely removed inside the spacecraft in about 16 minutes. Boots and gloves could be removed, the hood unzipped and folded back as a head rest.

The new suit had two layers of material; an inner layer with pressure-restraining neoprene-coated nylon bladder and an outer layer of six-ounce high-temperature-resistant nylon. Link net sections sewn together with the direction of expansion carefully matched to the normal movements of the human torso improved the astronaut's mobility. Elimination of the large metal neck ring reduced weight and improved comfort. External ventilation was provided by ducts down the outside of the legs and arms of the pressure bladder at the extremities. There were fewer pressure points than in earlier suits, and after the 14-day flight of Gemini 7, the crew reported they felt comfortable wearing the suit; they slept better and perspired less because they were able to remove the suit entirely.

For the Gemini 8 flight in March 1966, the outer protective cover was reduced and the thermal protective fabric in the gloves incorporated into the glove design. The flight of Gemini 9 in June 1966 presented yet another new challenge to the suit designers. The Astronaut Maneuvering Unit (AMU) developed in-house under the directions of Richard Johnson, (Chief of the NASACrew System Division) which the astronaut used outside the spacccraft required that changes be made in the lower portion of the EVA suit. The high-temperature fire plume from the AMU could damage the suit, so a stainless steel fabric outer covering was developed to serve as protection. A high-temperature super insulation used below the outer cover and alternate layers of double aluminized film and lightweight fiberglass. The helmet visor was also changed to give more protection against impact. The Plexiglas pressure visor was replaced with a coated polycarbonate pressure visor. This also permitted use of a single lens sun visor. During the EVA, the helmet's pressure visor fogged; raising the sun visor helped to melt the frost on the inside of the clear visor, but the problem did cause the operation to be cut short.

By the time of the Apollo flights, the culmination of 40 years of experience went into the environmental and life support systems that enabled men to go to the moon and return to the earth. The moon explorers were exposed to the harshest environments ever encountered by man. On the lunar surface, temperatures ranged from 212°F. down to -240°F. and the almost complete lack of atmosphere allowed the full solar flux to reach the moon's crust. Cosmic radiation and meteoroid particles pelted the surface continuously as the men moved about in a gravity one-sixth that of earth. Crater-packed areas covered with dust were subjected to

245

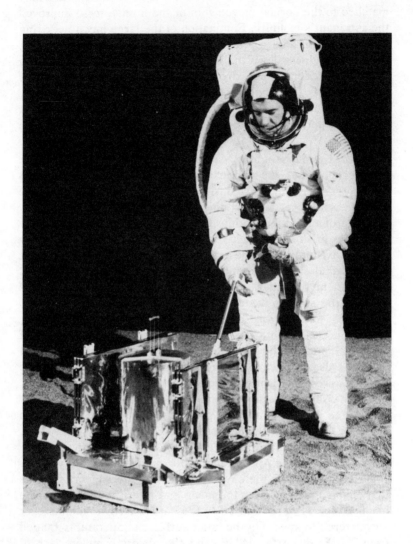

The Passive Seismometer Experiments Package (PSEP) was a self-contained 100-pound seismic station with its own transmitter, powered by solar cells. It was designed to detect motions of the lunar crust and interior and help clarify the origin and structure of the moon./*NASA*

meteoroid storms; the difference between life and death was the artificial environment in which the astronauts were encased.

The astronauts on their long journey had been able to don and doff their suits and much of their time had been spent in "shirt sleeves;" only at critical mission periods such as launch, docking with the lunar excursion module (LEM) and lunar operation, was it necessary to wear the heavy protective suiting.

But the array of equipment, including the portable life-support system (PLSS) did, in a sense, represent a roundup of what had gone on before. In the beginning, there was the armor-like suit reminiscent of the deep-sea diver gear, then the partial and full-pressure suits, the Mercury and Gemini outfits, and finally the Apollo systems designed for lunar scientific excursions.

To TV viewers, the Apollo systems looked pretty much like their predecessors in the shiny suit, bubble helmet, Frankenstein monster boots, and thick gloves; reporters described the insulative overgarment, the micrometeoroid protective garment and the backmounted portable life-support system. This PLSS weighed four pounds, but testers could not feel the weight even in normal earth gravity when their suits were pressurized to 3.5psi.

The main function of the PLSS was to condition and replenish the atmosphere inside the space suit during lunar excursions. It maintained a suit oxygen pressure at 3.7 plus or minus 0.2psi and controlled temperature, carbon dioxide, odor and moisture levels inside the suit. Each of the two PLSS units carried to the moon was rechargeable from spacecraft supplies, could operate up to four hours without recharging, with three hours for nominal excursion, reserving one hour for contingency operations.

Originally, the PLSS for Apollo provided cooling and ventilation by circulating oxygen through the space suit, as was done in Project Mercury. But because of the high metabolic heat rates produced by the lunar explorer, the gas ventilation system relied almost entirely upon evaporative cooling which caused the astronaut to perspire profusely.The problem was solved by switching to a liquid cooling system, pioneered at the British Royal Aircraft Establishment in Farnborough, England. This unique concept relied on the circulation of cool water through a network of tubes built into the space-suit undergarment in such a way that the tubing came into contact with the astronaut's skin. The skin was

247

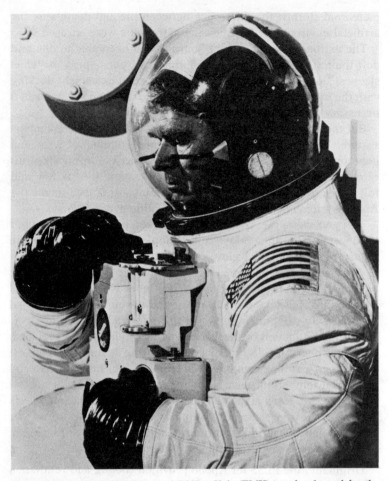

The Space Shuttle Extravehicular Mobility Unit (EMU) can be donned by the astronaut himself. The suits, available in small, medium and large sizes were designed in anticipation of work to be done outside the Orbiter. The two-piece suit has an upper torso made of rigid aluminum, with the life-support pack permanently attached./*NASA*

cooled by direct conduction, thus resulting in little or no perspiration.

The astronauts' eyes were given special protection. This was required because there is no atmosphere on the moon to disperse or reduce the sun's rays; not only are eyes exposed to visible, infrared; and ultraviolet rays, but the solar reflections from the spacesuit, the lunar module and other equipment produce a blinding glare.

The astronauts wore an adjustable visor, similar to the sun visor of an automobile, which reflected about 90 per cent of the visible light, and infrared as well as nearly all ultraviolet rays. The inner and outer visor arrangement kept the visors from fogging during extreme temperature changes.

The gas circulation system provided pressurization, breathing oxygen and removal of carbon dioxide and other gaseous products during lunar operations. Oxygen was circulated by an electrically powered centrifugal fan into the suit through a gas disconnect.

Although a number of suit proposals were made and worked on, the final selection, the A7L, was influenced by NASA's Apollo 204 Review Board which investigated the fire that killed the three astronauts in January 1967. Flammable materials were replaced in the redesigned suits with non-flammables, and non-flammable fiber glass was used for the outer layer. It was more comfortable, fire-resistant and mobile than any of its predecessors.

The A7L suit was used in all manned Apollo missions during prelaunch and launch phases and during re-entry into the earth's atmosphere. The rest of the time the crew wore unpressurized flight suits. The A7L was worn for the lunar landing, exploration on the moon's surface and rendezvous of the lunar module with the command module in lunar orbit.

Today, ordinary travelers reap the benefits of aviation medicine laid down by Paul Bert, Harry Armstrong, W. Randolph Lovelace and many others when they book passage aboard the Supersonic Transport (SST), Concorde. For the first time, aeromedical advice was sought, according to Group Captain Peter Howard of the Royal Air Force Institute of Aviation Medicine in Farnborough, England. Designers took human factors into consideration for both crew and passengers.

The Concorde flies at 25 miles a minute, spans an ocean in an hour and comes to life in the tropopause. "...and it is there that the new aviation medicine begins...."*

*The Harry G. Armstrong Lecture, 1977, "Aeromedical Research and the SST," by Group Captain Peter Howard, Royal Air Force, RAF Institute of Aviation Medicine.

To date, most SST headlines have featured the environmentalists protesting the noise. According to Dr. Howard, "The whole subject is bedeviled by politics, tinctured with emotion and obfuscated by the logarithmic properties of the decibel..."

Opponents of the SST worried about altitude and its effect on crew and passengers, but in actuality, it makes no difference whether the cruising altitude is 20,000 feet or 200,000 feet. "Concorde and Skylab are under the same skin as the DC-3." The absolute pressures of the cabin atmosphere have long since been determined by the physiological requirements, thanks to the early researchers. Nevertheless, the British did conduct a series of hypoxia studies with the SST in mind. The result was a formal recommendation that the maximum cabin altitude for normal operations of the Anglo-French SST should be 5,000 feet, and although the advice did not become part of the final specification for the aircraft, it was accepted and followed.

The greatest potential hazard of the Concorde was the possibility of decompression. Flight surgeons were particularly concerned about the safety of crews flying the prototype at a time when the cabin conditioning systems were still being developed. Oxygen masks and demand regulators, which had long been standard equipment for airline flight decks, were useful only to 40,000 feet, with a pressure breathing mask adding another 5,000 feet. It was clear that pressure suits would be needed as emergency back-ups; not as complicated as those worn by the astronauts, but life-support systems nonetheless. Those suits finally used were the type developed by the French and British Air Forces for high-altitude flight tests and were considered sufficient to get the crews down to a safe altitude, should decompression occur. Each crew seat had a three-stage parachute assembly, an emergency oxygen supply and a personal survival pack, along with such items as smoke goggles and electrically heated gloves. Personal equipment included an immersion suit and life-preserver because the most dangerous phases of flight were over water. An air-ventilated suit was also worn in case the temperature conditioning system at supersonic speeds failed. Said Dr. Howard: "All this equipment was intensively tested for an emergency which never occurred—a common fate for aeromedical research, but one that is gladly accepted by its practioners."

250

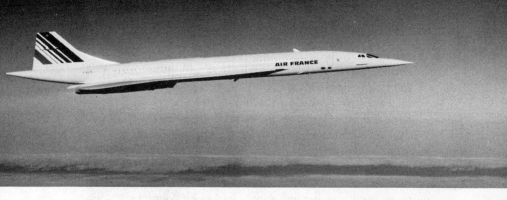

The Concorde SST flies at 25 miles a minute, to span the Atlantic ocean in an hour, but when due respect is paid to the environment in which it operates, and proper safety precautions are taken, flight at supersonic speeds in the stratosphere is safer than it was in barn-storming days./*Air France*

But what of naive passengers who could hardly be expected to wear pressure suits and space helmets? Again, a large number of experiments were carried out, using monkeys and baboons as subjects. Physiological and behavioral patterns were studied under varying conditions of decompression. The results of the investigations were crucial to the question of passenger safety. Again, to quote Dr. Howard: "In the worst case considered to be consistent with continuing structural integrity of the pressure cabin, a sudden decompression from the loss of a window six inches in diameter, followed 30 seconds later by descent to a safe altitude would expose the occupants to a maximum height of 36,000 feet. The time spent above 20,000 feet would be six minutes, and 30,000 feet would be exceeded for about three minutes. This dose of hypoxia...would, in a passenger totally unprotected by oxygen, lead to unconsciousness but it would be insufficient to cause lasting cerebral damage. A considerable measure of consciousness would have been restored before descent was complete; the victim would be confused and would probably have a merciful amnesia, but his brain would be undamaged and his recovery total..."

Although the "drop-down" oxygen masks and life jackets have long been common in airlines, few experts believe passengers would use them properly in an emergency. To cope with this, engineers "over-engineered," the cabin system; small windows (six inches in diameter) reduced both the risk of decompression and its rate and multiple redundancy of air supplies ensured that decompression would be slow and limited and more than one failure could be accommodated.

Oxygen masks would be provided the passengers and crews should cabin pressure drop to an equivalent altitude of 14,000 feet. These requirements are at least as stringent and in their implementation are at least as efficient, as those stipulated for subsonic airliners. Special precautions were provided the crew to prevent any loss of motor function or judgement. Oxygen masks containing an undiluted oxygen supply had to be donned with one hand within five seconds; training in pressure breathing was required for pilots and crews, and separate and independent supplies were to be provided for passenger cabin and crew compartment.

But donning an oxygen mask in five seconds with one hand was no simple matter. According to Dr. Howard: "The problem is similar to that faced by a one-armed theatre nurse attempting to put on a cloth surgical mask against the clock." The problem was solved with the engineering of a new type of mask and harness—and a device that resembles a skeletal bowler hat. "Although this equipment does not have the aesthetic appeal of standard oxygen mask assemblies, it is extremely effective in use. After a minimum of training, Concorde aircrew are able to don the mask and restore communication well within the five seconds demanded by the regulations. Many of them indeed reach the three second limit..."

There was considerable research on the effects of the SST on the ozone layer, effects of radiation on passengers and thermal conditions in the stratosphere at supersonic speeds. All were methodically investigated by the aeromedical specialists and although there will probably continue to be protestations from the alarmists, each of these areas of investigation have shown that given due respect to the hostile elements and proper precautions taken, the ordinary passenger can safely fly at supersonic speeds in the stratosphere. Said Dr. Howard: "For all the controversy that surrounds it, Concorde is but the first of its breed, and it is significant that the possibility of an American SST has recently been re-opened at Congressional level. When that aircraft is built -

and I say 'when' with a confidence that dismisses 'if' - it, too, will rely upon the principles and practice of aviation medicine..."

Ten years have passed since the first men landed on the moon. Altogether, 12 astronauts have made the trip and returned safely, thanks in part to exact control of their environmental surroundings in the spacecraft, the lunar landers and their portable life support systems. That phase of the space program has now ended, and it is most likely that the Apollo space suits, their usefulness ended, will wind up in the National Air and Space Museum along with the NC-4, the first aircraft to fly the Atlantic, and other relics of the colorful past in the air.

In another 10 years there will be more men—and women—in space, perhaps for weeks and months at a time, as they work in orbiting spacelabs. There will be no bulky helmets or PLSS outfits, for the labs will provide a "shirt sleeve" environment, drawing on solar energy for power, and quite likely recycling the atmosphere through banks of green algae to keep the oxygen supply fresh and clean. In the years to come after that, as technological advances pyramid one on another, space stations may have established environmental conditions so suitable to human existence that instead of people going up to a space station for a few weeks, some space station workers may be at the point where they could consider coming down to visit the earth for a few weeks.

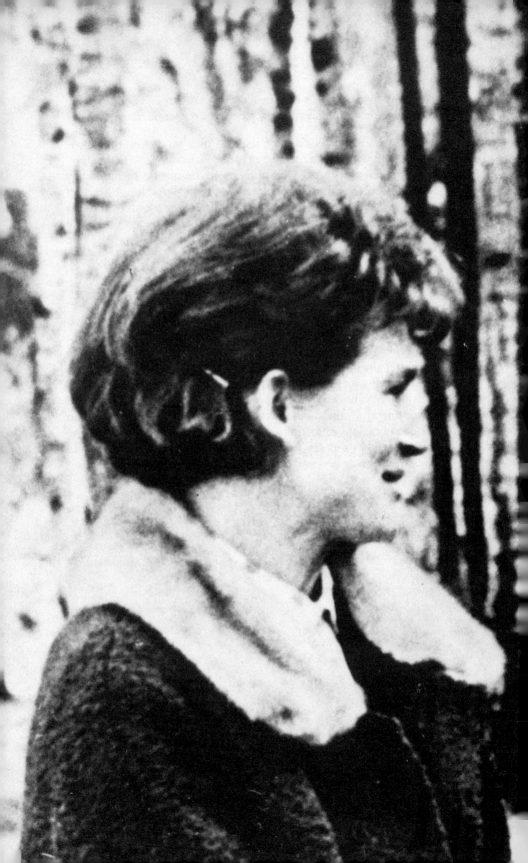

9
High, Hot and Hazardous

About two and a half hours after liftoff from earth, a moon-bound spacecraft fires its booster rockets for a minute or so in a maneuver to take it out of earth orbit and into trans-lunar trajectory. The "burn" begins at an altitude of perhaps 175 miles, and when it is finished the craft is nearly 700 miles away from earth, in cislunar space. In those few short moments, it completes one of the most critical parts of the flight as it passes through a region of dangerous—and until 20 years ago unknown—ionizing radiation, an invisible Sargasso Sea of the sky, as it were, except it nearly surrounds the earth, and can well spell disaster for those who enter it unprepared. Unlike the Sargasso Sea, it was discovered long before men reached it, through the brilliant reasoning of physicist James A. Van Allen of the University of Iowa. The world-girdling band of protons, neutrons and high energy electrons wich which all astronauts are familiar, is named the Van Allen Belt after its earthbound discoverer.

The only space-age mother in the world, Valentina Tereshkova flew 48 orbits of the earth in 1963, and later married Colonel Andrian G. Nikolayev who had flown 64 orbits. Despite fears of the damage cosmic rays may do to the human biological system, their daughter, born in 1964, was normal in all respects./*Smithsonian Institution*

But above and beyond the Van Allen Belt, space is filled with more radiation: gamma rays, which may originate in extra-galactic sources such as super novas; X-rays from binary star systems; radio waves from neutron stars and pulsars; and all the elements of the solar electromagnetic spectrum, which also includes gamma and X-rays, ultraviolet light, visible light, infrared rays, and radio waves.

The existence of cosmic rays was discovered in 1911, in Switzerland, when Victor Hess was measuring high-altitude ionization changes by carrying an electrometer aloft in a balloon. Actually, the rays had been detected earlier, at lower levels, but they were supposed to have originated in radioactive materials in the earth. Hess then realized the rays were of extraterrestrial origin; he was awarded the Nobel prize in 1936 for his discovery. At that time the radiation was called *Hohenstrahlung*—high-altitude radiation.

Radiation connected with solar flares was first discovered in 1956 when there was a worldwide change in ground-level cosmic background radiation. Solar flares produce mainly protons of various energies, and a small percentage of helium ions. They have been divided into four classes, according to intensity. So far, no extremely large flare has occurred during a manned spaceflight, although a fairly large one took place in 1974 during a Soviet spaceflight. That flight was in a low orbit, and most of the flare was deflected by the earth's magnetic field. If the flight had been outside that field, the cosmonauts could have received a heavy radiation dose.

It is estimated that during a series of 100 15-day spaceflights, there would be the probability of one major Class 1 solar flare, two Class II and two Class III flares, and 32 Class IV flares. The radiation dosage of the Class I flare of 1956 was 34rem, while that of a Class IV flare of 1960 was a mere 0.3rem. A spacecraft traversing the inner Van Allen belt would subject its crew to a dosage of only seven rem. On the other hand, a spacecraft that remained in an equatorial orbit about the earth for from 30 to 60 days would meet a calculated dosage of 50 to 100rem.

A solar flare is a vast explosion of energy that may leap out hundreds of thousands of miles from the surface of the sun in no more than 20 minutes. High-energy protons thrown out in the explosion will reach the upper atmosphere of the earth in only a few minutes, disrupting short wave radio communications in the hemisphere facing the sun. During the last complete sunspot cycle—1956-1970—there were ten large flares.

An intensely powerful series of flares occured in August of 1972, lasting about five days. During that period, high-energy protons severely disrupted radio communications. An astronaut exposed to radiation at that time might have received a dosage of 350 to 800rem on his body, up to 180rem in his eyes, and from 3 to 12rem in bloodforming organs.

In actual space operations, average dosage has been very much less. Figures compiled from thermoluminescent dosimetry data for the entire series of Vostok, Voskhod, Soyuz and Salyut flights by the Russians, and all American flights from Gemini 3 to Skylab—a total of 38 flights—showed the average dosage for all crew-members for all fights to be a mere 272mrads. As some of these flights lasted only a few hours, most of them were no more than ten or twelve days, and only the Skylab and Salyut missions extended over many weeks, the average appears higher than if applied to flights of equal duration. For the eleven Apollo missions, average radiation dosage ranged from .16 in two cases to a high of 1.14, with an average of .40 per mission.

Every day of his life, a person on earth is hit by some sort of radiation—solar particle rays during the day, and galactic cosmic rays at night. There is a perfect rain of solar particle radiation; an area the size of a person's palm is hit about 50 times a minute, and even the tip of one's nose is hit a couple of times a minute. Cosmic rays do not hurt when they hit, but about 20 hours after a solar flare, the effect shows up in a form of irritation or scars. But solar particle rays have their use; their increased penetration into the atmosphere triggers rain. Solar flares reach their maximum during peak sunspot activity, which runs in a cycle of about eleven years; a side effect of this is that the rings marking a trees growth are larger every eleven years of so, marking maximum solar flare activity.

In some ways, studying the effects of cosmic radiation was like trying to determine the effects of longterm weightlessness. It was impossible to simulate such space conditions on earth. But there

257

were experiments along those lines. During the period 1958 to 1962, six artificial radiation belts were produced by the United States and three by the U.S.S.R. by exploding nuclear fission bombs at high altitudes. Radioactive fission products injected into the magnetic field created a temporarily trapped population of charged particles. The most intense, produced by the U.S. in 1962, was known as Starfish. This was a hydrogen bomb with the equivalent of about 1,500,000 tons of dynamite, exploded at an altitude of 250 miles over the Pacific Ocean. It produced an intense radiation belt at an altitude ranging from 1,800 to about 3,600 miles, in the plane of the equator. A spacecraft flying through that radioactive belt would have encountered a dosage of from 5 to 50 rad. Most of the injected electrons disappeared within a year but there were some traces five years later. Such tests are now forbidden by international agreement.

The possibility of trapping, or confinement, of electrically charged particles in the external magnetic field of the earth was first shown theoretically by the Norwegian mathematician Carl Stoermer in 1907. He had become fascinated by the aurora borealis and actually produced similar effects in his tiny laboratory.

The existence of two bands of trapped radiation was discovered in 1958 after the satellite Explorer I, sent into orbit by the Army, carried Geiger counters into the exosphere where they detected "hits" from particles before they were absorbed or thinned out by the lower atmosphere.

These hits were then broadcast as radio signals, taped at a ground station, transformed into an oscilloscope trace, and "read" by Van Allen and other experts. The "hit" line was then plotted against the orbit of the satellite, which had an apogee of 1,500 miles and perigee of 114 miles. As the satellite increased altitude, the signals from the detector showed an increase in the number of particles hitting it. But instead of the increase continuing as the satellite got further away from earth, the detector registered practically nothing at all. Then, when it swung towards earth again, the count rose as if it had never been interrupted.

Scientists had been certain that as a spacecraft moved deeper into space, it would encounter more radiation paricles. But the instruments indicated either that the scientists were wrong, or else the instruments were faulty. They did not produce the results anticipated.

Convinced that heavy radiation did exist at those extreme distances, Dr. Van Allen decided that perhaps the radiation was so intense that the instruments then in use were incapable of measuring it. The team went to work, and put two detectors on the next satellite sent into orbit. One instrument, such as used in the first test, monitored low-order radiation, while a newly designed instrument with much greater capacity was used to monitor radiation of very high order.

The men anxiously followed the satellite's course as the low-powered detector faithfully recorded particles, but suddenly at a certain distance, the counters jammed. The second instrument took over. Although most of the particles were absorbed by the protective lead coverings of the counters, scientists could still judge that there was far more radiation in nearby space than anyone had known before.

American and Soviet satellites made hundreds of orbits to gather information about the radiation belts. The first living creatures to penetrate that mysterious region were three black mice named Sally, Amy, and Moe (quite obviously on the staff of the School of Aviation Medicine) who rode an Atlas nose cone 700 miles into space on 13 October 1960. They returned to earth safely after experiencing the fringe radiation for a very short period.

Experts soon learned that there are two belts of charged particles circling the earth. The inner belt starts as low as 300 miles above the surface in some places, and reaches out from about 2,000 to 4,000 miles in the same doughnut shaped magnetic field that holds the particles in its grasp. The trapped particles are mostly protons and high energy electrons, a significant part of which were, at the time, debris from the high-altitude tests of nuclear weapons.

Before the outer belt starts, about 12,000 miles out, there is a gap called the slot in which there are fewer particles, mostly electrons. The outer radiation belt extends almost to the edge of the magnetosphere, some 40,000 miles from earth.

In 1961, Explorer 12 showed that there are two quite distinct regions in the outer belts. The section farthest from earth has only a few electrons but these few are moving much faster than those in the nearer part and have more energy than they could have received from the sun. It is now believed that such particles are of extra-galactic origin.

Being toroidal (doughnut shaped), the Van Allen belts are thickest on the plane of the equator and nearly non-existent in the "funnels" of the magnetic north and south poles. The safest way for a spacecraft to navigate through them is to remain below the inner belt while in earth orbit, then to escape as quickly as possible to space through the area of low-radiation intensity near the poles, and, when possible, keeping clear of the South Atlantic Anomaly, an area of unusually intense radiation which draws particles closer to earth than any other region.

An isodose profile of the earth's surface from latitude 80 north to 80 south shows that in general, from 40 degrees north to 40 degrees south, the reading fluctuates from 5 to 10. It gets no higher anywhere in the northern hemishpere, but in the ocean area between Cape Horn and the Cape of Good Hope, it reaches 20, and along the prime meridian, at about 60 degrees south latitude, it reaches a reading of 40. And, although the extent of the Van Allen belt is known, and the location of the South Atlantic Anomaly has been definitely charted, it is impossible for a spacecraft to avoid flying through it.

The Apollo spacecraft, flying trajectories inclined 50° from the equator, each made approximately five traverses through the anomaly every 24 hours, and absorbed dosages of from 156 to 600mrads, except for Apollo 14 which absorbed 1142mrads. That mission received the largest dosage experienced on any manned flight to that date, presumably because the outward bound trajectory of the craft took it through the heart of the trapped radiation belts. As solar flares were at a minimum then, the dosage was largely due to relatively higher cosmic ray activity.

By contrast, the earlier Russian spacecraft flew at an inclination of 65 degrees to the equator, and received much lighter doses of radiation, ranging from a low of 2.0mrads to a high of 80.

On all Apollo missions, each crew member carried a personal radiation dosimeter, which monitored the overall radiation as the mission progressed. In addition, they wore passive dosimeters at the ankle, thigh, and chest areas.

Once a spacecraft leaves the earth's geomagnetic field, it encounters more intense and frequent particulate radiation than would ever occur on earth, because the earth's magnetic field and atmospheric envelope protects it from most of such radiation. Exposure to such radiation results in various effects; changes in the blood render men more susceptible to disease; ionizing radiations can cause injury to the lenses of their eyes; their reproductive systems can be damaged and in extreme cases complete sterility could result. Besides the radiation from solar or galactic sources, there is also artificially produced radiation, originating in the radioluminescent panels of the spacecraft.

Because a spacecraft passes through the Van Allen belt in only a few moments, both going and coming, any cosmic radiation observations by astronauts must be limited in scope. But on the earth, a constant space radiation surveillance network has been arranged by NASA. It is manned by experts who have a thorough knowledge of space radiation, who can recognize any sudden change in radiation activity, and who can recommend necessary preventive measures.

Despite all the research on cosmic radiation, no one yet knows where it originates; a considered opinion is that such radiation comes from extra-galactic space, perhaps from the explosion of novas in the distant past. There is also the problem of solar-particle radiation—subatomic particles thrown into space by a solar flare at such speeds that they reach the earth in about eight minutes. Exact forecasting of such radiation storms is not yet possible, although statistical prediction is possible, based on the sunspot cycle.

For spaceflights, NASA provides the astronauts with estimates of particle dose and visual or radio frequency confirmation. In addition, there are solar monitoring stations; the Solar Particle Alert Network (SPAN) made up of three multiple-frequency radio telescopes and seven optical telescopes. SPAN provides information to NASA as to the severity of solar-particle events so that the astronauts can take appropriate action to protect themselves. But the Apollo Command Module was so well shielded that even when the largest solar-particle display on record occurred, on 4-9 August 1972, there would not have been any concern for the safety of the astronauts or spacecraft.

For the first time, whole-body counting and neutron-resonant foil were used for measuring neutron doses. And although neutron doses are less than anticipated, these measuring methods will be kept for later space missions.

Long-term exposure to cosmic radiation has not, of course, been experienced by men, nor biological specimens. In *Bioscience* in 1968, R. S. Young and J. W. Tremor described an experiment in which frog eggs were fertilized in space under zero g conditions because such eggs respond to disorientation of normal gravity by abnormal development. However, the eggs that did develop were normal in all respects, indicating that the low level of cosmic radiation reaching earth at that particular time apparently had no effect on them.

So far, the only living proof that cosmic rays, at least in limited quantities, have no effect on the human system is the first child (now a teen-age girl) born to parents who had both been in space. Her father, Andrian G. Nikolayev, a colonel in the Russian air force, made 64 orbits of the earth in Vostok 3 in 1962. Her mother, the only woman to have flown in space, was Valentina Tereshkova, who made 48 orbits of the earth in Vostok 6 in 1963. The two cosmonauts were married later that year and in 1964 became parents of a perfectly normal baby girl.

The problem of protecting space voyagers against cosmic radiation was recognized long before man was able to reach the most hazardous zones. Laboratory animals and insects, riding in rocket nose cones, and in high-altitude balloons, were exposed to limited radiation, but at the most, no more than a few minutes in rockets, several hours in balloons. A few mice returned to earth with gray hairs, the result of cosmic radiation, but none were exposed sufficiently long to furnish scientifically satisfying results. As men began to explore the upper limits of atmosphere they were exposed to radiation for very short periods. Orbital flights subjected them to longer periods of radiation. Even after the longest space missions to date, in Skylab and Salyut 6, no ill effects have resulted from radiation exposure which must be, considering the possibilities, of limited value.

Careful evaluation of radiation hazards involved on missions lasting months or years, however, must take in several

Radiation terms and measures

Roentgen—The basic indicator of quanity of radiation. Specifically, that amount of radiation required to produce 0.001293 grams of air ions carrying one electrostatic unit of either positive or negative electricity.

Rad—Radiation absorbed dose. Most common measure of exposure; one rad = absorption of 100 ergs per gram of any medium.

Rem—Roentgen equivalent, man. This refers to the absorbed dose of any ionizing radiation which produces the same biological effects in man as those resulting from the absorption of 1 roentgen.

considerations: length of mission, type of radiation, and amount of exposure. The next consideration is the calculation of levels of effective dose an astronaut might receive, balanced against the allowable dose levels. In a paper presented at the fifteenth meeting of COSPAR in Berlin in 1973, it was stated that a flight of one year would result in absorbed dose of 100rads; 2 years, 200rads; and 3 years, 300rads. For the longer period, the effective dose at the end of the flight was estimated to be 142.5rads.

As to permissible dose levels, estimates vary. The Russians calculate the allowable dose for flight up to 30 days in length as 15rem, with 125rem being considered critical. For long term spaceflights preliminary estimates of maximum allowable dosage are: for 1 year, 200rem; for 2 years, 250 rem; for 3 years, 275rem. Yet other estimates consider a dose of 300rads per year of flight permissible. Behind all such estimates, there is the sobering thought that eventualities could create a vast difference between estimate and actuality—by which time it would be too late to go back to the computer for a new printout.

Protection against radiation presents intensely complex problems, and can be achieved only through equally complex solutions.* In a planetary mission, astronauts would be exposed to

*The essence of the discussion on this subject is derived from a 98-page paper published in Moscow in 1973 by R. P. Saksanov, of the Institute of Biomedical Problems, Ministry of Health. The title translates as "Protection Against Radiation (Biological, Pharmacological, Chemical, Physical).,,

Short-term effects from acute whole-body radiation

Dose (rads)	Probable effect
10-50	Probable minor blood changes.
50-100	Vomiting and nausea for about a day; fatigue, but no serious disability.
100-200	Vomiting and nausea for about a day; 50 per cent reduction in white blood corpuscles.
200-350	Vomiting, nausea, loss of appetite, diarrhea, minor hemorrhage. About 20 per cent deaths in 2-6 weeks.
350-550	Same as above, with about 50 per cents deaths within 30 days
550-750	Vomiting and nausea within 4 hours in 100 per cent o personnel; up to 100 per cent deaths; few survivors convalescen for about 6 months.
1000	Vomiting and nausea, all personnel, within 1-2 hours; 100 pe. cent deaths within days.
5000	Incapacitation within minutes, to hours. Total fatalities within week.

radiation in the inner Van Allen belt, proton fluxes from solar flares, and galactic cosmic radiation. Physical protection against radiation would involve passive protection—shielding by structural components of the spacecraft—and active protection—either electrical or magnetic fields set up about the spacecraft to deflect charged particles away from the crew quarters.

Physical protection has proved successful so far in American and Russian spaceflights, but they are still of short duration. Also, early orbital flights were at comparatively low altitudes—below 115 miles. Solar flares could have caused problems at higher altitudes because shielding was limited.

A spacecraft, to have ideal physical protection from radiation, should have a shield with the effective density of earth atmosphere and of the same magnetic field as that around the earth at the equator. But to achieve this in a spacecraft, instead of using the 600-mile-deep atmospheric layer, would require either a water barrier 10 meters thick or a solid lead shield a meter thick. Any such shield would weigh hundreds of tons and no rocket could lift it.

Active protection against radiation, either in the form of

electrical or magnetic fields, is possible with current technology, but so far no actual systems have been developed. The advantage in active protection, as compared with passive protection, is that the weight involved should be about a hundred times less.

Biologic protection against radiation might be required in certain unfavorable radiation situations, such as strong radioactive chromosphere flares on the sun, extended exposure in the inner Van Allen belt, or flight through an artifical radiation belt. Among the most effective substances are liquid extracts of such plants as ginseng (once considered an effective aphrodisiac by the Chinese) and Chinese magnolia vine, and certain vitamin complexes. Russian experimenters have also used bone marrow in treating radiation sickness, and it has been suggested by Professor J. F. Thomson that for spaceflights, specimens of bone marrow be taken from each astronaut, frozen in glycerin, and replaced in the event of exposure to radiation.

Before man went into space, many of the world's most respected scientists thought that cosmic radiation would be the killing factor that would prevent space exploration, and keep him earthbound. The successful completion of the Apollo flights proved that radiation was not an operational problem. Dosages experienced were within acceptable limits; there were no major solar-particle events during the entire program. Some minor radiation was detected by a sensor outside Apollo 12, but there was no increase in radiation exposure to the crew members inside the craft.

Of course, solar flares are random events, unpredictable, and it is always possible that such flares, with their accompanying high-energy nuclear particles, might hinder future flights beyond the magnetosphere of the earth. Obviously, the monitoring of cosmic radiation will be increasingly critical as missions become longer. Constant monitoring of sun-spot cycle activity, during any planetary mission, will be necessary in order that scientists may predict solar flares in sufficient time to allow astronauts in space to take such measures—active, passive, or biological—as developing techniques may have made possible by that time.

Despite the invisible threat of cosmic radiation, man has moved into space. Space shuttles will soon be hauling scientific and technical personnel into the sky to continue the research that made it possible for them to work in space. That "first small step" was only the first of many larger ones.

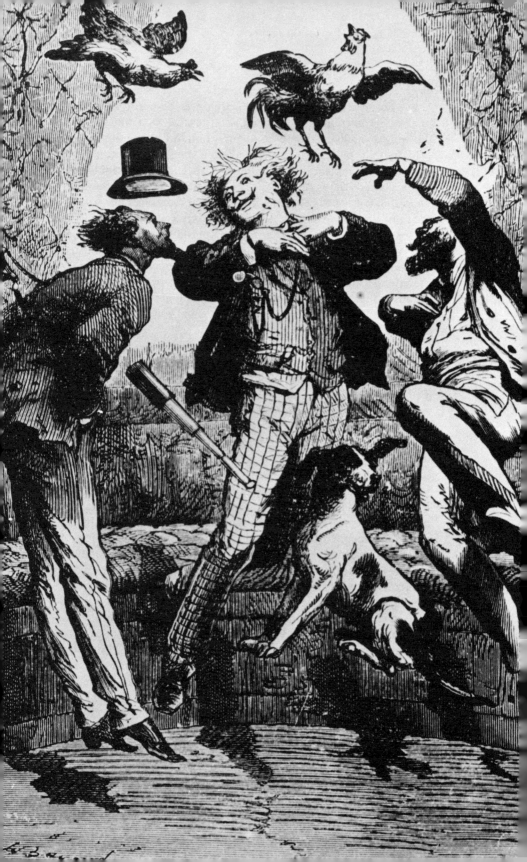

10
Up's the Other Way from Down

From the very beginning of terrestrial life, when one-celled creatures swam in the primeval seas, until the crew of Apollo 8 left the earth behind on man's first flight to the moon, everything on earth has been subject to the unseen and mysterious force of gravity. Man evolved in a constant gravity, and every moment of life is affected by gravity, but most people are aware of it only when they step on the bathroom scales.

The force of gravity is immutable, measurable, and exactly determinable—Newton's apple, a high punt in the Rose Bowl, or the proverbial ton of bricks, all fall to the surface of the earth at exactly the same initial velocity--32.2 feet per second.

Yet the same force that totals a breakfast egg all over the floor just one-tenth of a second after it rolls off the kitchen counter reaches out to the remote rim of the solar system, nearly four billion miles into space, to keep the planet Pluto swinging in its vast orbit, around the sun once in every 284 years.

Jules Verne anticipated some of the problems of spaceflight in his science fiction novel, *From the Earth to the Moon*, published in 1865. This illustration from the first edition of his book depicts his happy adventurers enjoying the freedom of weightlessness/*NASA*

As gravity has affected all human development, the mysterious force has been the subject of speculation and experiment by philosophers, astronomers and scientists for many centuries. The Greek astronomer, Aristarchus, about 300 BC, concluded that the planets revolved around the sun, as if held on invisible leashes. He was right—the leash is gravity, and it holds the solar system together. A clear understanding of how the solar system was put together, with the sun at the center (in marked disagreement with the time-worn Ptolemic theory of a universe centered on the earth) was reached about 1530 by the Polish mathematician Nicholaus Copernicus. His findings were published the year of his death, and set off a fifty-year argument involving theologians and theoreticians—at least one Roman philosopher, Giordano Bruno, was burned at the stake for insisting that Copernicus, not Ptolemy, knew what he was talking about.

Then, in 1609, Galileo Galilei of Padua, using a rude telescope copied after that invented by Hans Lippersheim of Holland, was amazed to see in the sky a miniature example of how Copernicus believed the solar system to be. Jupiter had four moons that were held in orbit around the planet by gravity.

A few years later Johannes Kepler published his famous three laws of planetary motion. These laws were then refined by the English mathematician, Isaac Newton, who first developed the theory of artificial satellites. Newton's work began with his realization that the same force that pulled a falling apple to the earth was that which kept the moon in orbit around the earth, and from his concept of gravitation an entire new science developed. Newton deduced that if a falling object had a known speed and force, an equal speed and force would be sufficient to propel it away from the earth and into space. Newton could compute the velocity required to put a satellite in orbit* but in his time, when the fastest speeds known—1,100 feet per second—were obtainable only by cannon balls, no scientist could conceive of anything that might go fast enough to leave the earth.

---

*At an altitude of 100 miles, a spacecraft must maintain a velocity of 25,000 feet per second to stay in earth orbit. It must accelerate to 35,000 feet per second to escape from orbit and move into space.

But man could dream of going to the moon long before there was ever any prospect of leaving the surface of the earth, and imaginative people described fantastic voyages into space from the comfort and safety of their studies. Serious thought about the problems of spaceflight were spurred by the advent of balloon flight, and in 1895 Konstantin Tsiolkovsky, a Russian high school teacher who was to acquire fame as the father of spaceflight, predicted the conditions to confront man in space: "We shall not have weight, only mass. We can hold any mass in our hands without experiencing the slightest weight...Man does not press himself against anything and nothing presses against him...There is no top or bottom."

Tsiolkovsky also predicted loss of spatial orientation and changes in motor and sensory functions in space, differences in blood distribution, and anatomical changes in the human body. Although he assumed that man would eventually adapt to weightlessness, he suggested that spaceships rotate in order to produce artificial gravity. The same idea was expressed later by Hermann Oberth, who commenced rocket research in Vienna just before World War II, in discussing the effects of zero-G on man during interplanetary flight: "If the prolonged state of lack of appression should have undesirable consequences, which seems doubtful, however, two such vehicles could be connected by cables a few kilometers long and rotated about each other." Oberth recognized the possible adverse affects of Coriolis forces produced in such an arrangement, even before it was investigated under laboratory conditions.

When post World War II technology made supersonic speeds possible, there was increased conjecture as to the effects on the human body when men were finally able to travel outside of the earth's gravitational field and become weightless. No human had ever experienced true weightlessness, so scientists could only guess. Would there be hallucinations, euphoria, or impaired psychomotor performance? What about bodily functions such as heartbeat, respiration, digestion, elimination, sight balance and orientation? Some scientists predicted death due to failure of the circulatory system; others insisted that man probably could not swallow.

269

Actually weightlessness was first experienced during World War II when German fighter planes made high-speed attacks on Allied bomber formations. They dove from high altitudes, made violent pull-ups for a firing run, then made steep dives as an evasive tactic. The pilots felt a high positive g on the pull-up and weightlessness during the pushover into the evasive dive. They later reported disturbed vision and weakness in their legs, plus insecure control movements during weightlessness. But after becoming accustomed to these maneuvers, some pilots said it was actually a pleasant flying experience. When German doctors looked into the phenomenon, Dr. Heinz von Diringshofen, Professor of Aviation Medicine in Berlin, noticed his legs were weak and his hand movements insecure, but once he got used to it, he too rather enjoyed the experience. However, when Dr. Hubertus Strughold, "flying by the seat of his pants," anesthetized his buttocks with novocaine before doing the parabola, he found it was decidedly unpleasant.

Although most conditions to which man is subjected in space can be reproduced in laboratories, there is no way on earth to create a long-time gravity-free environment. *Increased* gravity is simulated in a centrifuge but there is no such "negative centrifuge" that can diminish the pull of gravity and its action on the human body. Actually, weightlessness is not produced by lack of gravity but by a particular kind of motion in a gravitational field. Gravity draws all objects toward the center of the earth, and the measure of attraction between any object and the earth is stated as its weight.

A parachutist is not weightless during descent because air fills the parachute and restricts his downward motion. He would not experience weightlessness even in a fall without a parachute because of the air resistance any falling body encounters. Efforts to achieve weightlessness by dropping down deep mine shafts or elevators failed for the same reason.

Space scientists the world over were fascinated by the challenge of what appeared to be an insurmountable problem. As early as 1946, doctors at the Aeromedical Center in Heidelberg, Germany, held a seminar to discuss "Man under Weightless Conditions." Much interest centered around the already established clinical findings that bedrest patients undergo major physiological changes because they have been exposed to a transverse 1g environment. In other words, the gravitational attraction of the earth was directed perpendicular to the long axis of the patients' bodies. The result was that all the adaptive and reflex mechanisms suffered, and when they were put in a vertical position (a vertical 1g) there were circulatory problems and sometimes fainting. In 1946, Doctors J. E. Dietrick, G. D. Whedon and E. Shorr published a paper on their experiences with normal volunteer test subjects whose pelvic girdle and legs were immobilized by casts. Even after only 10 days' confinement there was significant deterioration; circulatory weakening, muscle wasting, loss of muscle tone, demineralization and nitrogen loss were observed. From the clinician's point of view, this meant that surgery patients ought to be on their feet sometimes within hours after their operations. For space researchers it reaffirmed troubles to be contended with in sub-gravity conditions.

Immediately after World War II, during the high-altitude rocket flights with small animals as test subjects, some preliminary data were collected. Then in 1950, German scientists Fritz and Heinz Haber, who had come to the U.S. via "Operation Paperclip," delivered a paper in which they explained how to achieve over 30 seconds of sub-gravity in aircraft flights. It required the aircraft to fly a parabolic arc, or Keplerian trajectory, in which the centrifugal force offsets the downward pull of gravity and the engine thrust counterbalances air friction. To fly a Keplerian trajectory, the pilot performs a special pushover maneuver in which he holds the needle of his accelerometer at the zero mark, goes over the top of the curve and speeds down, very much like a carnival roller-coaster.

Several prominent American test pilots flew Keplerian trajectories in 1951; Scott Crossfield made some 30 flights in an F-84, experiencing weightlessness for from 15 to 40 seconds. He first reported "befuddlement" during the transition but after his fifth flight he could handle it well. He had no sensation of falling and no loss of muscle coordination other than a tendency to over-reach with his arm; there was some vertigo on the pull-up after a run. Dr. E. R. Ballinger of the Wright Air Development Center experimented with several test subjects who reported sensations similar to Crossfield's but added that if they had been blindfolded and not restrained in their seats, they would have been severely disoriented. Major Charles "Chuck" Yeager, at the end of 15 seconds of weightlessness became "lost in space" but with returning weight, his orientation was restored.

Little by little, data were gathered that revealed the effects of sub-gravity on various organs and systems of the body. Dr. Harald von Beckh, who had left Germany for Argentina shortly after the war, experimented with South American water turtles. He found a turtle whose vestibular function had been injured accidentally, tested it on a sub-gravity parabola and found it was better coordinated and oriented than its normal companions; it learned to compensate visually for lack of normal gravitational cues. Von Beckh also tested human volunteers in a series of eye-hand coordination tests on sub-gravity flights and learned that the tendency to overreaching was reduced with practice.

Dr. James Henry of the Aeromedical Laboratory at Wright-Patterson Air Force Base studied the behavior of mice in weightlessness.* Photographs showed the animals virtually floating through space. Then on returning to normal gravity, they behaved in their usual way. The following year, Dr. Henry, and Air Force officers Captain E. R. Ballinger, Major P. J. Maher, and Major D. G. Simons, published more encouraging data. They used anesthetized primates in seven rocket flights during which sub-gravity lasted from two to three minutes. The animals' pulse, respiration, electrocardiogram and arterial and venous pressures were telemetered to earth during the journey, leading the doctors to conclude, "...there is no evidence of a significant disturbance of the cardiovascular or respiratory systems..."

On 1 July 1955, Captain Grover J. D. Schock, the first scientist to receive a Ph.D. in space physiology, was assigned as task scientist at Holloman Air Force Base where he made many sub-gravity flights in the F-94C aircraft. These aircraft fly a sub-gravity trajectory of more than 30 seconds and more than one trajectory or "run" could be scheduled for a single flight—a considerable advantage during that very economy-minded era before the "race for space" created unlimited budgets. There

*Journal of Aviation Medicine, October 1952: "Animal Studies of the Subgravity State during Rocket Flights,"

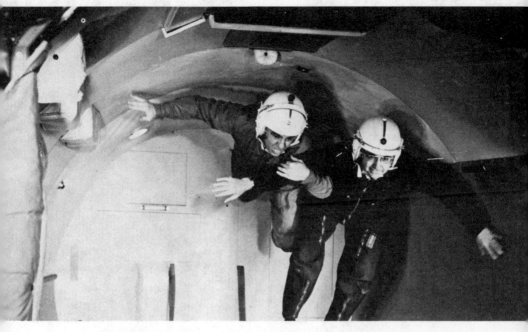

Major General Oliver K. Niess, (left) Air Force Surgeon General, and Colonel John Paul Stapp experienced weightlessness in a parabolic flight of a C-131. Both doctors fared well during the 15 seconds of zero gravity./*U.S. Air Force*

were improvements, too, in flight techniques and test instrumentation. Captain Schock devised a golf ball gadget which dangled on a string in the cockpit to show when pure weightlessness had been achieved. They later developed a combination of differently placed accelerometers which instantly relayed information to the aircraft pilot.

Nevertheless, all was not smooth flying for the experimenters. Problems with loss of oil pressure, hydraulic fluid and "sticking" of the trim tab motor, along with the presence of extra equipment mounted inside the aircraft, made the flights worrisome from a flight safety standpoint.

There was difficulty with the standard microphones in the F-94 and earlier in the F-89 because clear messages could not be transmitted between the pilot and test subjects. With research and

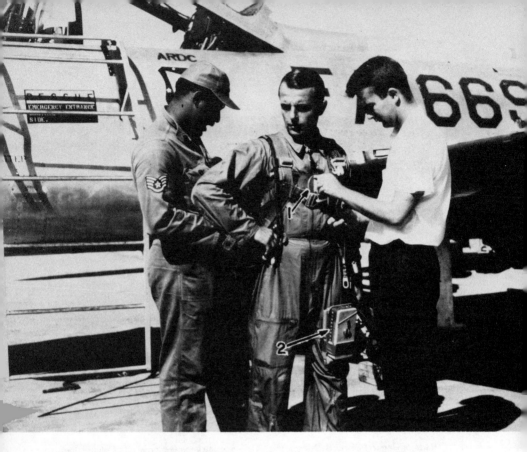

Many types of aircraft flew Keplerian trajectories to study the effects of weightlessness. Shown here is Dr. Harald von Beckh as he prepared for a F94C flight. He was able to prove that tolerance to G loads decreased after exposure to weightlessness./*U.S. Air Force*

the installation of a more satisfactory microphone, Captain Schock could safely say, "Voice communications in future space vehicles should present no problem."

Some test subjects actually enjoyed the gravity-free state. Dr. William Douglas who later became the personal physician to the Original Seven astronauts and went through the selection and training process with them loved the zero g state. "My heavens, the most thrilling experience of my life is to get in the back of a big old KC-135 and be at the rear of this tremendous long fuselage and have it push over into a weightlessness parabola and just literally float, fly from one end of that thing to the other. It's the most exhilarating experience you can imagine. That's only for 30

274

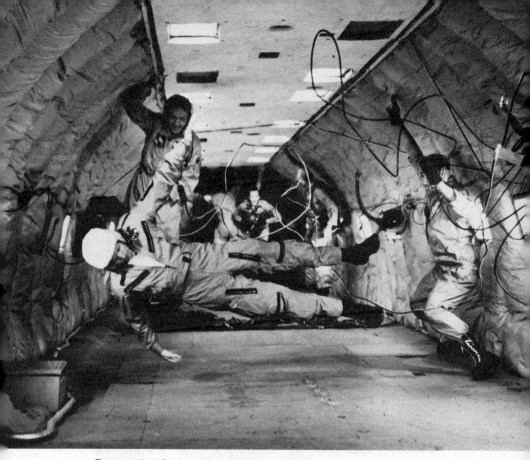

Everyone had fun but the pilot when a plane pushed over into a weightlessness parabola. "...the most thrilling experience of my life," Dr. William Douglas called it./*NASA*

seconds or so, but if you multiply that by hours, what a glorious experience that must be."

But there were other test subjects who had nausea and vomiting. Those who had little or no difficulty were invariably experienced test pilots. The conclusion could then be drawn that with the apparent wide variations in human tolerance, one criterian for the selection of space crews ought to be a comparison of monitored responses during sub-gravity flights. But at that time, more definite information on pilot reaction was needed. Could the discomfort have to do with high acceleration and deceleration during the plane's entry to and exit from the parabola? And how much more than 30 seconds could the experienced subjects endure?

The flights made at Holloman Air Force Base had a variety of sensorimotor performance tests which indicated a subject would have little difficulty in touching his nose with a fingertip or marking Xs in a row of squares—if he hadn't been sick, that is, and if he had a visual frame of reference. Eating peanut brittle during weightlessness was also possible so long as it was chewed and forced to the back of the mouth where the swallowing reflex went into action. Drinking required a squeeze bottle, with the water being forced to the back of the mouth by the tongue.

By mid-1958, almost 100 people had participated in experiments on the effects of weightlessness. Dr. Gerathewohl, working in the program, also did extensive experiments on the labyrinth righting reflex of cats during the trajectories, as did Captain Schock.

Although many weightlessness worries were dispelled during this period, there was still serious concern about the effects of long-term exposure to spaceflight; the progressive deterioration of gravity-compensating muscles, bones and circulatory reflexes when the pervasive influence of gravity was no longer present. A major threat appeared to be man's ability to safely return to normal gravity following prolonged zero g exposure, especially with the high g decelerative stresses and the demand for functional effectiveness during recovery.

What was needed now was research to study this adaptive process, define its elements and ultimately develop protective measures to counteract zero g adaptation. Questions such as, would space travelers wind up with jelly bones and be unable to stand upright even temporarily after return to earth, bothered just about everyone. According to Dr. Hamilton Webb, the continual fight against gravity takes an enormous amount of energy. "The g force must be opposed with an equal and opposite muscular force, and it has been estimated that of man's total energy production, one-third is utilized for this."*

Hoping to solve the mystery of no weight in space before man actually got there, experimenters simulated zero g with ground-based procedures. Dr. Duane Graveline (later to be named as scientist-astronaut with the fourth group of NASA astronauts)

*"Speculation of Space and Destiny," From *Human Factors in Jet and Space Travel*, ed. S. B. Sells, Ph.D., and Charles A. Berry, M.D., The Ronald Press Co., New York.

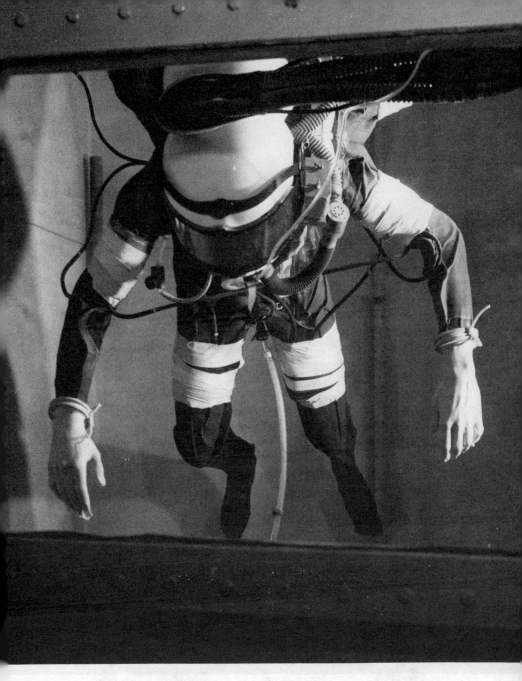

No frogman, Dr. Duane Graveline suited himself up as a test subject for water immersion experiments to study various physiological effects of this simulated weightlessness./*Duane Graveline*

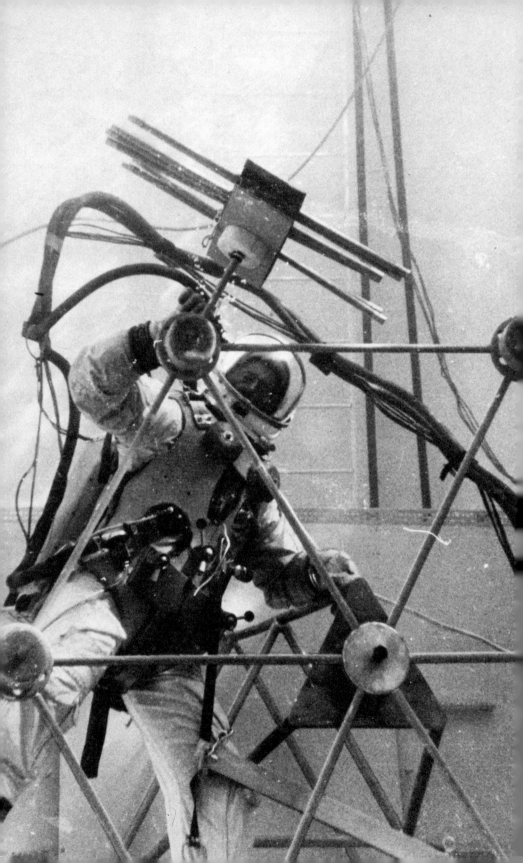

studied four healthy male volunteers in a two-week bedrest deconditioning experiment. He recorded a loss of gravity compensating mechanisms, particularly in the cardiovascular and musculoskeletal systems, as evidenced by impaired performances on tilt table and treadmill testing.

But what would happen without the strict immobilization of bedrest? It was known that Italian doctors had experimented with water immersion, keeping subjects who wore "wet" suits dunked in water for various lengths of time. Dr. Graveline decided to use himself as a subject in a week-long water immersion experiment to study body fluid redistribution, hematological and biochemical changes, ability to stand upright, tolerate g stress on the centrifuge and work on the treadmill. Although recognizing the possible experimental bias induced by altered thermal balance in the water, and the possible alteration of breathing mechanics induced by immersion, Dr. Gaveline noted that the changes were identical to those previously observed in bedrest experiments. Even so, after a full week of water immersion which robbed him of substantial functional capacity, he could still undergo rigorous testing on the centrifuge and the treadmill.

Dr. Graveline was a strong proponent of using water immersion for this kind of research, the reason being that hydrostatic pressures in the body, particularly those of the cardiovascular system were neutralized. Also, research subjects could remain reasonably active and assume any body position they wanted, as would be the case in a true weightless state. The hydrostatic forces on the long columns of blood in the arteries and veins were thus nullified—an approximation of what was anticipated in a zero g condition.

Dr. Graveline spent two years further defining man's adaptive mechanisms, and developing possible counteractive measures. Elaborating on the oscillating bed principle to maintain cardio-vascular responsiveness despite prolonged bedrest, he developed the extremity tourniquet, later used on two Gemini flights. In these experiments, interconnected tourniquets placed around all

This technician simulates an astronaut performing EVA in the weightless environment of space while working under water. Weights attached to his body provide neutral buoyancy. A restraining line around his waist prevents him from floating away./*NASA* four extremities were periodically inflated enough to inter-mittently obstruct the return flow of blood to the heart, thus simulating the tendency for venous pooling which naturally occurs during standing in a normal gravity state. The scheme was highly effective in minimizing body fluid redistribution; test subjects' ability to withstand tilt table testing after the experiments were markedly improved.

In 1957, Captain Schock staged a series of experiments at the indoor pool of the El Paso YMCA with a blindfolded test subject in a rotating seat in eight feet of water. They also used the pool of the New Mexico School for the Visually Handicapped in Alamogordo. The idea was to measure orientation in weightlessness when visual cues were absent.

Many people were studying subgravity, one way or another. The School of Aviation Medicine had its program under the direction of Dr. Gerathewohl using jet parabolas, as were the Russians, who claimed weightlessness of 40 seconds. Researchers at the University of Illinois assisted Captain Schock's study of the vestibular mechanism in cats by performing the special operations on the animals. They also worked on techniques for attaching a recording device directly to the vestibular portion of the eighth cranial nerve.

The Yellow Springs Instrument Company developed an airborne galvanic skin resistance meter to continuously record resistance to electric impulses under subgravity conditions. The Cornell Aeronautical Laboratories made theoretical studies of animal experiments that might be performed both in existing test vehicles and in more advanced vehicles yet to come.

American scientists were progressing quite well in spite of budget problems. Many doctors look back on that period as being one of the most exciting of all because *everything* was new and each question had to have an answer squeezed out of it. Doctors Rufus Hessberg and Stanley White both agree, however, that it was a step-at-a-time process, that the building blocks were being stacked up little by little. But many of these projects had to be worked on furtively, buried in an acceptable terminology or they might be cancelled from "above." "Silly time at the Pentagon," they called it. Finally, a directive issued on 27 August 1957 ordered "cessation of work," effective immediately. "Cessation,"

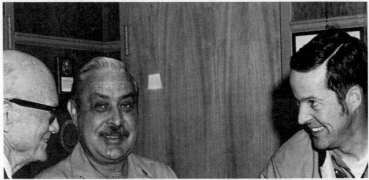

Pioneers in aerospace medical research: Captain Ashton Graybiel, (MC) USN (Ret.) (left) still heads the research laboratory in Pensacola as a civilian, Captain Robert C. McDonough, USN, was head of the Naval Aerospace Medical Institute at Pensacola, Captain Joseph Kerwin (MC) USN, (right) is the first American physician to go into space./*U.S. Navy*

of course meant stopping any work that involved money such as the F-94C parabola flights, which cost $63 an hour. This left Captain Schock having to content himself with tossing cats around in the laboratory—and going swimming. Then came the headlines that announced the beginning of the space age. Russia launched Sputnik, and the U.S. ended budgetary restrictions on the space program. The word was, "go!" but the time lost could never be wholly regained.

Investigations became more detailed as scientists looked into the effects of weightlessness on the larger of the two saclike cavities in the membranous labyrinth of the inner ear—the utricular mechanisms. Explored too, were the possible loss of reflexes and problems of prolonged sensory deprivation (true weightlessness could be considered a sensory-starved environment). And "motion sickness" somehow had to be tied down etiologically. Was it autonomically controlled or psychologically induced? There were also the effects of launch accelerations and re-entry deceleration to be explored.

A critical need at this time was a means of measuring the astronaut's cardiovascular adaptive change while still in space. Dr. Graveline, along with co-workers at the Air Force School of Aerospace Medicine developed the prototype for a lower body negative pressure (LBNP) device. This technique, which simulated standing erect, isolated the lower half of the body from the waist down; varying degrees of negative pressure were then induced. Observers could note any serious changes in the astronaut's cardiovascular capacity, particularly those that might compromise his ability to tolerate recovery stresses. Such a device could conceivably be incorporated into a sleeping chamber; properly designed it could be used long enough during a 24-hour period to offer significant protection. Exercise devices, both isometric and isotonic, also had to be developed and readied for inflight use.

At this time, and on the basis of these and many other similar experiments done by others, Dr. Graveline was able to say, "The great bulk of information currently available to us indicates that for long-term exposure to orbital situations, adequate artificial gravity will be highly desirable, if not mandatory. For intermediate exposure, relatively simple countermeasures may be adequate. For short-term exposures, no special consideration appears necessary."

By the time the Gemini and Apollo flights were scheduled, Dr. Berry had enough data to proceed cautiously, subjecting astronauts to subgravity conditions in step-by-step increments. It was seen, for example, that man could be exposed for 90 hours, so doubling that time was the next logical step. Even when the heart no longer had to battle 1g force as it does on earth, exposure to re-entry deceleration proved to be no problem; the astronauts readapted to earth's gravity quickly with no permanent physiological damage. Within two or three days they were as good as new.

One extremely important pre-Apollo flight was that made by Gemini 7, which lasted two weeks. It was designed to be enough longer than a trip to the moon to provide a reassuring safety factor, and as astronaut Michael Collins would later say, "a medical orgy of experimentation..."

In his book, *Carrying the Fire,* Collins devoted several pages to his opinions of what he considered medical highjinks, objecting to the situation that allowed someone on the ground to determine whether the astronauts were ready to perform. This, he maintained, required "decisions to be made by the wrong people (the medics), in the wrong place (the ground) with the wrong information (brainwaves)." Said Collins: "If a simple thing like taking a pee requires twenty steps, consider what might be involved in complying with the whole array of Gemini medical experiments.'' To be exact, there were seven of them, plus a near dozen scientific, technical, or military experiments to be carried out, and some did take considerable time.

Certain medical experiments, set up to determine the effects of weightlessness, required compilation of data taken before, during, and after flight. Astronauts in Gemini 5 and Gemini 7 wore inflatable rubber thigh cuffs designed to squeeze the thighs in a crude imitation of gravity. This was expected to stimulate the autonomic nervous system and to help readjust to normal on returning to earth. The only problem was, astronauts had no control over the devices—they were programmed to inflate automatically, at intervals, day and night, no matter what their wearer might be doing at that time.

In order to study calcium balance, the medical experimenters controled the astronauts' intake of food and liquid for several weeks before a flight. They measured, not only what the men ate and drank but their leftover food and drink as well. They also measured the output—feces, perspiration and urine—which required astronauts to turn in their sweaty underwear and dirty bathwater. For travel by commercial airlines, they carried ice cream containers and bottles in special attache cases for their personal use.

One particular experiment, which Collins insisted would "infuriate any crew," was a research program to determine whether an electroencephalogram of electrical activity of the brain could provide the medics with information on the astronauts sleep-wakefulness cycle, alertness, and readiness to carry out their duties. It required the subject to wear electrodes fastened to shaved spots on his skull, along with wires and electronic amplifiers, in what was at best a complicated situation. This, Collins maintained, was a classic case of the tail wagging the dog.

Although Collins was disenchanted with medical experiments*, it was quite obvious that the results of these experiments were

*Some of the early astronauts, primarily test pilots, wanted to *fly* and objected, not only to detailed medical examinations, but to extensive ground control during their missions. Later astronauts, with engineering or scientific backgrounds, were more receptive to such "interference."

urgently needed if the Apollo program was to proceed as scheduled. Dr. Berry recalls that he had to fight someone every step of the way: those who said he was too conservative and too cautious, and those who almost called him a murderer for sending men to certain death. But the astronauts would not have landed on the moon when they did, had it not been for the intensive work and data-gathering that made their achievement possible.

The effects of weightlessness are no longer the mystery they once were, although some problems remain to be solved. The dire consequences predicted—hallucinations, euphoria, and impaired psychomotor performances—never materialized. By taking certain precautions such as maintaining a controlled high potassium diet, carefully controlled work loads, and work-rest cycles, and having cardiology consultation service at hand, weightlessness can be tolerated longer than was thought possible. For example, the Apollo 15 astronauts worked on the lunar surface for 18½ hours, twice as long as those on the Apollo 14 flight. For the first time, however, irregular heartbeats were noted during lunar activity and on the return flight. Postflight, it took the men 13 days to return to normal, but the culprit wasn't zero-g. The reason they didn't bounce back was that they were simply exhausted; too much work, not enough rest, and insufficient potassium in their diet.

The Apollo 16 flight corrected the earlier conditions. There was a high potassium diet, along with the establishment of cardiology consultation, made possible by telemetry of electrocardiograms from space to earth-based specialists. Additional metabolic and cardiac data were collected preflight during simulation, for comparison with postflight results.

The Skylab missions provided a much broader base of information on prolonged weightlessness than did the Mercury, Gemini and Apollo projects. Those earlier spacecraft were so cramped for room the astronauts had little opportunity to become disoriented. But Skylab, with its relatively commondious accomodations, was another story. Some crew members fared better than others, but each mission added to the store of knowledge.

Skylab I carried the first American physician astronaut, Captain

Joe Kerwin (MC) U.S. Navy.* During the 28-day mission, he observed the weightless state both objectively and subjectively. On motion sickness, he said: "I liken it to a person going on an ocean cruise for the first time. He either gets his sea-legs promptly or not. In any event, 99 per cent of us adapt to that in a few days and press on. In our case, it took probably five minutes. Then going on through the mission, I had sort of briefed myself to look at five or six indicators that I thought would give me a clue as to how well we were wearing in the environment; were we really under stress? Were we showing it?"

"Number one is your individual feeling of well-being...as for the group, we exercise a lot and feel healthy. I found along about day six or seven (and so did my crewmates), that we had that feeling up there...I was waking up in the morning and feeling great. That's a subjective thing. We had objective measures too. Diet and hunger; are we taking on as much food as we thought we would? We are taking on more. Water intake, urine output, body weight. Is it being maintained, is there a loss, is the loss progressive? Based on inflight measurements, we did have a rather immediate loss and then we almost leveled off, plateaued." Once the crew learned to exercise in zero g, "it was fun, and we were able to do them with approximately the same physiological costs as we had on the ground."

Inflight, Kerwin observed that there is a constant feeling of fullness in the head which does not seem to be a matter of trapped secretions. "...I think it is a cardiovascular thing, a fullness of the blood vessels, all of them rather than an increase in venous pressure. Neck veins are always full and so forth." Dr. Kerwin noticed too, that the voice has a nasal twang, which he attributes to soft palate movement. And, "you have a strange kind of posture... you notice you are going around with your shoulders hunched. You notice Pete (Conrad) is going around with his hunched, and you look down and sure enough you are the same. You pull it down but it doesn't want to stay there. These anti-gravity muscles just relax and really power down. One of the most impressive things in doing

*The Soviets lay claim to the first medical doctor aboard a spacecraft. Dr. Boris G. Yegorov flew in Voskhod 1, 12 October 1964. He studied the condition of the cardiovascular and nervous systems of crew members.

285

the brief physical examinations I conducted was how soft, almost dough-soft, like a baby's arms, all the muscles of my crewmates were and my own, when they weren't using them. The abdominal muscles, the muscles of the upper extremities get flaccid when they are not in use." There was also a sluggish feeling—getting sleepy when he wasn't tired.

Pinpointing the long-term exposure further, a report prepared at the LBJ Space Center referred to "Anthropomorphic Changes," or more lightly termed, "the beanpole effect." Puffy faces, stuffy noses, engorged veins in the head, low back discomfort, and of all things, increased height, or, "bird leg."

One of the pilots on the Skylab 4 mission gained two inches in height, and lost four around his middle. Another, who was not quite so tall as his wife, grew just enough to change that situation, but on return to earth lost it all and a bit more besides. Heights change because of the reduced load on the spine due to loss of thoracolumbar curvature, and expansion of the intervertebral discs. The most immediate effect of sudden increase in height is that space suits and other essentially tailor-made gear will no longer fit.

There is also a marked change in body form, as reported by studies prepared at the Texas Institute for Rehabilitation and Research, and the LBJ Space Center. There was a reduction in the volume of abdomen, buttocks, calves, and somewhat less in the thighs. About a third of the loss was due to atrophy of leg muscles; the rest because of a deficit in body fluids.

Measurements of leg size made in the Apollo 16 crew showed postflight decreases in both calf and thigh, with volume decrements from 100 to 800 millimiters. These decrements persisted beyond seven days in the postflight period.

Such changes are not permanent; most men returned to normal in about 30 days, with much of the recovery made in the first four days after landing. All astronauts had relatively small losses in their arm volume as compared to legs; this was simply because there was more work for their hands and arms to do than for their legs, which, except for periodic conditioning exercises, got no effective loading.

Spaceflight, involving long periods of weightlessness, produces still other changes in the human body, the causes of which are as yet undefined. Among both American astronauts and Russian cosmonauts, there have been small but detectable changes in the musculoskeletal system in the form of slightly reduced bone optical density. Functional underloading of the skeletal muscles may be to blame, along with decreased energy expenditure during work or exercise.

And just to prove that biomedical science has not yet solved all its problems, studies of preflight and postflight blood volume of the Skylab astronauts, made at Baylor College of Medicine, showed that in all flights, all personnel experienced reduced red blood cell mass volume. The decrease in volume ranged from 3.5 to 5.0 per cent. There is, as yet, no explanation at all for this.

As for the vestibular system, Dr. Kerwin was amazed at their immunity to motion sickness. "We had an experiment designed to elicit motion sickness, to find out what our threshhold was. It had to do with getting into a rotating chair at a fixed rpm and making head movements which on the ground will elicit motion sickness in any individual unless he is a labyrinthian defective. We all know our thresholds very well. All I can say from the inflight experience is that physiologically we were labyrinthian defective up there. My own feeling is that the unloading of the gravity receptor, the otolith organ in the head, must inhibit the symptoms of motion sickness being elicited by rotation and head movement. You can feel vertigo. You can feel all the movements and motions of moving your head."

On return to earth, Dr. Kerwin's otolith was "back on," and he did experience motion sickness. "But all of us, motion sickness aside, felt that we were conscious of sensations which are normally unconscious, moving the head and changing one's posture back in the gravity environment was associated with very conscious sensations of rotation which in aviation medicine we describe as vertigo. They are not the same as the dizzy vertigo clinicians used to describe, but they are there."

The third Skylab crew did not have nearly so merry a time of it during their three-and-a-half months in weightlessness as did the first two. In fact, Edward G. Gibson, Gerald M. Carr, and William R. Pogue, instigated the world's first "space strike," in protest to

287

the heavy work loads heaped upon them by the Houston flight directors.

They got off on the wrong foot, at the beginning when, in spite of the flight surgeon's protest, Mission Control allowed the three men to enter 13 hours earlier than originally planned. There was work to do, the men were excited and wanted to experience zero-g as soon as possible. But getting used to it proved troublesome moreover, nausea struck. Nausea pills floated every which way when released from the bottle so a chase had to be made. In the large open spaces of the space station, the astronauts realized they had been trying to do too much too soon, and, "O1' sweaty-palm time," or, "stomach awareness," was upon them. Pogue threw up, and according to the rules, he was supposed to freeze-dry his vomitus and bring it back to earth for medical analysis. But the men decided against it on the grounds that the adverse effects of weightlessness might put a crimp in NASA's future space funding. "We won't mention it," said Carr, the commander, "and we'll just throw it down the trash airlock."

Gibson concurred, saying, "They're not going to be able to keep track of that."

Pogue said, "It's just between you, me and the couch."

Carr agreed. "You know damn well every manager in NASA, under his breath, would want you to do that."

The tape recorder for the B channel was, of course, live and the whole conversation was neatly typed, duplicated, and distributed back at Houston. The severe reprimand that followed, affected the crew's morale from then on. Capsule communicator, Dr. Story Musgrave, himself an astronaut, later said the incident plus the reprimand were doubtless responsible for things that went wrong later.

All of the Skylab astronauts experienced the sometimes pesky, sometimes pleasant aspects of living and working in zero-g. It is generally agreed that it took them about a month to get the hang of it. Even the simplest tasks had to be learned. Their clothing, for example, had pockets in the sleeves, chests, flanks and all the way down the legs and if the flaps weren't kept tightly fastened, the contents would float away. They learned to put on their shoes last because this was the hardest part of dressing. Without gravity, they had to force themselves to bend and use their stomach muscles to pull their feet up. Sometimes this included a backward somersault before the shoes were tied. Their canvas-top gym shoes had aluminum soles coated with rubber to which they could fasten one or two types of cleats. Many parts of Skylab's floor had triangular metal grids to which the cleats could be attached, thus keeping them from floating away. On the lower deck where the ceiling was low, they learned to shove themselves sideways off the wall, so that they glided as though on ice skates. They walked by pushing against the ceiling, then stepping with both their arms and legs. In order to stay put, they wedged their bodies into corners or crevasses to free their arms for working.

The astronauts were immediately confronted with what they called the "jack-in-the-box" aggravation of compartments or cabinets. Open the door and everything flies out; toothbrush, toothpaste, extra razor blades, screws, nuts, hammers...everything not fastened down. The solution was the use of the adhesive fabric Velcro. Nevertheless, a lot of time was spent corraling floating objects.

Eating wasn't easy and not particularly pleasant. For one thing, nothing smelled very good because smells, like sound, don't travel readily in space. And the congestion in the astronauts' heads prevented them from smelling or tasting much. Salt and spices didn't improve the flavor and often floated away (as a blob when mixed with water). Keeping food from flying off the silverware was a problem because if the diner were to stop midway with a forkful of scrambled eggs, the eggs would continue their own trajectory into his face. In the beginning, they adopted the Japanese style, getting their mouths close to the food and shoveling it in. Later, they developed a smooth, arc-like motion upward, keeping their mouths open to catch the food. All of them made a point of consuming a lot of water to offset the false impression that their bodies contained too much liquid. This was because of the pooling around the heart. Coded water hoses kept track of water intake for later study.

Everything it seemed had to be weighed and measured. During the flight, blood was drawn with a syringe and whirled in a small centrifuge to follow the loss of red cells and establish when that trend started and stopped. The flight surgeons would also check on the change of shape in red cells; normally they looked like tiny red checkermen, concave on both sides. But as time went on, a large fraction of them distorted, becoming thin, attenuated, and flat.

The astronauts were required to weigh their leftover food by placing the cans in a wire mesh box and pressing a button to make the box rock back and forth. The amount of rocking indicated the can's mass. The same principle was used for weighing the astronauts themselves.

There was a great deal of exercise, particularly on the bicycle ergometer, but it was hard work because there was no weight to help out. To keep himself on the bike, Pogue put a pillow on his head and braced himself against a pipe on the ceiling. He gripped the handlebars tightly and locked the triangles on his shoes to the pedals. The effort was tremendous and the heat rose suffocatingly around him he later reported. Cleaning up after these exercises could take up to 25 minutes because it had to be done with a wet cloth.

The "space strike" of Skylab 3 occurred six weeks into the flight when the astronauts found themselves not only behind in their assigned chores and experiments, but their meals were interrupted as well. Carr told Mission Control, "There's nothing worse than having to gobble your meal in order to get some task done that really should have been scheduled at some other time, so please loosen up!"

The astronauts began to feel they were nothing much more then inputs for a computer. There was no time for privacy and reflection because their schedule was so packed. Carr kept reminding the flight controllers, "On the ground, I don't think we would be expected to work a sixteen-hour day for 85 days, and so I really don't see why we should even try to do it up here."

Flight surgeons and capsule communicators tried to stop the pressure, but it took some doing. A major obstacle for the flight surgeons was the fact that many of the extra experiments were medical ones which actually made them among the chief offenders. Dr. Jerry R. Hordinsky, the crew surgeon for the third mission said later, "At conferences, when we were on the side of easing up, of saying that the flight plans were too much, the engineers couldn't understand what we meant. We witnessed Mission Control getting off on the wrong foot, but there was no place to blow the whistle. And communications between us and the flight planners was not good. They told us that 'the flight schedule was a nonmedical duty,' so there was a bad interface. It took us three weeks to see what was going on; then we went to bat..."

After the crew went on strike, they did exactly what they wanted to do. Gibson went to the solar console and Carr and Pogue sat in the wardroom looking out the window, sometimes taking pictures of sights they liked. Carr, realizing that Mission Control was probably under pressure from NASA administrators to get more and more results of the flight said, "I imagine you guys are probably caught right smack in the middle of it, and the question that arises in my mind is, are we behind, and if so, how far? Or is all this hassle over our time the result of people coming out of the woodwork with new things to be done?...That's essentially the big question, where do we stand?"

The controversy was finally resolved with the astronauts being given more time to do their experiments, and fewer of them to work on. The crew's performance picked up and finally equalled and in some areas surpassed that set by the Skylab 2 crew.

In weightlessness, many astronauts slept most comfortably curled up in a fetal position—a situation that later produced backaches. Future missions will probably include restraints to keep the voyagers in a "posturepedic" position, giving the spine support where needed. On the other hand, one of the Russian cosmonauts, reported that after several days he adapted beautifully, sleeping for seven to nine hours, awakening fresh and in good humor. "Crewmembers fell asleep rapidly in about the same manner as on Earth. One crewmember appeared to adapt so well to sleeping in the weightless condition that he preferred to sleep without being tied into his cot."

Under conditions of weightlessness, there was concern that the semicircular canals and the otolith apparatus of the inner ear might not act to keep the body properly oriented, but there appeared to be no notable vestibular dysfunctions. However, the relationship between the gravity-dependent vestibular apparatus and motion sickness soon became evident and both the Americans and Soviets were deeply concerned with the problem.

Soviet cosmonauts suffered from space sickness in nearly every Vostok and Vosknod mission, as well as having illusions of being

291

inverted. Such symptoms disappeared on meeting reentry acceleration. The Soviets first thought that their cosmonauts were at fault, when in reality spacecraft stabilization was the problem. Meanwhile, they intensified their pre-selection vestibular testing procedures, bearing in mind that pilots are less subject to motion sickness than non-pilots. (See Chapter 9)

Metabolism, put simply, is biochemical change. It is the chemical and physical process continuously going on in living organisms and cells, comprising those by which assimilated food is built up (*anabolism*) into protoplasm and those by which protoplasm is used and broken down (*catabolism*) into simpler substances for waste matter, with the release of energy for all vital processes. The question for the space scientists was, how could this process be measured? Next, how many calories per day do astronauts need for living and working in weightlessness for two weeks or so? Do they burn up more energy or less?

"All energy used by the body (except that for outside work) finally appears as heat," said Dr. Berry. "Since oxygen is used in the process of breaking down nutrients to yield carbon dioxide and water, oxygen consumption and carbon dioxide production are useful indices of metabolic rate."

Dr. Berry explains that direct metabolic measurements have not been made during actual spaceflight, but inferences could be made from telemetry data. To learn about thermal balance, doctors compared the inlet and outlet temperatures in the water cooled undergarment during lunar surface work. They measured oxygen use from the portable life-support system and also compared heart rates with those they had collected preflight with bicycle ergometry.

Dr. Berry concluded: "The techniques used for determining metabolic expenditure inflight admittedly are gross. Nevertheless, the expenditures calculated by this technique indicate that the diet provided for missions is more than adequate for living and working in space up to two weeks..."

As to neuromuscular changes, doctors expected deterioration of the body's muscles during weightlessness. The bedrest study made by Deitrick, Whedon and Shorr in 1948 showed an increased urinary nitrogen excretion and muscle atrophy in the arms and thighs of test subjects, so when the time came for astronauts to experience true weightlessness, there was great concern as to their reactions. According to Dr. Berry, "We tried everything. We tried compressing the skeleton with springs, and things like elastic suits where you always have to move against pressure. The Russians have what they call a penguin suit but it doesn't work. It doesn't prevent calcium loss to the skeleton nor protein loss from the muscles..." Exercise of course helps, but the problem was, how much would be enough? Astronauts had to do something besides exercise all the time.

As matters turned out, actual exposure to weightlessness for 14 days produced no muscular atrophy or impairement in coordination, but there were losses in nitrogen that persisted postflight in spite of nitrogen intake. The cosmonauts on the Soyuz 9 flight of 18 days reported radical changes. They said their limbs felt extremely heavy and they had difficulaty walking or lifting ofjects for days afterwards. When they lay down, they felt "pressed" into their beds and between the second and fifth day postflight they felt muscle pain. Doctors Cherepakhin and Perushin blamed it all on weightlessness *per se* because the body has no need to maintain a posture and that those muscles subjected to a lesser load showed the greatest change.

But, as missions became longer, more attention was paid to diet and exercise; it appeared that man could adjust to weightlessness remarkably well. Said Dr. Berry, "We showed that man got better after an 84 day mission than he was after a 25 day one. And he was better after 59 days than after 25..."

To minimize muscle and skeletal deterioration, Soviet cosmonauts and American astronauts kept vigorous exercise schedules. During the Soyuz 9 flight of 18 days, the Russians exercised for an hour, twice a day, with rubber bungee cords which provided for increased load during simulated walking and running exercises. A similar routine was worked out for the Americans.

Both groups, however, lost bone mass, showing that despite vigorous and operationally barely acceptable exercise schedules such exercise simply could not compensate for all the pervasive influence of gravity on the skeletal systems.

It's easy to see that hair and fingernails are alive and constantly growing, but a person's skeleton is another matter. The old adage, "out of sight, out of mind," certainly pertains here because it too is a living, though nearly forgotten part of the body, constantly undergoing change—a dynamic system that renews itself just as the skin does. Studies on animals have shown that their bones increase in density if they are subjected to more than normal gravity. Dr. Graveline, at the School of Aerospace Medicine, raised one litter of mice on a small animal centrifuge which simulated a 2g environment and their litter mates in a normal 1g. X-rays showed that the skeletal density and bony definition of the mice exposed to 2g far exceeded those raised in the normal envrionment. "They were Herculean in their build, and unusually strong..." Graveline reported.

But what happens if the skeleton is placed in a condition of zero gravity? According to Dr. G. D. Whedon, Director of the National Institute of Arthritis, Metabolism and Digestive Disease at NIH. "The body reasons in weightlessness, or in bedrest, that it doesn't need the calcium. Calcium is important to the skeleton to keep it strong and hold our weight up. Well, whatever the impulses are that keep calcium being pushed into the skeleton from the diet just aren't there. A certain amount is lost anyway because bones turn over. Calcium is going in and out of your bones all the time..."

In the Gemini and Apollo missions, bone mass loss was measured with a bone desitometric X-ray technique. Althoug the loss varied from person to person, and from site to site, a pattern emerged that indicated bone demineralization had a way of correcting itself on longer voyages. Dr. Berry reported on studies made by Dr. John Vogel: "In contrast to earlier findings, Apollo 14 bone mineral content determinations did not reveal bone demineralization. Pre- and postflight examinations of the left central os calcis and the right distal radius and ulna by means of a monoenergetic photon absorption technique revealed no significant losses during the 10-day mission..."

For longer flights, however, any loss at all continues to worry scientists. Exercise does not prevent it and apparently the body must have real weight bearing—be on its feet for something like three hours in 24 in order to stem the outflow of minerals. According to Dr. Whedon, "We were a little concerned as pure

294

experimentalists in the Skylab program that the exercise program the astronauts were going to do might cloud the answers that we were after. But the degree of change in the Skylab studies were such that even though the exercises they were engaged in were quite vigorous in the second and third flights, they couldn't have had much effect on the loss of calcium. They really weren't bearing weight in the degree enough to prevent this loss..."

The Skylab study on mineral and nitrogen balance was carried out for a total of 909 man-days. In all cases, urinary calcium excretion peaked out during the latter part of each flight, and was from 80 per cent to double the rate of bedrest levels. The rate of actual calcium loss was from 0.3 to 0.4 per cent of total body calcium per month—small in relation to total skeletal weight, but of great significance when projected over the duration of a planetary mission, and indicative of the need for developing rigorous protective measures—the importance of direct physical longitudinal stress (weight bearing) to the integrity of the bone, and the possible value of increased weight-bearing stress as a deterrent to or aid to correction of this condition.

As to predictions for future flights, Dr. Whedon states that "...flights up to six to nine months could be safely conducted as far as bones are concerned. But sometime after that, this mineral loss could be a really serious matter. And this has some reality when you realize that to go to Mars and back, which is really the next place to go after you've gone to the moon, will take anywhere from 18 months to 36 months. And you'd want to spend a little time there, of course. That time is variable because it will depend on how far we are from Mars at the time of flight. So, based on the losses we saw up to three months, then you have to be concerned about it..."

Artificial gravity could be produced in a rotating space station but it would have to be a very large one to avoid other problems connected with spinning, such as the Coriolis effect. As for a moon colony, Dr. Whedon feels that with one-sixth weight bearing, a period of six months in such a station would be feasible.

NASA wisely began supporting studies to find some protective regimen or diet or hormone or procedure that might at least reduce the amount of mineral loss. Most of these studies have been carried out in the Public Health Service hospitals in San Francisco,

295

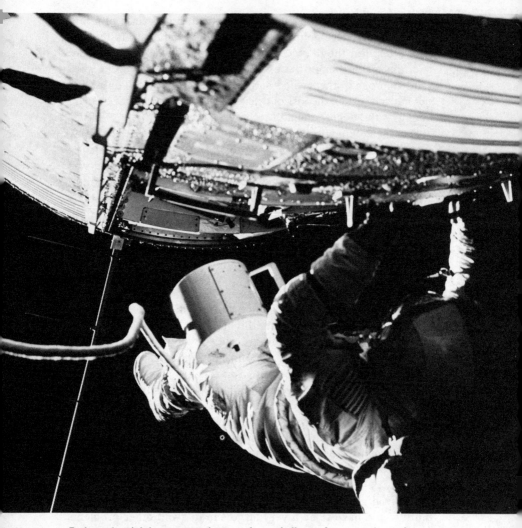

Prolonged weightlessness continues to be a challenge for researchers of many disciplines. Here, performing EVA during the flight of Apollo 17, Navy Commander Ronald Evans collects film cannisters/*U.S. Navy*

which are well equipped for studying bedrest and more specifically studying the effects of various procedures to try to counteract this calcium loss. Although the primary purpose is for the space program, if the researchers can find a workable solution it could be applied to bedrest patients on earth. It could be used for treating patients who have demineralizing diseases such as osteoporosis—literally porous bones—that affect 14 million people in the United States. This disease, said Dr. Whedon, "...affects 30 per cent of women over 50. Men get it as well, but they don't get it to the same degree or frequency. So, these studies are a legitimate spinoff..."

At present, specialists are focusing on finding some means of applying the equivalent of weight-bearing while an individual is in bed. This involves a suit with elastic straps which will apply pressure too, so other straps press against the shoulders. The effect is to compress the body either in a static fashion, or with alternate pressures, as in walking. These devices are being used on volunteer test subjects—healthy unemployed young men—who are free to discontinue the experiment and leave anytime they want to. Some of them have done exactly that.

In addition to skeletal deterioration in long-term weightlessness, problems with the cardiovascular system still haunt the researchers. Because of all the background research and experience, doctors were not surprised nor alarmed over the speeded up heart rates at *launch* time. "Command pilot syndrome," they called it, and they were not particularly concerned about the individual differences; the lunar module pilot on Apollo 16 had a heartbeat of 130 beats per minute at launch time, while the mission commander had a rate of 108—understandable because he was making his fourth spaceflight and was thus relatively calm. But *returning* from orbit can be quite another matter.

Should there be a malfunction of one or more cardiovascular control loops responsible for hemostatic regulation, the astronauts could not tolerate the heavy g load connected with re-entering earth's atmosphere. According to Dr. Graveline: "Orthostatic intolerance was noted postflight in all astronauts and cosmonauts. If those men had returned from orbit under less favorable conditions and had been forced to endure survival stresses, their relative tachycardias (fast heart beats) and hypotensive tendencies might have been decisive."

Fortunately there were no malfunctions of the system. Reduced orthostatic tolerance was noted in postflight examinations, but these symptoms disappeared within two or three days (except for the Apollo 15 crew).

The most serious aberrations in cardiac electrical activity were noted during the Apollo 15 mission, when both the lunar module pilot and mission commander were affected. Uneven heart beats were first noted at 177 hours into the mission. The electrocardograph tracings revealed premature ventricular contractions (extrasystoles), a condition which on earth is seen in overworked or exhausted people.

Experts have examined the results of Mercury, Gemini, Apollo and Skylab flights and have concluded that the road to the planets is open. That man not only can tolerate weightlessness but can work hard and productively in this exotic environment for periods of a few months is no longer in doubt. It is certain that a sizeable number of physiologic responses to the unloading from the force of gravity, many of which are poorly understood, take place fairly promptly and are reversible when the space traveler resumes his accustomed place on the surface of the earth. Yet is equally clear that some of the physiologic adjustments are slow, and do not reach completion even after 84 days of continuous exposure to weightlessness. Furthermore, there is valid concern that a few of these continuing processes, if they go long and far enough, may result in irreversible pathophysiology..."

Optimism, of course, can have its set-backs. What is the difference between the 84 days in space by the Americans and the 96-day flight of Salyut 6 by cosmonauts Yuri Romanenko and Georgy Grechko? A mere 12 days longer. When the Soviet space travelers returned to earth on 16 March 1978, they had trouble walking, picking up a cup of tea and even turning a radio dial. The crew's doctor, Robert Dynakonov explained, "Their organisms had gotten too used to freedom from weight. Now, every step is work..." The men tried to "swim" out of their beds in the morning instead of getting up the normal way.

An entirely different picture emerged in November 1978 when cosmonauts Vladimir Kovalynok, 36, and Alexander Ivanchenkov, 38, returned safely to earth after nearly 140 days in space. The Russians withstood their ordeal well, keeping in shape with rigorous exercises and the use of vacuum suits that forced their blood to circulate as if they were standing upright on earth. Encouraged by the results, Flight Director Alexei Yeliseyev contended that the Soviets could now send out manned space expeditions of practically unlimited duration. Besides eclipsing the earlier mark of 96 days, they chalked up two other feats by playing host to two visiting ships, one carrying an East German, the other a Polish cosmonaut. They were resupplied three times by remote-controlled ferry craft which carried such homey items as a guitar, fur boots, strawberries, fresh milk, onions and garlic.

The space flight director reported that the only physiological barrier to extremely long space flights seemed to be psychological conditions. "Man finds himself in a small collective, extremely far away from home, relatives, friends. It is more difficult to solve the psychological loads." He added that much is being learned on this score and that he is certain more longer flights can be made.

Prolonged weightlessness continues to be a challenge for researchers of many disciplines. Said Dr. Pace: "For the biologist, a whole new class of experimentation awaits spaceflight opportunities. The study of the physiologic and morphologic characteristics of successive generations of animal and plant species raised in continuous weightlessness is a truly important and exciting prospect for the future. Finally, by increasing understanding of the effects of removal of man and other earth organisms from gravitational loading under carefully controlled experimental conditions, knowledge of the interaction of gravity and the life process as it affects all on earth throughout their lives will also be improved."*

*Quoted from *The New England Journal of Medicine,* July 7, 1977

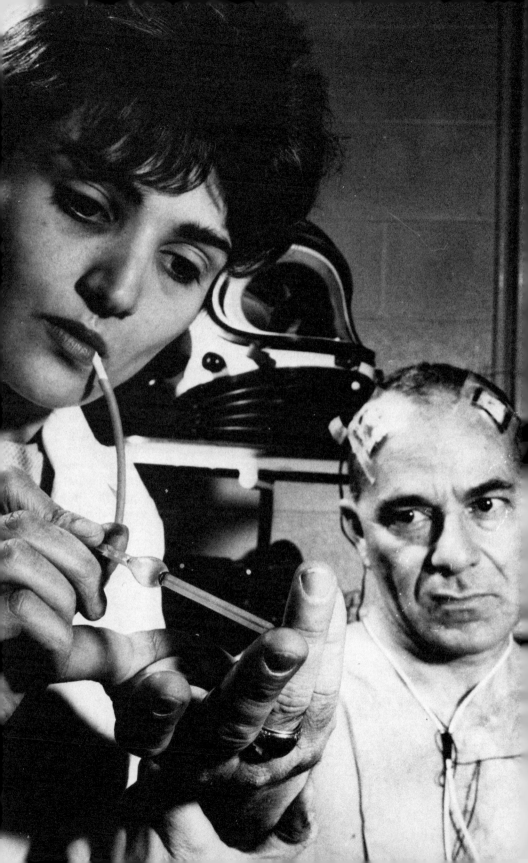

11

Physiological Aspects of Spaceflight

The first step on the way to the moon, made nearly two centuries ago in France, merely lifted a few venturesome men a mile or so into the sky where their flimsy craft floated no higher than the green hills of Auvergne, and gave them a new perspective on a pastoral world. And in that sea of air, they gradually reached higher and higher, until no more than three decades ago they had reached the discernable top of the earth's atmospheric envelope. Perspective had been left behind; on the very verge of space they faced new hazards and experienced physiological effects unknown to earthlings.

Then the World War II weapon, the V-2 rocket, was converted to a vehicle able to leave the earth completely behind. In rapid succession, men reached the edge of absolute space, orbited the earth, and finally, reached and landed on the moon. The view of the earth was new, the experiences of the few men destined to walk on the moon were unique, and a great new insight into the

The physiological factors involved in spaceflight have been determined, in many cases, to relate to conditions of the cardiovascular system. At the Republic Aviation Corporation plant where such factors were studied in designing the Apollo space suits, environment engineer Arnold Beck submits, unhappily, to that ubiquitous laboratory tool, a sharp needle./*NASA*

301

physical and physiological requirements of men in space became available. Yet these latter developments did not come over night; researchers, scientists, and doctors had been exploring and examining such aspects of spaceflight long before men left the earth behind.

Along with the physiological and biomedical aspects of spaceflight, men in space experienced many psychological demands, depending in part on the problems encountered, and the individual role in a spaceflight mission. The psychological requirements were concisely stated by Dr. Randall Chambers* of the Naval Air Development Center, Johnsville, Pennsylvania, who pointed out the diverse nature of the duties demanded of a man on a space mission. Besides being a flight systems monitor and scientific observer, he may also have to act as a scientific specimen, observer and monitor, information processing unit and decision maker, flight controller, test conductor, and research scientist.

While performing those duties, a man may face "many psychologically adverse conditions in spaceflight which are potentially disruptive to perception, performance, and personality. These include high acceleration and deceleration stress, prolonged weightlessness, transitions between high g and zero g, prolonged confinement (involving restraint and restriction of movement), psychological isolation and deprivation of needs, altered physiological and psychological diurnal cycles, sensory deprivation (input underload stress), sensory overload (input overload), fatigue, boredom, and prolonged work; disorientation, prolonged exposure to extreme hazards; uncertainty and fear of the unknown."

For the layman, the best place to enter such a quagmire of technical and scientific terminology is to consider the aspect of visual perception. Visual perception, man's ground-based navigational system, depends on the highly perceptive "Mark I eyeball," which defines color, detects motion, and through steroscopic vision measures distance. But once an astronaut climbs into his pressure suit, he will never use his eyes "naked"

*In "The Psychology of Spaceflight and Centrifuge Training," Journal of the British Interplanetary Society, v. 21, 1968.

as on earth; he will see everything through face plates, ultra-violet excluding visors, and space-craft windows. And in space, there is very little for the astronaut to see. The sky is perpetually dark, and the stars—mere pinpoints of light, may appear side by side with the sun. They will not twinkle until he returns to earth. The sky is not completely black, nor is it especially light; the illumination level is about one-tenth that of the sky as seen from earth on a moonlit night.

In deep space, there will be nothing to provide a reference point for visual observations, except the interior of the spacecraft. Stereoscopic vision outside the craft will not be possible, because there will be nothing to see except stars, and for all practical purposes, they are at infinity. A man gazing into space will be subject to ''empty field myopia,'' a condition in which his eyes focus automatically at a point about 9 feet distant. Under conditions of empty field myopia, it is possible for a pilot to fail completely to see objects as close as 100 feet. At such times, if a satellite or another spacecraft entered his field of vision, he would be unable to determine its distance or size.

Illusory sensations experienced by pilots flying prop or jet planes ranged from confused ideas of altitude to that of flying upside down. Experiments at the Naval School of Aviation Medicine at Pensacola by Graybiel and Clark showed that 96 per cent of all pilots had had such sensations. When Friendship 7 made its orbital flight, John Glenn experienced a sensation of tumbling forward when the rocket engines cut off and acceleration suddenly dropped to zero, much as he had experienced during simulation on a centrifuge. When his retrorockets fired on reentry, he had the sensation that he had suddenly commenced flying backwards. Other astronauts—Shepard, Grissom, Carpenter and Schirra—also experienced such sensations.

High-altitude flight sometimes results in a feeling of being detached, isolated, and separated physically from the earth—a condition termed the "break-off phenomenon." Nearly half of all Navy and Marine jet pilots interviewed in a 1957 experiment reported that they had experienced the effect, when flying alone, flying at high-altitudes, and flying with a minimum of activity required. They variously experienced feelings of remoteness, loneliness, anxiety, exhilaration, or euphoria. High-altitude balloon flights also produced this effect. Major David Simons, writing in the *Air University Quarterly Review* in 1958, said he felt an identification with the space above, rather than the earth below, and in his 1959 report on the flight made in Man High II, said "...it seemed right that I should be going toward space, as if that was where I belonged...I experienced a separation of emotional ties and interests from the earth below and felt an identification with the void of space above..." First American sub-orbital flights did not produce this effect in pilots, possibly because they were of such short duration.

As Apollo 11, its moon mission completed, coasted earthward across the black reaches of cislunar space, both Neil Armstrong and Edwin Aldrin saw something they had never seen before— strange flashes of light. They were not seeing the "fireflies" noted by some astronauts during orbital flights, nor were they seeing bits of insulation or other debris trailing along with their spacecraft, as in the case of the dead dog tossed out of the fictional moon craft by Jules Verne's adventurers. Neither were they experiencing the hallucinations which Dr. Berry had predicted as one of the physiological aspects of spaceflight.* The flashes were inside the spacecraft cabin, and they could see them whether their eyes were open or closed.

In postmission debriefing, Armstrong and Aldrin said the lights appeared as faint spots or flashes, seen when the cabin was dark and their eyes had become dark-adapted. Astronauts on all subsequent Apollo missions reported seeing the same flashes, more frequently en route to the moon than on the way home. Generally they were described as white, or colorless, although Edgar D. Mitchell in Apollo 14 saw them as "blue with a white cast, like a diamond." Three types of flashes were reported. Sixty-six per cent of the flashes were described as a "spot" or "starlike," similar to a photo flash seen from several hundred feet away. Sometimes they came in pairs, both in the same eye, or one in each eye. About twenty-five per cent of the flashes were

*In the paper delivered to the 10th Plenary Meeting of the Committee for Space Research, in London, in 1967, summarizing medical knowledge resulting from the Gemini flights.

described as streaks; the rest of them were said to resemble a lightning discharge seen behind clouds.

After crew members on the Apollo 12 and 13 missions also reported seeing light flashes, definite periods were set up on the missions by Apollo 14, 15, 16, and 17, during which the men wore simple blindfolds for an hour; their comments and descriptions of each light flash were transmitted to tracking stations on earth and taped in the spacecraft. Richard F. Gordon, in Apollo 12, said "There were big bright ones all over." He had not seen the flashes during earth orbits in the Gemini program.

Subsequent to the Apollo missions, astronauts and scientists who flew the three Skylab mission also saw the light flashes. They appeared most often as Skylab crossed through the South Atlantic Anomaly.

Investigations conducted at the University of Houston by W. Zachary Osborne, Ph.D., and Lawrence S. Pinsky, Ph.D., and at the Lyndon B. Johnson Space Center by J. Vernon Bailey resulted in the conclusion that the light flashes were the result of high energy, heavy cosmic rays penetrating the spacecraft structure, and producing visual sensations through interaction with the retina. The fact that the light flashes could be "seen" even with the eyes closed indicated that cosmic radiation was penetrating the optical nervous system; the fact that the flashes were noted only after the eyes were dark-adapted suggested that the retina, rather than the optic nerve itself, was involved.

Light flashes were one of the lesser physiological aspects of spaceflight, and their occurrence had no effect on the success of the Apollo missions. In space, other sensations are experienced. The oculogravic or vestibular visual illusion occurs during definite changes in acceleration rate, and has the effect of giving immobile objects an apparent motion in the direction of the resultant force of gravity.

Autokinetic illusion, also the subject of studies at Pensacola, occurs when a pilot keeps his eyes on a stationary light source outside his cabin; eventually the light appears to move slowly in a random direction. In tests conducted by Graybiel and Clark, subjects could not differentiate between apparent motion of a light, and its actual motion. This could be dangerous during landing operations, or in space maneuvers such as will be common when the Space Orbiter commences operations, resupplying satellites.

What an astronaut sees—or thinks he sees—governs actions which at times require split-second reaction, but at earth orbit escape velocity, a spacecraft moves several miles in a split second. Such velocities adversely affect human ability to respond appropriately to visual stimuli; the determining factor here is the time response related to visual recognition. This was studied, before the advent of rocket-powered spaceflight, as early as 1951, and reported on by V. A. Byrnes in "Visual problems of Supersonic Speed." The greater the velocity, the less likely the chance that human response can be translated into appropriate reaction.

Once a man is in space, orientation becomes a problem, because of the lack of normal vision cues, such as a definite horizon, and distant objects. In the earth's atmospheric envelope, light is scattered by molecules of air, dust, and moisture, but as altitude increases, light distribution changes. The contrast within the visual field is much greater than that to which the human eye is normally accustomed, resulting in what some scientists refer to as the "searchlight effect."

Visual acuity—the measure of what or how much the unaided human eye can perceive from space—is the subject of considerable disagreement. In "Visual Surveillance and Reconnaissance from Space Vehicles," written in 1963, Muckler and Narva determined that a visual angle of ten minutes was the operational minimum, and that minimum resolvable object length (MROL) at an altitude of 113 miles would be 1730 feet. A year later the limits of acuity were revised to 0.5 second of arc for an extended contrasting line and 15 seconds of arc for minimum separation of two points sharply contrasting with the background. Existing camera systems can resolve objects down to 0.4 seconds of arc—about five to fifty times better than the human eye. But the camera merely photographs, and can not use inference or interpretation.

In earth orbit, at an altitude of 100 miles, one can see the horizon 900 miles away. Gordon Cooper in Faith 7 was disbelieved when he said he saw smoke from a locomotive, but he was correct. In

Skylab, orbiting at 237 miles, it was possible to see the entire east coast of the United State, from Canada to the Florida Keys, and pick out such details as a bridge 500 feet long.

Said John Glenn: "You can see something that crosses a river and you assume that it's a bridge. As far as being able to look down and say that it is a bridge, I think you are only assuming that it is a bridge more than really observing it." In checking reports of visual sightings by various astronauts, it was considered that many of them were based on inference (one prime difference between the camera eye and a human eye with a brain attached); roads could be seen where the map indicated there were roads, or buildings might be seen because the area looked like a place where buildings should be.

When an astronaut is moving at the rate of miles per second, and involved in the multitudinous tasks of astronavigation, communications, attitude control, and other aspects of spaceflight, he may become subject to sensory overloading—when too many tasks require simultaneous attention, the requirements may exceed his capacity, and his performance level is lowered.

Said Dr. Berry, in comparing predictions with results of the Gemini flights, "Each individual apparently has an optimal level of input over acceptable periods of time. Whereas an individual may be able to perform adequately at a very high level for a short period of time, it would not be expected that he could continue at the same level indefinitely. Repeated, continuous sensory overloading leads to a variety of emotional and psychiatric problems."

At the other end of the scale from sensory overloading is sensory deprivation, a condition facing a man with little to do and with limited sensory stimulation. Early astronauts, trained as test pilots, objected to the "man in a can" concept of riding around in orbit with little control over their movements. Sensory deprivation was at one time considered a major problem in lengthy spaceflights, but the experiences of Skylab crews—as long as 84 days—and the even longer Russian flight—proved that fears of sensory deprivation were groundless. Men on these extended flights were in constant communication with earth, and it is unlikely that any manned interplanetary mission would ever get out of range of their friendly flight controller on earth.

307

The effects of prolonged isolation were studied extensively in the years immediately preceding the first orbital flights, and much literature resulted. Isolation studies included observations and reports on the actions of explorers, shipwrecked sailors, prisoners in solitary confinement or concentration camps and, more to the point, crews of test pilots enclosed in a spacecraft cabin simulator for as long as 15 days. Experiments with animals maintained in isolation for long periods during which they did not have use of normal sensory cues showed that they developed abnormalities in perception and behavior. The chief effects of long isolation on humans were perceptual distortions, illusions and hallucinations, changes in motivation, attitude and temperament, and reduced powers of memory, reasoning, and thinking.

The conditions under which astronauts performed in flight, up through the Apollo and Skylab missions, were not exactly like the laboratory conditions under which earlier assessments of isolation effects were based. Most orbital flights were comparatively short, and even on the Apollo missions the requirements for navigation, communications, scientific observation and general housekeeping routines kept men busy enough so they were spared long periods of sensory deprivation and inactivity.

Limited physical motion, a problem of sorts in the Mercury and Gemini missions, was not quite so critical in the Apollo missions because there was a little more room. In the Skylab, of course, people had great freedom of movement, and could either work with others in the crew or withdraw from them if they desired. A three-month flight in Skylab is about a sixth as long as the shortest possible round trip to Mars, but with the experience gained so far in space, and the expected progress in the art before such a flight leaves earth, there is every expectation that the first flight to Mars should be as successful as the first flight to the moon.

Crews on the three Skylab missions were so busy that they reported sleeping less in space than they did on earth, and found their work so interesting they "overworked." Scientists Owen K. Garriott, in particular, became so engrossed in an experiment with spiders that he carried it on beyond the termination period.

Noise and vibration may also affect the physiological conditions of astronauts, although perhaps not to the extent feared before the Apollo and Skylab missions were flown. Both can produce anxiety, choking, fatigue, difficulty in breathing, some bodily pain, headaches, and, if sustained long enough, deafness. The noise generated by a Saturn-5 at liftoff reaches 165 decibels, as compared to 130 decibels for a wide open jet engine on the ground, or 130 for a pneumatic chipping hammer at a distance of five feet. However, on liftoff the astronauts are inside, and do not hear nearly as much as ground observers.

Vibration can be a bigger problem; in Gemini flights astronauts had difficulty reading the instrument panels when vibration reached 50 cycles per second, as their eyeballs began resonating and blurred their vision.

In deep space, of course, there can be no external noise, and a spacecraft, much like a submarine, operates in a state where it can "run silent, run deep." But even so, the on-board complement of pumps, fans, motors, and other equipment is either in constant or intermittent operation. Anyone distracted by a humming fluorescent tube or a dripping faucet for several hours could appreciate the fact that a man who had listened to a clicking relay for ten months on the way to silent Mars might at least briefly consider staying there to miss the ride back.

In space, too, astronauts miss the slow progression of the sun and stars across the sky that mark terrestrial day and night. While a spacecraft is in earth orbit, it completes a circuit of both the day and night side of the earth in approximately 90 minutes. On a lunar or planetary trajectory, the sun is always visible, but only as a white disc against a black sky filled with stars—day and night have been left behind in the atmospheric envelope of earth. There is no longer any variation in levels of illumination and temperature which mark sunrise and sunset on earth, and thus set up the environmental cycle that induces periods of wakefulness and sleep in diurnal creatures such as man.

This physiological cycle is related to the physical cycle of day and night, caused by the earth's rotation, and is referred to as the circadian cycle (from *circa* and *dies* = about one day), or circadian rhythm. The circadian cycle affects certain behavior of all humans and animals, as well as plants. It has been studied for at least a hundred years, but only recently has it attracted public attention because of the fact that high-speed travel makes it possible for a person to move half around the world in a very short time and experiences a phase shift of their accustomed day-night cycle, commonly known as "jet lag."

The result is that people become hungry or sleepy at the wrong time for their new locale, until they can adjust to the change. It takes a person from three to four days to adjust after a transcontinental flight, and up to five or six days to adjust after a trans-Atlantic flight. A trip half way around the world may require as much as 10 to 12 days to adjust to the new time. Most people adjust more easily to the new time when flying eastward, but some find it easier to adjust after a westward flight. Colonel William Douglas, U.S. Air Force, the first physician for the Mercury astronauts, determined that in adjusting to a new time zone, it took about a day for each hour's change in time.

But astronauts in earth orbit crossed a new time zone about every four minutes, and in general they observed the wakeful-ness-sleep pattern to which they were accustomed on earth: the Russian cosmonauts usually went to sleep on Moscow time, and American astronauts went to sleep on Houston time. Skylab missions kept the same routine as observed by their control center on earth. Even a mission to Mars will observe a sleep, rest, and work schedule that corresponds to their physiologic circadian rhythm on earth. (Incidentally, the circadian cycle of people observed in laboratory experiments is not exactly 24 hours, the period in which the earth rotates on its axis. Rather, it is just enough longer to coincide with the rotational period of earth's nearest neighbor, Mars. This, according to Dr. Hubertus Strughold, may give science fiction writers a slight hold on the belief that flying saucers did indeed visit earth, thousands of years ago, bringing our ancestors from Mars. Considering conditions on Mars now, as determined by space probes, one can well understand why they left.)

Actually, the circadian cycle seems closely related to as yet undefined earth-moon relations. Experiments both in Russia and the United States with laboratory subjects established that the time cycle is either a little more, or a little less, than the 24-hour solar day, depending on illumination intensity and local environment. In Russia, W.B. Tshernyshev kept beetles in a chamber that was half in light, half in darkness. True to their built-in beetle schedule, they occupied the lighted part of the chamber during the day time, but moved to the dark area at night, with a cycle of 24 hours. If the chamber was kept constantly lighted, they began seeking shelter as evening time approached. If the chamber was kept completely dark, they set up a time cycle of 22 hours 18 minutes.

The lunar day is 24 hours 48 minutes in length, and people under laboratory conditions will establish a sleep-wakefulness period almost exactly that long. At the University of Minnesota, F. Halberg noted that seven women who spent two weeks in a cave established a cycle of 24 hours 42 minutes, as did a man who spent six months underground.

According to Dr. Strughold, the normal circadian cycle of 24 hours plus is not an inborn, instinctive action. During the first few months of life, infants act like both nocturnal and diurnal animals in their eating and sleeping routine. They finally adjust to the 24-hour cycle after they have learned to walk, when about two years old.

It is possible to shift the sleep-wakefulness cycle, as is required for people who work graveyard or swing shifts in factories, or for astronomers who must be wide-eyed during the night hours. And the cycle can be shortened to about 18 hours or extended to about 28 hours. But the cycle can not be changed quickly, or broken; it appears that astronauts on future planetary voyages, though they may be a long way from home, will still remember "the old home town," whether it be Moscow or Houston, when it's time for bed or breakfast.

Time disorientation, the inaccurate or false perception of the duration of time, or its rate of passage, has been the subject of much experimental work. Obviously, exact orientation in time is an absolute necessity for space travel. An astronaut must be aware of four kinds of time: clock time, geographic time, physiologic time, and psychologic time. Near instant communications with space control centers take care of the first two. Physiologic time is a complex cycle based on the metabolic reactions of the body and various organs, and is better understood as circadian rhythm or cycle. Psychologic time, the awareness of the passage of time, and the ability to determine the passage of time, is based on normal work-rest cycles, and to some extent on a person's past experience.

Before the Mercury and Gemini spaceflights, there was concern that operations under zero g conditions—weightlessness—would result in functional disruption of the vestibular system. All the components of this earth-bound navigational system as it were, normally function without any conscious effort on the part of their owner, but their inherent limitations in adjusting to abnormal conditions can create the acute distress known as motion sickness.

It is of interest to note that astronauts in the Mercury and Gemini missions experienced no vestibular dysfunctions, although they flew in various attitudes and could see the earth moving above or below them as the case might be. It was apparent that operation in a weightlessness state did not prevent the otolith organs from carrying out the integrative processes of the central nervous system that influenced spatial orientation.

Instances of vestibular dysfunction during the Apollo missions were believed to be due to the fact that the Apollo spacecraft permitted greater physical freedom, and thus astronauts could move their heads about before they had adapted to orbital flight. Later, during lunar landings, it was found that, while zero g could cause vestibular dysfunctions, men moving about under one-sixth g on the moon suffered no disorientation or vestibular dysfunctions. This established that while man had evolved under normal earth gravity, the otolith organs could still provide sensory guidance under limited gravity and control bodily posture.

One unexpected condition of flight under zero g conditions was first encountered during the Gemini program, when astronauts reported a feeling of "fullness of the head." Some men stated that it was accompanied by a feeling of hanging upside down. The effect was due, not to spatial disorientation, but to rapid bodily redistribution of extravascular and intravascular fluids—an active demonstration of the effect of Pascal's law on the human system.

An assessment of vestibular dysfunctions during all Apollo missions was made by J. L. Homick, of the Lyndon B. Johnson Space Center and Earl F. Miller of the Naval Aerospace Medical Research Laboratory. They reported that of the 33 men involved,

312

eleven experienced apparent vestibular difficulties; nine of these men had positive motion-sickness histories. However, of the 27 who had positive motion-sickness histories, 18 had no inflight problems. They also noted that of 15 men making their first spaceflights, 40 per cent developed inflight symptoms, while of 18 veteran pilots involved, approximately 28 per cent developed such symptoms. Thus, while previous flight experience is a deterrent in motion-sickness, it can not be a sure preventive.

So far, actual experience with vestibular effects has been limited to relatively short term flights—two weeks to the moon, about three months in Skylab. With a view to determining the role of the vestibular system in manned space missions of long duration, such as a voyage to Mars, when the vehicle might be kept in a slow-rotation status, partly to induce some slight effect of artificial gravity, and also to set up a "barbecue effect" to eliminate continuous solar heating on one side of the vehicle, extensive experiments have been conducted at the Naval Aerospace Medical Center, Pensacola, especially by Ashton Graybiel. There, a slow rotation room (SRR) allows subjects to walk on the "wall" and carry out their tasks while horizontal with respect to the vertical pull of gravity.

Tests in the SRR lasted as long as four or five days, with the room rotating at 4rpm, while the subjects spent part of their time in a horizontal position, part of the time in a vertical position, and the rest of the time in a bunk. On leaving the SSR mild sensations of motion-sickness were experienced. Even in a test lasting 12 days at 10rpm, any indications of subsequent motion sickness were trivial or absent. However, a man might say "I'm all right," and then walk head-long into a wall.

After several thousand man-hours in space, some of the pre-space fears and conjectures had been allayed. Men were able to work in a weightlessness state, spatial disorientation had presented no problems, and vestibular dysfunctions, while experienced to some degree, had not reduced the efficiency of astronauts in any of the many missions. Most medical problems of spaceflight, and for that matter, jet flight, turned out to be cardiovascular in nature. Despite all the black boxes, no astronaut was effective unless his system performed the vital function of

313

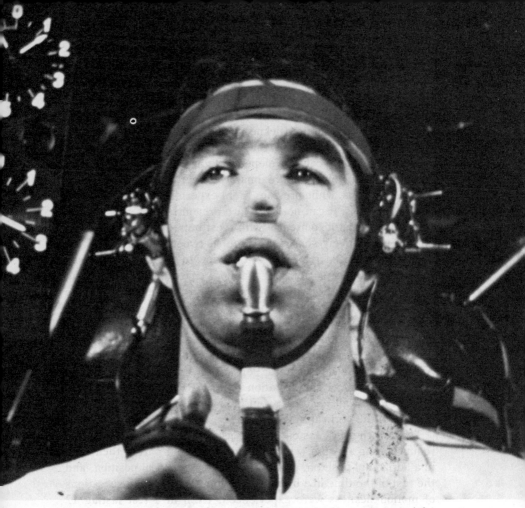

Countless hours of tedious and sometimes strenuous laboratory work ensured the safety of astronauts in space. Dr. Earl Wood, who worked with the human centrifuge at the Mayo Clinic, is shown here undergoing a centrifugal force of nearly 3G. Over the entire series of experiments, he experienced a total of 15 minutes with zero blood pressure in his head./*Mayo Clinic*

delivering oxygen to his body cells and transporting carbon dioxide to the lungs for disposal. It was a matter of physical logistics—the circulatory system was the transport mechanism between the source of supply and point of demand.

Concern over the ability of the cardiovascular systems to withstand flight stress began long before spaceflight. In World War II the Air Force School of Aviation Medicine commenced a wide range of studies including altitude decompression sickness, hypodynamia, and lower body negative pressure (LBNP) and developed tests on which to base an astronaut's physiological readiness for spaceflight. As actual spaceflight operations commenced, it was apparent that engineering and operational complications severely limited inflight physiological studies of those measures considered vital to crew safety and health assessment; accordingly, only examinations believed to have the greatest relevance to the understanding of physiological responses to spaceflight were undertaken.

An early finding of cardiovascular response to spaceflight came with the Mercury-Atlas 9 mission, when Gordon Cooper showed moderate orthostatic hypotension after only 34 hours in orbit, and nearly fainted on the deck of the recovery carrier. A later indication of the "C-V deconditioning" or loss of orthostatic tolerance effect came after the Russian Soyuz 9 completed an 18-day orbit flight, and the crewmen had to be assisted from their craft on landing because they had difficulty in standing.

Tilt table tests for orthostatic tolerance were made a part of all subsequent preflight and postflight evaluations, and confirmed consistent but variable losses of orthostatic tolerance after flights ranging from three to fourteen days in duration. Increased heart rate, lowered pulse pressure, and increased pooling of fluid in lower body extremities were all noted in postflight periods, but usually normal conditions were established within 50 hours after landing, no matter how long the flight.

Of all the various cardiovascular measurements obtained from crew members during the Apollo missions, heart rate was the most easily measured and yielded the most accurate and predictable values. Individuals were tested under three conditions: resting supine, under the highest level of LBNP, and passive standing. In general, heart rates increased in most of the individuals tested, under all three conditions. During postflight evaluations, more crew members demonstrated a larger heart rate increment over preflight rates during LBNP stress than during resting control; significant group differences disappeared by the third postflight evaluation.

While heart rates showed decreases during weightlessness conditions of space missions, the fact that the heart had less work to do had a direct effect on its size. Cardiothoracic (C/T) ratios

315

were calculated for all Apollo astronauts, through posterior-anterior chest X-rays both preflight and postflight. Comparisons showed that 80 per cent (24 out of 30) of the men showed a mean cardiothoracic ratio decrement of five per cent. The others showed no changes of clinical significance, except for one member of the Apollo 17 crew who wore a special antihyposensitive garment from splashdown until LBNP evaluation was complete five hours later—he showed about a five per cent increase.

With the initiation of the Apollo program, new questions and problems confronted the medics. The changing acceleration stresses of lunar descent and ascent were expected to have unfavorable reactions on the cardiovascular system; there was also the expectation that postflight tests would show important differences in cardiovascular responsiveness between those astronauts who had experienced one-sixth gravity on the moon and those who had remained in lunar orbit under zero gravity conditions, but in fact there has been no such finding.

LBNP in conjunction with fluid loading and whole body exercise offers a partial therapeutic technique against the effects of zero gravity on the cardiovascular system, eliminating some speculation early in the space program that planetary voyages could never be attempted for fear that the crewmen would, after months of zero gravity, be reduced to a "jellyfish" condition.

Once a spacecraft lifts off the launching pad, its occupants are cut off from the world except through electronic communication. No one leaves the craft until they return to earth, but there is always the possibility that invisible and sometimes highly dangerous passengers will appear in their craft unexpectedly. The mysterious riders have been identified by the medics as *hyperoxia* (too much oxygen), *hypoxia* (not enough oxygen), and *hypobaria* (reduced barometric pressure).

Astronauts traveled in a closed, controlled environment (see Chapter 8) but it did not reproduce normal earth atmosphere. They lived in a single-gas system of 100 per cent oxygen at 5psi which is better than the partial pressure of oxygen at sea level, but the equivalent of a pressure altitude of 27,000 feet. The maintenance of proper cabin pressure is critical. Each time the pressure increases by 1 millimeter of mercury, at 37 degrees centigrade, the oxygen content of the blood plasma will increase by 0.003 per cent. If cabin pressure were to increase to an indicated altitude of 12,310 feet while the content was 100 per cent oxygen, the upper limit of oxygen tension, or saturation,—considered to be 425mm Hg—would be reached. Continued exposure at such conditions would result in irritation of the lungs, thickening of the alveolar membranes, causing a decrease in the oxygen content of arterial blood.

The reaction in the blood system, after breathing pure oxygen at sea level, is rapid reduction in the number of red blood corpuscles and hemoglobin—five per cent in 10 minutes. The normal level is regained after 50 minutes, but then again there is a prolonged and extensive reduction in the red blood cell components. As the hemoglobin supply is reduced to compensate for the excessive oxygen, there follows a stage of inadequate oxygenation of arterial blood; next come extensive muscle damage to the left ventricle of the heart.

Demonstrations have proved that short term exposures to hyperoxia at tensions below the critical level of 425mm Hg will not result in either temporary or permanent damage, but the results of long exposure under such conditions are still unknown. As spacecraft such as Skylab are engineered to permit astronauts to work in an oxygen-nitrogen mixture, that particular problem will be eliminated—like so many in the past—by cooperation between aerospace medicine and engineering.

An unexpected reaction to hypoxia is that an organism greatly increases its resistance to radiation. Laboratory experiments in Russia, as reported by P. P. Saksanov of the Institute of Biomedical Problems, showed that rats exposed to radiation doses of 1400 R in a normal atmosphere all died, but when other rats were exposed to similar doses of radiation in an enviroment of only five per cent oxygen, their survival rate was 29 per cent. Russian experimenters consider that hypoxia can be recommended as protection from ionizing radiation, but only when the radiation dose is extremely powerful and of limited duration, as might pertain when an aircraft was forced to fly through a radioactive cloud.

Silent and invisible, hypoxia is insidious; it can grab a man before he knows it. An individual may develop symptoms without being aware of them; he may become euphoric, display poor judgment, and show inability to perform normal tasks. It is this aspect of hypoxia which makes it particularly dangerous to astronauts. Fortunately, engineering has virtually eliminated its possibility, and biomedical telemetry enables ground monitors to detect its persence long before it affects an astronaut.

Hypobaria, the third invisible hazard that can manifest itself suddenly in a spacecraft, is the result of diminished barometric pressure, and can exert profound influences on the physical condition of astronauts, varying from simple discomfort to death.

Changes in barometric pressure are a part of everyday life. That often used, and not quite so often understood expression, "the barometer's dropping," predicts a change for the worse in weather. Apart from knowing that in some way the barometer* is related to "30 inches of mercury," the subject of barometric pressure is a mystery to many people. Simply stated, during periods of good weather there is high atmospheric pressure, and accordingly, a "high" barometer. Low air pressure that indicates approaching poor weather conditions is marked by a "low" barometer.

Much of the early knowledge concerning the medical aspects of barometric changes were gained from experiences with man working below sea level—sand hogs in tunnel building and divers in salvage work. In such conditions, men were exposed to increased barometric pressure, called *hyperbaria*. Only after men began to fly and reach heights far above sea level did they experience the opposite of *hyperbaria*, or *hypobaria*. Both conditions are a form of *dysbarism*, which is the result of differences between the atmospheric pressure and pressure of gases within the body.

Dysbarism, as first experienced by sand hogs and divers, was known as the "bends," and was caused by formation of nitrogen

*The first barometer was devised in 1644 by Evangelista Torricelli, a student of Galileo, who discovered that normal atmospheric pressure would support a column of mercury 30 inches high in a glass tube. That figure is now commonly expressed in millimeters of mercury as "760mm Hg."

bubbles in the blood vessels of the knee joints, wrists and shoulders, after a man who had been working in higher than normal atmosphere again returned to normal air pressure.

In flight, the effect of reduced barometric pressure is to cause expansion of any trapped gas within the body. Gas in the gastrointestinal tract will expand so long as the barometric pressure is reduced through gain in altitude, and produces acute abdominal discomfort. There may also be cardiopulmonary reactions—circulatory shock, and pulmonary irritation and coughing—the "chokes"—caused by small nitrogen bubbles in the lung capillaries. This can, in turn, cause pulmonary hypertension and even heart dilatation and failure. Accordingly, preparation for any spaceflight involves strict attention to diet, abstention from known gas-forming foods, and regulation of bowel habits.

The last and most common example of the effect of change in barometric pressure is one experienced by passengers in commercial jet liners that make a rapid descent into an airport control area. The increasing barometric pressure will result in negative pressure in the middle ear, if the eustachian tube is not "clear" or patent, there may be retraction of the ear drum and severe pain.

One need not be an astronaut to gain relief—all the small fry at the local swimming pool know how to "pop their ears." The medical term for it is the *valsalva maneuver*—pinching the nostrils shut while attempting to breathe out, thus increasing pressure to the middle ear.

One of the first effects of hypobaria observed after spaceflight commenced with a simple skin itch, usually on the body, which sometimes produces a fine red rash. While its cause is not yet known, it may be due to gas evolving from subcutaneous fat tissue.

Despite a recitation of the many physiological aspects of spaceflight, the results of the space program to date indicate that man generally adapts well to, and functions effectively in, the space environment. Some potentially serious problems have been discovered, but they are not insurmountable. Considering the achievements of aerospace medicine at this stage in the conquest of space, there appears to be every prospect that biomedical scientists will meet each new challenge with success.

319

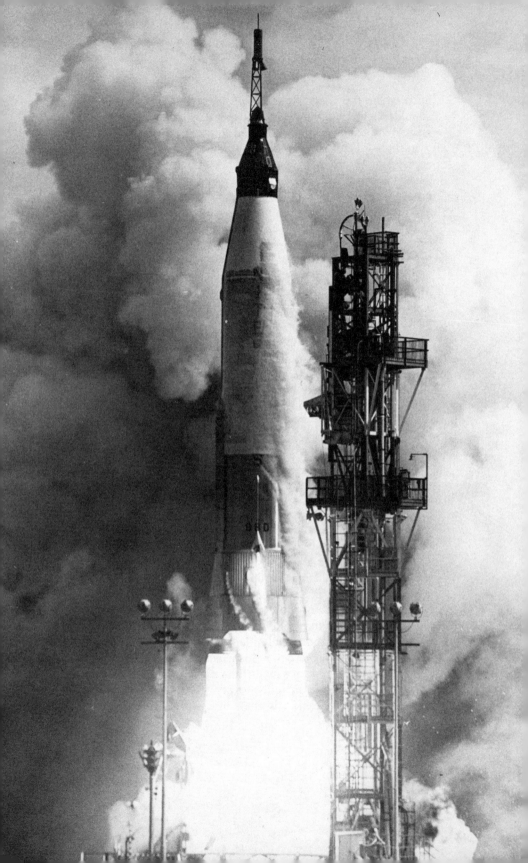

12

The Fiery Chariots

Standing on the launching pad at Cape Canaveral on 16 July 1969, the Saturn rocket with its payload—three astronauts, a lunar lander, a computer with a vocabulary of 138,000 words, and enough meals for three men for nine days—was a white spire, coated with hundreds of pounds of ice, as it towered into the morning sky.

More than a million people, for various reasons, had gathered at the Cape to watch the countdown and liftoff. In front of TV screens around the world, in every nation but Albania, China, North Korea and North Vietnam, an estimated five hundred million more waited to see the big bird climb a tower of fire into space. Nearly 3500 newsmen, including 812 from 54 foreign countries, were there to cover one of the biggest stories of the century.

If events transpired as advertised, they were about to see the commencement of a voyage that would eclipse the travels of Marco Polo, and Magellan: Apollo 11 was going to land two men on the moon.

The long trip to the moon begins here, on the launching pad at Cape Canaveral. This is the liftoff of Apollo 17, the flight which terminated the Apollo program, on 7 December 1972./*U.S. Navy*

At 7:02 Central Daylight Time that morning, Apollo 11 Mission Control went on the air with the first of the 582 transmissions that would describe the moon mission:

"This is Apollo-Saturn Launch Control T minus 1 hour 30 minutes 55 seconds and counting. All elements are GO..."

This was not the first rocket off the Cape, nor would it be the last. Other men had already flown around the moon, and still others would follow Apollo 11 across space. But this was to be the "giant leap for mankind" that would fulfill the dreams of philosophers, scientists, and astronomers of centuries past. The moon had filled the night with mystery and wonder ever since Peking Man gazed at it across the camp fire, a million years ago. On nights when the moon was full, one might feel that he could reach out and touch it. No one knows who first decided that the moon could be reached, but here will follow the named of men who have done so.

The sun was less mysterious; it was right there every day, where it was needed. In Greek mythology the god Apollo typified the sun, and Pegasus, the winged horse, left the earth to mount into the skies. Icarus followed Pegasus toward the sun, but its heat melted his wings of wax. The Old Testament describes how Elijah was carried up to heaven in a fiery chariot.

The moon though, was another matter; it waxed and waned, and disappeared completely at times. Crops were affected by the moon, as were tides and sleepless dogs. By the time the Christian era began, men believed the moon to be a solid body in the sky, and near enough—it moved around all the while—for there to be some hope of reaching it. So, the first journey to the moon was described in 160 AD by a Greek satirist, Lucian of Samosata. His *Vera Historia* came closer to modern "space opera" than some current Hollywood productions, and it is probably just as well for the advancement of science that it was more or less forgotten for some fourteen hundred years. A man headed for the moon was going to need more than a whirlwind to make the trip.

"This is Apollo-Saturn Launch Control at 1 hour 7 minutes 25 seconds and counting, countdown still proceeding satis-

322

factorily...The estimate is more than a million persons are in the immediate area in Brevard County to watch the launch..."

Among the spectators that morning was Lyndon Johnson, President of the United States, come to see the fulfillment of the goal announced by President J. F. Kennedy on 25 May 1961, that of landing a man on the moon before the end of the decade. Kennedy's announcement was made only 20 days after Alan Shepard had become the first American in space by riding Freedom 7 to an altitude of 115 miles in a short 14.8 minute flight, and despite the fact that the newly created National Aeronautical and Space Administration (NASA) had advised Congress that a lunar landing would cost from twenty to forty billion dollars.

Presidential interest in flight was nothing new. The first balloon flight in the United States was witnessed by the first president. What Washington had seen was a balloon ascension by the "bold aeronaut," French-born Jean Pierre Blanchard, from the Walnut Street Prison in Philadelphia, the morning of 9 January 1793. Although credit for the first flight over American soil went to a Frenchman, Blanchard was accompanied by a small black dog who was undoubtedly a native American and thus claimed at least part of the resulting publicity.

"This is Apollo-Saturn Launch Control. We are now less than 16 minutes away from the planned liftoff...At the 2-second mark we'll get information and a signal that all engines are running...We will have some 716 million pounds of thrust pushing the vehicle upwards...We are now 14 minutes and 30 seconds and counting..."

Based on past performance—Apollo 8 and 10 had made orbital flights around the moon, and Apollo 10 had sent a lunar module down to within 47,000 feet of the lunar surface—Apollo 11 looked a fit ship for the trip. In sheer size alone it was monumental—363 feet overall, as big, far more powerful, and infinitely more complicated and expensive than a World War II destroyer. The whole assembly, comprising 15,000,000 parts, weighed close to 6,500,000 pounds—3,250 tons. The three stages of the rocket

323

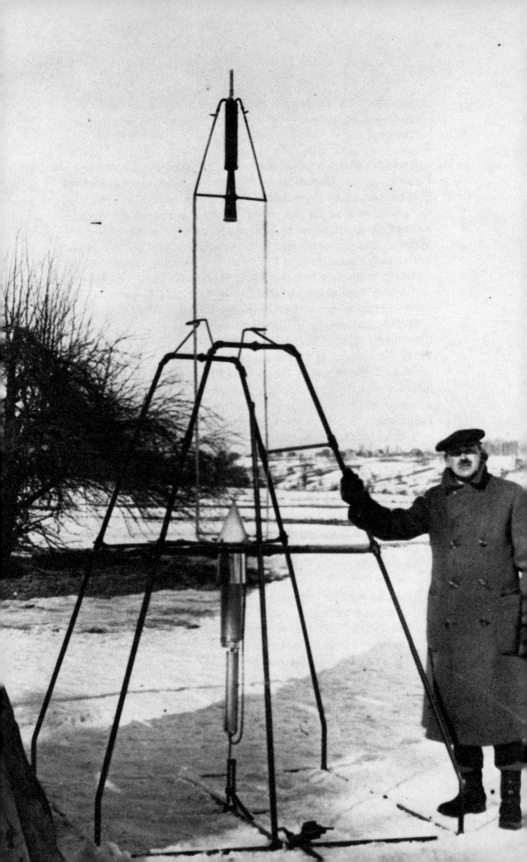

contained more than a million gallons of liquid oxygen and kerosene and hydrogen fuel.

Few people watching the countdown would know that Saturn's great grandfather had been a primitive affair, weighing a little over five pounds empty and twice that loaded, and that it had made the world's first flight with a liquid propellant—liquid oxygen and gasoline—on 16 March 1926, at Auburn, Massachusetts. No one at all would have been impressed by its performance—altitude, 41 feet, and length of flight, 184 feet, to a crash landing in a cabbage patch.

That rocket marked the end of twelve years of study and experimental work by Robert H. Goddard, the noted American pioneer in rocketry. He had gained some publicity in 1919 when the Smithsonian Institution published his 69-page paper titled *"A Method of Reaching Extreme Altitudes."* and then issued a press release inviting attention to his speculations on a rocket shot to the moon. A year later Goddard published a short, 23-page paper in which he discussed most of the principles of modern space flight—the use of gyros and in-flight course corrections by small rocket motors, retro-rockets, and an ablating heat shield for reentry.

Newspaper staffs in those days being far less blessed with scientific writers than they are now, the New York Times gave Goddard the benefit of its editorial opinion, stating that as a professor of physics he should know better than to propose space flight, as the whole idea violated a fundamental law of dynamics.

There was nothing new about the idea of rocket propulsion and space flight—it merely deviated from the fictional concepts of Jules Verne and H. G. Wells, and actually was much older than either of them. The Chinese, who invented gunpowder, credit a legendary mandarin named Wan Hu with the first rocket flight. He had a chair fitted with a bank of rockets, and after coolies lit them all at once, he took off and was never seen again.

"This is Apollo-Saturn Launch Control...Two minutes, 32 seconds and counting...The target for the Apollo 11

Dr. Robert L. Goddard, the "Father of American Rocketry," poses with the great-grandfather of all rockets, at Auburn, Massachusetts, on 16 March 1926. The Goddard Space Center honors this pioneer of the space age./*NASA* astronauts, the moon, at liftoff will be at a distance of 218,096 miles...We're approaching the 60 second mark..."

After the introduction of gunpowder into Europe, considerable effort was devoted to writing about rockets, but not much practical work ensued until the beginning of the 19th century. Then the British found themselves beset by rockets used against them in India. William Congreve went to work to produce something better, and by 1805 was firing rockets with a range of little over a mile. Throughout the rest of that century, various national powers experimented with military rockets, using them much as the Germans did against London during the latter part of World War II. Copenhagen was nearly burned to the ground by a massed rocket attack in 1807; Danzig surrendered after a rocket bombardment in 1813; and in 1814 the British use of rockets in their attack on Fort McHenry, at Baltimore, aside from the resulting noise and damage, resulted in their being given prominent mention in *The Star Spangled Banner.*

All such rockets, of course, burned gunpowder which required oxygen for combustion and could not have functioned once they left the earth's atmospheric envelope. The answer to space flight was a rocket fuel not dependent on an outside oxygen supply, and thoughts along this line occupied the minds of several men, other than Robert Goddard, at about the same time. In France, Robert Esnault-Pelterie had seen the possibility of space travel by 1908, and in 1913 published a paper describing the force generated by a hydrogen-oxygen mixture.

In France, also, Louis Damblanc began work on multi-stage rockets which burned solid fuels, and between 1935 and 1939 he had launched 360 of them.

Herman Oberth, in Germany, read Jules Verne, and the writings of Konstantin Tsiolkovsky, and by 1917 had proposed a long-range rocket fueled by ethyl alcohol, water, and liquid oxygen. He also corresponded with Goddard, began firing tests in 1928, and by 1930 had successfully demonstrated the first European rocket engine powered by gasoline and liquid oxygen.

In 1928, in Breslau, Germany, a few scientifically-minded men had formed a society with the intent of furthering the idea of planetary travel. They called their group *Verein fur Raumschif-fahrt* (Society for Space Travel) but usually referred to it as VfR. Within a year it had over five hundred members, including Herman Oberth and Robert Esnault-Pelterie. One of the younger members was named Wernher von Braun. By 1930 von Braun was experimenting with liquid-fuel rocket engines, as was Goddard in the United States and A. I. Polyarny in Russia. The V-2 rockets which terrorized England during World War II were developed at Peenemuende under von Braun's direction, and when some of them were brought to the United States by the U.S. Army after the war, von Braun came along to serve as technical advisor.

After working on the development of guided and ballistic missiles for many years, von Braun became the director of the Development Operations Division of the Army Ballistic Missile Agency in 1956. When that agency was absorbed by NASA and redesignated the George C. Marshall Space Flight Center, von Braun became its director. Each time a space shot thundered into the sky at Cape Canaveral, von Braun could remember back to his younger days in Germany, when a rocket developed a mere 15-pound thrust.

One American development of rocket power which provided valuable experience in metallurgy, pressure suits, and supersonic flight involved the X-15 research aircraft built by North American. Three of the craft were ordered in 1955, for joint work with the Air Force, Navy, and NASA. They began operations in 1959, and set several speed and altitude records before they were withdrawn from service. On 3 October 1967 the X-15A-2 with Air Force Major Pete Knight as pilot flew at a speed of 4,534 miles per hour, or mach 6.72. An all time altitude record for aircraft was set by NASA's chief test pilot Joseph Walker who reached 354,200 feet on 22 August 1963. The X-15 developed skin temperatures as high as 1,320 degrees Fahrenheit, and had a rocket powerplant producing 58,700 pounds of thrust. But the craft, although rocket-powered, could only strain at earth's gravitational pull. No matter how high they went, they had to come down again.

"This is Apollo-Saturn Launch Control...We are approaching the 60 second mark on the Apollo 11 mission. T-60 seconds

327

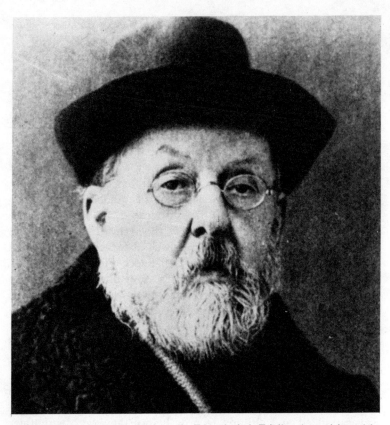

Born far ahead of his time, Konstantin Eduardovitch Tsiolkovsky anticipated by fifty years the flight of his country man, Gagarin, into space when he wrote: "Man will not stay on earth forever...." The Russians have named a huge crater on the far side of the moon in honor of Tsiolkovsky./*Smithsonian Institution*

and counting...55 seconds and counting...Transfer is complete on internal power with the launch vehicle...40 seconds...All the second stage tanks now pressurized..35 seconds and counting...T-25 seconds. 20 seconds and counting. T-15 seconds, guidance is internal. 12, 11, 10, 9, ignition sequence starts, 6, 5, 4, 3, 2, 1, zero, all engines running, LIFTOFF. We have a liftoff, 32 minutes past the hour. Liftoff on Apollo 11."

328

Apollo 11 was on its way to the moon, fulfilling the dreams of Konstantin Eduardovitch Tsiolkovsky, an obscure Russian school teacher born in 1857, as he had expressed them over half a century earlier. A man with a solid knowledge of physics, Tsiolkovsky, in Russia, ranks as high in the history of rocket propulsion and space flight as do Goddard and von Braun in the United States. By 1880 he was known for his aeronautical theory and in 1898 he published his theories of rocket-powered space flight. The Goddard experiments, and the subsequent American liquid-fuel reaction engines which sent the Mercury, Gemini, and Apollo astronauts on their missions, all were working examples of his theories.

Far ahead of his time in his concepts of powered flight, Tsiolkovsky wrote in 1911: "Mankind will not stay on Earth forever; in pursuit of flight and space, it will take first timid steps beyond the atmosphere and then conquer the whole space around the Sun." It was a Russian, Yuri A. Gagarin, who took that first timid step on 12 April 1961, when in Vostok 1 he became the first man to orbit the earth.

A fitting memorial to Tsiolkovsky, who died in 1935, has been established on the moon. The Russian lunar probe, Lunik III, first photographed the moon in October, 1959, and revealed a huge crater, 150 miles in diameter, which has been named for Tsiolkovsky. The crater is on the far side of the moon, where only those astronauts who have helped make Tsiolkovsky's dreams come true will ever see it.

After the first few Apollo missions, space shots at the Cape had become more or less routine. Starting with the first suborbital flight by Alan B. Shepard, Jr., a brief 15-minute jaunt aboard a Mercury-Redstone rocket—there had been 19 more flights before Apollo 11 took off. The pre-launch preparations had been standardized into hours-long check-off lists. People who tuned in for the exciting final minutes of the countdown and liftoff were unaware of the many tedious hours of painstaking drudgery by numberless people that had already passed. At the moment, most visible at the top of the personnel pyramid was Christopher C. Kraft, Jr., Director of Flight Operations at the Manned Spacecraft Center. But from coast to coast, border to border, in some 20,000 laboratories, shops, and factories, about 350,000 scientists, technicians, and workers had been involved in the ten-year space program—Mercury, Gemini, Apollo—in which the United States had spent twenty-five billion dollars in a determined effort to put the first men on the moon.

Those men—Neil Armstrong and Edwin Aldrin, along with Michael Collins who would remain in lunar orbit while they were on the moon—had begun their long day at 4:15 a.m. (EDT) that morning, with the usual astronaut's low residue breakfast of orange juice, steak, scrambled eggs, toast and coffee. They had checked out their suits—individually crafted to fit each man, and designed to protect them from the hazards of extreme cold in space, at a cost of $100,000 each—and taken an eight-mile, 27-minute ride to the launch pad. The rest of their trip would go considerably faster.

After liftoff, the big bird rose majestically, then flashed out of sight as Launch Control, and Space Center at Houston, called out the stages of its progress:

"...downrange 70 miles, 43 miles high, velocity 9,300 feet per second."

"Downrange 140 miles, altitude is 62 miles, velocity 10,300 feet per second."

"Downrange 270 miles, altitude is 82 miles, velocity is 12,472 feet per second."

"Downrange 530 miles, altitude 95 miles, velocity 17,358 feet per second."

"Velocity is 23,128 feet per second, Downrange 1,000 miles, altitude 101 miles."

"Apollo 11, this is Houston, at 10 minutes you are GO."

In ten minutes, Apollo 11 had passed all the mileposts to space established during two centuries of flight. In a minute it had passed the 18- to 20,000-foot level at which critical hypoxia struck balloonists, and the even more critical level at 63,000 feet, the

330

"Armstrong Line,"* at which, in an unprotected environment, barometric pressure drops to 47mm, equal to the pressure of water vapor at body temperature, and a man's blood and body fluids boil. Fifty miles up, it had passed the von Karman Line, the level at which the tenuous atmosphere makes aerodynamic navigation (flight with airfoils) impossible. Above that level, control surfaces must be replaced by reaction control—jet thrust—and spacecraft follow ballistic trajectories. The other levels   governing atmospheric or space flight have technical or biomedical significance, but the von Karman Line may eventually have some legal standing, as some law experts consider it the limit at which national authority over airspace terminates.

At 62 miles Apollo 11 had passed the official demarcation line between atmosphere and space, as established in 1946 by the *Federation Internationale Aeronautique* in Geneva. The next step—up and out, as it were—comes at 120 miles, the mechanical zero line of air resistance. There spacecraft enter the so-called "Kepler Regime" where the laws of celestial mechanics, unhindered by air resistance, become fully effective, and astronomical space begins.

"...Apollo Control at 36 minutes...We have a report on the launch rates now from the flight surgeon. Commander Neil Armstrong's heart rate 110, Command Module pilot Mike Collins 99, Lunar Module pilot Aldrin 88. These compare with their first Gemini flights...Armstrong's heart rate was 146 at that time, Collins was 125, Aldrin was 110..."

Biomedical telemetry, which enabled Dr. Berry at the Control Center in Houston to keep his finger on an astronaut's pulse even while he was on the moon, had come a long way since Dr. Barr first began working with it in 1948. The Apollo 11 flight was the 33rd manned flight, in the conquest of space, that began when Yuri Gagarin had first proved that it was possible for a human to survive and function in space. Russian telemetry for that flight was

*Named for Harry G. Armstrong, Surgeon General of the Air Force, who discovered it.

331

very limited in scope, but by the time Enos, the first American astro-chimp went into space a few months later telemetering technique had been improved to the point where Berry could read an EKG on a subject moving at high speed in space.

When the Mercury program began, continuous monitoring of any physical data while a pilot was in flight was a new concept. Equipment standards had to be established, mission rules developed to aid in flight control were necessary in medical areas as well as engineering. Finally, the evaluation and judgment of the medical officer flight controller had to stand as the prime determination in making a decision. Doctor Berry stated that "the condition of the astronaut as determined by voice and interrogation rather than physical parameters alone became a key factor in the aeromedical advice to continue or terminate the mission." In this connection, voice transmissions were an especially valuable aid. To insure that medical monitors were familiar with an astronaut's normal voice, tapes of mission simulations were sent to all the tracking stations in the network before each mission.

One of the basic objectives of the Mercury project was to evaluate human response to the space-flight environment, including the wearing of full-pressure suits (although not pressurized in flight) confinement and restraint in the Mercury spacecraft with legs elevated to a 90-degree position, the 100-per cent oxygen atmosphere at 5psi pressure, variations in cabin and suit temperatures, excessive g forces met in launch and reentry, weightlessness, vibration, high decibel noise, sleep schedules, diminished food intake, and dehydration. Data obtained during the missions showed that peak physiological responses were closely related to critical inflight events.

It was determined that some weightlessness fears were unfounded. The astronauts were able to conduct complex visual-motor coordination tasks, and experienced no dysfunction of any body system. Urination continued normally, and there was no evidence of difficulty in intestinal absorption under zero gravity. As the Mercury flights were at a level below the Van Allen belt, radiation was not a problem. During the Mercury 8 and 9 flights astronauts wore dosimeters which showed they received no greater radiation than they would have experienced on earth.

Several valuable lessons were learned, regarding the pattern of medical care, and general handling of astronauts. There was need for many practice runs. A medical countdown was developed with specific timing of events. Initial consideration was given to isolating flight crews before a mission to prevent exposure to communicable disease, but this proved impractical because the men had too many last minute activities with a great number of people who had essential duties in the launch routine. Also, care had to be taken to prevent fatigue during final preflight preparations and postflight activities, with minimum postflight rest after a 34-hour mission established at between 48 and 72 hours.

The successful completion of the Mercury and Gemini programs provided a valuable store of biomedical information gained through telemetry, and led to greater confidence in the next stage of spaceflight, the Apollo missions.

In a summary of the manned space program printed in the Journal of the American Medical Association in July, 1967, Dr. Berry stated:

"Nineteen men have flown 25 manned flights, giving us a total weightless experience of some 2,000 man-hours...

"This massive flight experience, while literally only scratching the surface of detailed space exploration, should provide some basis for comparing the predictions concerning man's support and his response to this environment with the reality of the findings from such experience.

"The medical objective in the manned space flight program, simply stated, is to provide medical support for man, enabling him to fly safely..

"In attaining this objective we find ourselves involved in tasks with different orientation...This calls for a constant interplay between the experimental and operational medical approach to these missions."

The interplay suggested by Berry was achieved—not always with the greatest of ease—as the success of the Apollo missions testified.

Biomedical telemetry not only let the astronauts' medical officer keep close check on their physiological conditions; it let those monitoring the flight from Houston keep tabs on the micro-environments in which the astronauts worked and slept. As Armstrong brought the lunar lander, Eagle, down to the first moon landing, his heart rate went up to 156; this was exceeded only during the period he was transferring geological specimens into the lunar module, then it topped out at 160. But while sleeping, on the moon, heart rates went as low as 50. Telemetry showed the lunar module then to have a temperature of 60 degrees—as compared to the -250°F existing outside, with cabin pressure at 5 pounds per square inch—one third of normal atmospheric pressure on earth.

"...Apollo Control at 2 hours 8 minutes into the mission...orbit changing slightly as the S-IVB third stage vents. We are showing an orbit now of 107 by 105.7 nautical miles in an orbital period of 1 hour 28 minutes 30 seconds..."

Apollo 11 was now circling the earth at 25,254 feet a second, following the paths marked in space by the Russians in their Vostok, Voskhod, and Soyuz missions, and by Americans in the Mercury-Redstone, Mercury-Atlas, and Apollo missions. Plus, of course, the first trails blazed by assorted dogs, rabbits, chimpanzees, and that first and most world-startling of all, Russia's Sputnik which began beep-beeping its way around the world on 4 November 1957 and started it all. Sputnik remained in orbit for only 22 days, during which it made 326 revolutions, but it added a new word to the English language—a small reminder that Konstantin Tsiolkovsky first used the word. In Russian, Sputnik means "travel companion."

The first Sputniks flew in uncrowded skies.* The United States planned to orbit a scientific satellite during the 1957 International Geophysical Year, using a 72-foot Vanguard rocket as the launch vehicle. The satellite, about the size of a grapefruit, made headlines but little history; in America's first space shot, on 6

---

*In January, 1979, the North American Air Defense Command announced that there were 11,247 pieces of manmade machinery and debris in space including 1,008 working earth satellites. There were 61 craft in deep space.

334

December 1957, the Vanguard lifted five feet into the air and then exploded in a ball of fire.

The next shot, on 31 January 1958, put the first American satellite into orbit; this was Explorer 1, which reached to 1,573 miles above the earth, and sent back radio data on the Van Allen Belt (See Chapter 9). Through the next ten years 36 Explorer satellites were launched, with one of them going beyond the moon. Bigger and better rockets—Redstone, Jupiter, Thor and Atlas—lifted heavier payloads with improved control, and made feasible the commencement of the manned space-flight missions which terminated with the successful Apollo programs.

On 27 October 1958, with Project Mercury still not much more than a name, a report issued by the Special Committee on Space Technology set the tone for all space research for the next couple of decades. It discussed, among other points, acceleration, high intensity radiation in space, cosmic radiation, closed cycle living, development of space capsules, and necessary concurrent biomedical and physical research to determine man's capability in space. The report included this far-reaching statement:

"The ultimate and unique objective in the conquest of space is the early successful flight of man, with all his capabilities, into space and his safe return to earth. Just as man has achieved an increasing control over his dynamic environment on earth and in the atmosphere, he must now achieve the ability to live, to observe, and to work in the environment of space."

Those words might well greet research scientists making their first trip to Skylab in the 80s, but they served, when written, as a strong incentive to get Project Mercury off the ground with all possible despatch.

Project Mercury was the first space program set up under NASA after it was created by the Space Act of 1958. The program was named for Mercury, the wing-footed messenger of the gods at the suggestion of Abe Silverstein, Director of Space Flight Development. The aim of Project Mercury was to design and develop a spacecraft capable of carrying a man in an orbital flight around the earth and return him safely, while at the same time evaluating his performance capabilities and functional efficiency

335

under conditions of high acceleration and deceleration, and zero gravity.

The matter of safe return to earth posed a fine problem in control of speed and rate of descent—too steep a descent at too great a speed would generate enough heat to incinerate the spacecraft, but too small an angle of descent could cause it to skip off the upper layer of atmosphere and keep on going. Also, as a spacecraft came down, the intense heat generated—about 5000°F a few seconds after it encountered atmosphere—caused a temporary "blackout" of communications. By the time of the Apollo flights, this phenomenon was understood and planned for in the mission. The first American experience with this came during the orbital flight of John Glenn in Friendship 7. As he returned to earth in his fiery chariot after his 17,544 mile an hour flight, voice contact was lost for about seven minutes of almost unbearable suspense. Dr. William Douglas, the physician for the astronauts during that program, was pictured by Time magazine as he stood, head bowed and hands folded, waiting...

One result of Mercury development was the blunt body shape used in all subsequent spacecraft; this was conceived by H. Julian Allen at the Ames Research Center, and involves a heat-ablation coating of phenolic epoxy resin on the base of the reentry capsule. A spacecraft returning to earth heats up within a few seconds after entering the upper layer of atmosphere, the heat is dissipated by the phenolic epoxy resin which melts and flakes away.

Project Gemini, named for the constellation of Gemini which includes the twin stars, Castor and Pollux, was planned to train two-man teams, in larger and more sophisticated spacecraft, for missions extending over a period of days—long enough to fly to the moon, land a scientific team, and return to earth. Twelve flights—two of them unmanned—were conducted during the Gemini program.

As set up by NASA, Project Gemini had specific mission objectives. These were: to subject two men and their supporting equipment to long-duration flights of up to two weeks in space; to achieve rendezvous and docking with another orbiting vehicle and develop efficient and reliable rendezvous techniques; to use target vehicle propulsion systems to maneuver the spacecraft in space after docking; to perform extravehicular activities (EVA) requiring one of the crew to leave the spacecraft for short periods of time while in orbit and develop the capability and techniques for EVA operations in space; develop a controlled reentry technique capable of bringing a spacecraft down to a specific landing area; and train crew members to fly in the subsequent Apollo missions.

With two men in a team, the Gemini flight missions became much more involved. For the first time, a man left a spacecraft in space while his team-mate remained on board. A flight of 14 days was made—nearly twice as long as needed for a lunar mission—and in preparation for the launching and later recovery of a lunar landing module on a moon mission, docking operations were conducted in space, and two spacecraft made a space rendezvous and flew side by side in formation.

The longer flight periods allowed more time for various experiments involving radiation, laser communications, celestial radiometry, photography, and spectrometer observations. Bio-medical experiments involved the effects of radiation and zero g on the blood, calcium deficiencies, bone demineralization, cardiovascular conditioning, and vestibular dysfunctions.

After the last Gemini flight splashed down in an outstanding example of pinpoint navigation—less than four miles from the recovery carrier, after 59 orbits of the earth, MSC Director Robert E. Gilruth explained the prime purpose of the Gemini flights: "In order to go to the moon, we had to learn how to operate in space...we have completed 10 manned flights in 18 months and have done all the things we had to do as a prelude to the moon."

"This is Apollo control. We are 10 minutes away from ignition on translunar injection. We want to add 10,435 feet per second to the spacecraft's velocity, looking for a total velocity at the end of this burn of about 35,575 feet per second."

This was where Apollo 11, following the procedures set up for the moon missions of Apollo 8 and 10, would speed up enough to leave earth orbit and head across space for the moon. Apollo 9, it should be noted, did not go to the moon, but the crew did

337

everything else required in a moon flight; while in orbit around the earth, they simulated operation of a lunar lander, descending to the moon, taking off, and rejoining the command module.

In the final orbit before it entered translunar injection (TLI) Apollo 11 was a hundred miles above the earth and about to move out into cislunar space—the zone between earth and moon and the edge of space, the Keplerian regime. Ahead of them waited the moon—the earth's only natural satellite. Besides establishing the laws of motion that governed the movements of planets and satellites—and spacecraft—Kepler also coined the word satellite, and wrote a fictional account of a trip to the moon, titled *Somnium* (Fantasy). He envisioned a mode of travel that was, to say the least, the most direct route from earth to moon—his astronomers were carried across space on the earth's shadow during a lunar eclipse.

Kepler and another of the great men who solved many of the riddles of the universe through mathematics, Isaac Newton, developed the basic principles of astronautics. Once the laws of motion and planetary orbits were understood, it was the turn of Karl Friedrich Gauss to work on the calculations of orbits, thus making it possible for any mathematician to determine that a satellite, to orbit at the surface of the earth, would need a velocity of five miles a second. The inability to attain such speed, a couple of centuries ago, was so overwhelming there was no point in further calculating that at an altitude of 1000 miles above the earth, a satellite would still need a velocity of 4.4 miles a second to stay in orbit. The concepts and calculations were all correct, but any prospect of seeing them carried out was impossible—*nothing* could move that fast.

"Apollo 11, this Houston. We are slightly less than one minute to ignition...We confirm ignition and thrust is GO...Velocity 26,000 feet per second...Velocity 27,800 feet per second...Velocity 32,000 feet per second...34,000 feet per second now...Cut out. We're showing velocity 35,750 feet per second. Altitude 177 nautical miles."

Apollo 11 had now attained escape velocity, the speed necessary to lift out of the earth orbit. If the departure speed and direction had been properly computed, they would be on a trajectory to the

338

moon. So far, in all recorded history, only six men, the crews of Apollo 8 and 10, had preceeded them—plus, of course, several shiploads of fictional characters. *Voyages to the Moon*, published in 1961 by Marjorie Hope Nicolson, listed more than sixty books written during the 17th century alone, describing extraterrestrial voyages.

The most famous moon voyage of all, before NASA began sponsoring them, was the classic *From the Earth to the Moon*, published just after the Civil War by Jules Verne, the noted French science fiction writer who later forecast the nuclear submarine in his equally classic *Twenty Thousand Leagues Under The Sea*. Verne came remarkably close to outlining the basic elements of the Apollo flights. He knew that the celestial mechanics involved required a launching spot within 28 degrees of the equator, and selected a spot on the west coast of Florida, just south of Sarasota and about 130 miles from Cape Canaveral, as the right spot.

Verne estimated 96 hours for the trip to the moon—the Apollo 11 astronauts landed after 103 hours, but had spent 24 hours in lunar orbit before they descended to the surface—and sent his three adventurers off in a 9-foot, 20,000 pound projectile not much larger than the Apollo reentry capsule. Verne described a pure ballistic flight; a projectile fired out of a 900-foot long gun barrel by 400,000 pounds of gun cotton. There could be no mid-course flight adjustments of course or speed, and as the aim was a little off, the fictional projectile went into orbit around the moon, leaving readers with a real cliff-hanger. In a subsequent book Verne wrote his men out of their predicament by having the projectile return to earth and splash down in the Pacific, just as American astronauts did a century later. There was another parallel with the Apollo 11 flight; one of Verne's characters was named Michael.

On 20 December 1968, Apollo 8, carrying Colonel Frank Borman, U.S. Air Force; Captain James A. Lovell, Jr., U.S. Navy; and Major William A. Anders, U.S. Air Force, blasted off from Cape Kennedy in a Saturn V rocket, a modern fiery chariot that in 11.5 minutes boosted them into earth orbit 118 miles high. After two orbits around the earth, they fired their third-stage rocket for five minutes, accelerated out of orbit and headed for the moon.

339

"You're on your way," said Christopher C. Kraft, Jr., from the MSC Houston, but it was really not so simple as all that. A good deal depended on heading in exactly the right direction, as no one knew better than one of the spectators that morning, Brigadier General Charles A. Lindbergh who, 41 years earlier, had set out on almost as daring a flight, from New York to Paris across the Atlantic.

Shooting at the moon is much like shooting a duck; one does not aim at where it is, but at the place where it is going to be. As the moon is circling the earth at better than 2200 miles an hour this requires exact determination of target angle and precise control of speed—an error of 0.1 per cent in the latter would result in a complete miss.

Another problem involved in space navigation is that after the vehicle breaks out of earth orbit at the required 35,000 feet per second, its speed constantly decreases. It is flying "uphill," as it were, until it crosses the invisible boundary of gravitational attraction between the earth and the moon. The moon, of course, is always within the gravitational field of the earth—that extends infinitely far into space, but as the gravitational force decreases as the inverse square of the distance, it becomes less and less effective. The *gravisphere*, the region within which the earth can hold a satellite in orbit, extends out about 900,000 miles, and the gravitational field is still influential several times farther than that. The moon's gravisphere extends to about 35,000 miles. About 190,000 miles out, a spacecraft crosses the line where the pull of the moon is greater than that of the earth, and the rest of the moon flight is "downhill all the way."

"Apollo Control at 61 hours 39 minutes...in less than 10 seconds now, we'll be crossing into the sphere of influence of the moon...at a distance of 186,437 nautical miles from earth and 33,822 nautical miles from the moon..."

After a spacecraft leaves earth orbit and enters its translunar trajectory, its crew spends the next three days checking navigation, taking photographs of the earth and moon, making TV transmissions back to earth, eating, sleeping, and performing housekeeping chores. A "shipboard routine" allowed two men to

340

sleep while one kept watch, but sleep was not deep or restful. Even Lovell, who had been in space twice before, had difficulty sleeping. Borman finally took a Seconal sleeping tablet, got some sleep, woke up with a headache, vomited, and began showing symptoms of acute viral gastroenteritis.

At the MSC in Houston, Doctor Berry diagnosed their problems as motion sickness, prescribed Marezine if they began feeling uneasy, and kept a close watch on their physiological conditions through biomedical telemetry.

As Apollo 8 climbed higher into space, farther away from the earth and its heavy gravitational pull, its speed was constantly reduced. By the time it entered the moon's gravitational field, it was moving at about 3,000 feet per second. Then it began to build up speed. So far the spacecraft had been heading toward the moon nose first, but now the astronauts turned it around so its rocket pointed toward the moon and prepared for the "burn" that would reduce their speed so they would enter a lunar orbit. The moon's pull had speeded them up to about 7500 feet per second; they would have to slow to about 5500 feet per second to make the maneuver, and they would do this after the spacecraft had gone around and behind the moon. All the spacecraft that followed them would go through the same procedure, while out of touch with and out of sight of anyone on earth who could help if something went wrong.

This is one of the most anxious moments of space flight. Going or coming: all communications are blanked off for 30 minutes while the spacecraft is behind the moon. If the burn is successful, monitors on earth still have to wait 20 minutes before they find out about it. Finally Jim Lovell's voice reached across nearly a quarter of a million miles to report "Burn complete. Our orbit is 169.1 by 60.5." This meant that apogee (the highest point of the orbit) would be 161.1 nautical miles above the moon as the craft passed in front of it, and the perigee (the lowest point in the orbit) would be 60.5 nautical miles above the moon as the craft passed behind it.

In the next 20 hours, Apollo 8 orbited the moon 10 times, during which the astronauts made hundreds of photographs of the lunar surface, described in great detail the features they could see, and sent back to earth the television pictures that let millions of people share the excitement of that historic flight. No one who watched that amazing "live" view of the moon on Christmas eve will ever forget hearing Borman, Lovell and Anders read from the Book of Genesis: "In the beginning God created the heavens and the earth. And the earth was without form, and void, and darkness was upon the face of the deep..."

Early on Christmas morning, Apollo 8 fired its main engine and broke out of lunar orbit for the return flight to earth. Again, the burn took place on the far side of the moon while the spacecraft was out of radio contact, a situation that caused nearly unbearable suspense. If the engine did not fire, Apollo 8 would remain in lunar orbit forever. Finally, there came Jim Lovell's voice again: "Please be informed there is a Santa Claus."

Apollo 8 was on its way home. At 10:51 a.m. Eastern Standard Time, 27 December, the spacecraft splashed down in the Pacific, within sight of the carrier *Yorktown*, only 45 seconds later than the flight plan had scheduled, after a historic flight of 500,000 miles to the moon and back.

On 3 March 1969 Apollo 9 went into earth orbit for a ten-day flight rehearsal of a lunar landing. The crew, James A. McDivitt, David R. Scott, and Russell L. Schweickart, were to evaluate the lunar landing module under space flight conditions, make an EVA contingency transfer from the lunar module to the command module, and demonstrate the capability to fly the two spacecraft on lunar landing type trajectories to achieve rendezvous and docking.

During the ten day mission, despite crew members suffering from colds, and Schweickart also suffering from nausea and vomiting, they conducted spaceflight operations. The lunar landing module was separated from the command module and the two flew for four hours, as much as 190 nautical miles from each other. Schweickart climbed out of the lunar module and was exposed to space for 47 minutes. The spacecraft splashed down in the Atlantic only three miles from the recovery carrier *Guadalcanal*; its crew had proved all systems to be nearly flawless, and had qualified the launch vehicle, the lunar lander, the portable life support system (PLSS) backpack, and the flight control techniques designed for manned lunar landing flights.

342

"Apollo Control at 75 hours into the mission. Apollo 11 is 2,241 nautical miles away from the moon. Velocity 5,512 feet per second. 41 minutes away from loss of signal as 11 goes behind the moon. We're 49 minutes away from the lunar orbit insertion maneuver no. I..."

"This is Apollo Control...at 78 hours 18 minutes into the flight of Apollo 11. Apollo 11 still passing around the far side of the moon. We are less than 5 minutes now away from time of acquisition on this second revolution..."

"This is Apollo Control at 100 hours 14 minutes. We are now less than 2 minutes from reacquiring the spacecraft on the thirteenth revolution. When next we hear from them the lunar module should be undocked from the command and service module. We're presently about 25 minutes away from the separation burn..."

On the far side of the moon, Apollo 11 and the lunar landing module separated, and as the two vehicles came around to earthside Neil Armstrong, flying the lunar lander, announced to MSC Houston:
"The Eagle has wings."

For Armstrong and Aldrin, it would indeed be downhill all the rest of the way if everything went well. Both vehicles would make one more orbit of the moon before the lunar lander commenced its descent, and back in Houston, at mission control, everyone who could crowded around TV screens to wait and watch—everyone from John Glenn, who made America's first orbital flight, to Wernher von Braun, who had been launching rockets before some of the astronauts were born. As Eagle came around the second time, still flying 50,000 feet above the lunar surface, everything checked out. Now was the time.

"Eagle, Houston. You are go...You are go to continue power descent."

It had been 102 hours and 38 minutes since Apollo 11 lifted off the pad at Cape Kennedy. Eagle began the burn that would drop

343

them to the moon, and Apollo Control in Houston called out the altitudes as they went down—40,000 feet, 33,500, 27,000, 21,000, 16,300, 13,500, 5,200.

Five minutes after Eagle started down, it was only 4200 feet above the surface of the moon, and Apollo Control gave them the green light:

"You're go for landing. Over."
"Roger, understand. Go for landing."

Armstrong called out his altitudes from then on as calmly as if he were riding an elevator:

"We're go. Hang tight. We're go. 2,000 feet...700 feet...600 feet...400 feet...300 feet...200 feet...40 feet...picking up some dust...30 feet...picking up some dust...faint shadow... contact light. Okay, engine stop...Houston, Tranquility base here. The Eagle has landed."

"Roger, Tranquility, we copy on the ground. You've got a bunch of guys about to turn blue. We're breathing again. Thanks a lot."

At the moment Armstrong set the Eagle down, Dr. Berry, in Houston, noted that his normal heart rate of 90 had gone up to 156. A good many other people showed the same reaction.

The lunar lander remained on the surface of the moon for 21 hours, during which time Armstrong and Aldrin spent 3 hours in EVA, performing the scientific missions laid down for the flight. Armstrong, the first man on the moon, climbed down the ladder from the lunar module and stepped off with the comment "That's one small step for a man, one giant leap for mankind." Next he completed the first and most important part of the mission; he collected a contingency sample of approximately a kilogram of surface material to make sure there would be some lunar samples aboard in case the mission had to be cut short.

Next Aldrin climbed down to the moon, and the two men uncovered a plaque mounted on a leg of the lander, which read:

"Here Men From Planet Earth First Set Foot Upon The Moon July 1969 A.D. We Came in Peace For All Mankind."

With both men on the surface, they set up a TV camera to transmit panoramic views of the landing area. They also set up an American flag, rigged so it appeared to stand out in a breeze; there is no atmosphere, and hence no wind, on the moon. The flag was left behind when they took off. But they brought back with them many other flags; they had carried three American flags, flags of all the 50 states and territories, and flags of all nations diplomatically recognized by the United States. Before the flight, messages from 74 nations, wishing the men Godspeed and good luck, had been reproduced by a microdot process to fit on a silicon disk about the size of a dollar, and this too was left on the moon.

The men described the moon as being light or dark gray, depending on the angle of the sun. With no atmosphere to filter the sunlight, it was too brilliant for them to face; on the other hand, in deep shadow it was difficult for them to watch their footing. They could not see the stars from the lunar surface, nor could they see far across the surface of the moon because of its markedly curved surface in comparison to that of the earth. Although they could step from a temperature of 180°F in the sun to -160°F. in the shadow, their life support suits kept them comfortable.

Next they set up the scientific experiments. First was a rectangle of aluminum foil suspended from a rod Aldrin forced into the lunar surface and aligned so it faced the sun to catch particles of energy carried on the "solar wind." On return to earth, it was sent to the laboratory of Professor Johannes Geiss at the University of Berne, in Switzerland, for analysis.

The astronauts also set up a Laser Ranging Retroflector (LRRR) which had a hundred silica corner reflectors mounted in an aluminum frame. The purpose of this was to enable observers on earth to determine lunar librations—the slight wobble the moon makes in its orbit around the earth—and measure its exact distance from earth. The latter is done at the Lick Observatory, Mount Hamilton, California, where the 120-inch telescope is used to fire a laser beam to the moon. Exact calculations on its time of

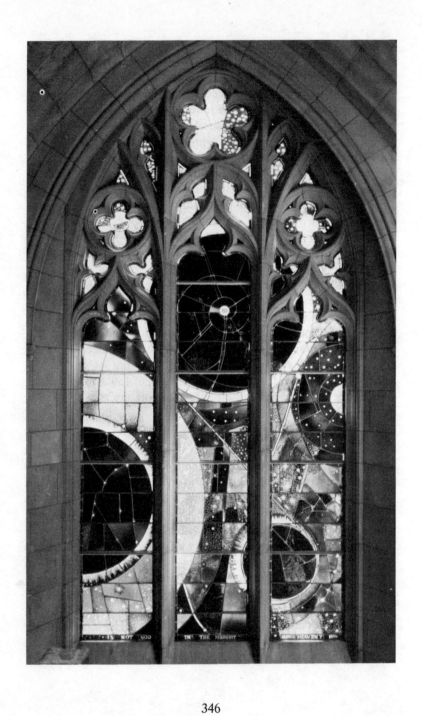

346

return—about 2.5 seconds—permit the moon's distance to be determined with an error of about 250 feet.

A Passive Seismic Experiment Package—PSEP—consisted of a self-powered seismometer which could transmit moon tremors back to earth. It was so sensitive that it recorded their footsteps, and the impact when they dropped backpacks and other equipment out of the lunar lander before they took off. A similar PSEP was left on the moon by the Apollo 12 astronauts; after they rejoined the command module, the lunar lander was allowed to crash on the moon. Although it landed about 40 miles from the PSEP, it set up vibrations which the PSEP sensed for more than an hour.

Finally, they loaded another container—they called them "rock boxes"—with more geological specimens. They brought back a total of about fifty pounds of lunar material; the amount was determined by the limited storage room and lifting power of the lunar lander. The moon rocks were worth their weight in gold, and prized far more highly by the 140 investigators around the world who were given samples of lunar material for scientific research. One small piece of "moon rock" has been mounted in the Smithsonian Institution's Air and Space Museum in Washington, D. C., where it has probably been touched by more people than ever kissed the Blarney stone. Another bit of "moon rock" is in a window in the Washington Cathedral.

On the completion of the Apollo program, there was enough lunar material on earth to satisfy the needs of all researchers everywhere. Apollo 12 brought 75 pounds, Apollo 14 brought 95 pounds, Apollo 15 brought 171 pounds, Apollo 16 brought 207 pounds, and Apollo 17 brought 243 pounds, making a grand total of 837 pounds. The age of the various samples ranged from an estimated 3.2 billion years to 4.7 billion years. The presence of gold, silver, and rubies in minute quantities was established, but not enought to cause a gold rush. The only person to cash in on the Apollo 11 voyage was a boy in London who had enough faith in the

On 21 July 1974, five years after the first moon landing, this Space Window in the Washington Cathedral was dedicated by the Very Reverend Francis B. Sayre, Jr. It was donated by Dr. Thomas Paine, a NASA administrator. The window depicts orbiting planets surrounded by stars. A small bit of moon rock from the Sea of Tranquility—the first moon landing site—is mounted in the window./*NASA* space program to bet a bookie that a man would reach the moon before 1970. He collected $24,000.

After 21 hours on the moon, Eagle blasted off and caught up with Apollo 11 on the far side of the moon during its 27th orbit. On the 30th orbit Apollo 11, with Armstrong and Aldrin aboard, fired its rockets, moved out of the lunar orbit, entered trans-earth trajectory, and started home. Apollo Control said all hands were asleep.

"Apollo Control at 148 hours 21 minutes...the spacecraft crossed from the moon's sphere of influence to the earth's sphere of influence...about 33,800 nautical miles from the moon and about 174,000 nautical miles from the earth."

In the next 40 hours Apollo 11 reached a point only 46,254 nautical miles from earth.

Seven hours later Apollo 11 was only 800 miles from earth—7 minutes away from reentry—and coming down at 33,000 feet per second. At reentry time it was making 36,237 feet a second, and went into a communications blackout for nearly four minutes. Apollo Control went off the air then to allow the recovery team in the Pacific, headed by the carrier *Hornet*, free communications.

"Apollo 11, Apollo 11. This is *Hornet, Hornet.* over."

"Hello, *Hornet*. This is Apollo 11 reading you loud and clear."

"Apollo 11 at 1,500 feet...Apollo 11 at 100 feet..."
"Splashdown, Apollo has splashdown."

Home Again!
Although Apollo 11 astronauts were treated as heroes by the press, they were handled as untouchables of the lowest cast in the Pacific, and all the way home to Houston. Once their command module had been opened, a swimmer in a protective suit tossed each one a biological isolation garment—a BIG outfit—and they sealed themselves into their new suits while the swimmer sponged them off with organic iodine, an antibacterial agent. A helicopter

348

lifted them to the *Hornet*, where they entered a mobile quarantine facility (MQF). They stayed in the MQF until the ship reached Hawaii, then—still inside—they were airlifted to Houston and moved into the lunar receiving laboratory (LRL), where they would spend the next 21 days. That period had been established in 1963 by the Interagency Committee on Back-Contamination (ICBC) set up by the Space Science Board of the National Academy of Sciences on the basis that most terrestrial disease agents were capable of invading a host and causing evident disease symptoms within 21 days after the host's exposure.

The lunar samples were handled in much the same way—opened behind absolute biological barriers under rigid bacterial and chemical isolation. All sample containers were emptied and the material was processed in a vacuum complex, and biological and chemical testing was done within biological cabinets. A secondary biological barrier surrounded the rooms in which the cabinets were handled, and a negative air pressure was maintained with respect to outside air to make certain nothing leaked out.

In the light of present scientific knowledge of conditions on the Moon—and Mars—such precautions may seem extreme, but at the time there was strong feeling about the necessity of strict quarantine. The ICBC working with NASA, developed the requirements and the guidelines which resulted in the Apollo quarantine program. The need for such a program was not universally accepted. In particular, Dr. Berry didn't believe in the quarantine and argued vociferously against it. He believed that enough data had come back from the lunar probes to prove that there were no living organisms on the moon. But the Academy of Sciences was of the opinion that "your data doesn't count. You haven't been there and you can't prove it."

However, fears of some sort of biological whiplash from a moon landing bothered many people, and before the Apollo 11 launching there was a flood of letters, some by university professors to their congressmen, and others from less-educated people whose understanding of the whole affair was far from accurate and possibly tinged by "moon bug" fiction of the 75-cent paperback variety.

Finally, Senator Anderson of New Mexico, Chairman of the

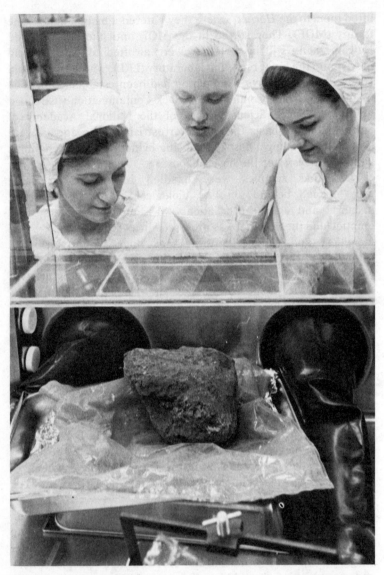

The most careful precautions were taken to avoid any possibility of earth contamination by lunar material. This piece of rock brought back by Apollo 14 is examined by technicians Linda Tyler, Nancy Trent, and Sandra Richards in the Lunar Receiving Laboratory. It was strictly a case of "look, but don't touch."/*NASA*

Senate Space Committee, called Colonel John Pickering at Brooks Air Force Base one evening and requested a statement from each member of the committee arranging the details of the LRL that they had taken every possible precaution to prevent any contamination. From seven that evening until four the next morning, Pickering phoned people all over the United States, arranging to get their statements to Anderson, who eventually had them printed in the Congressional Record. The results of the experiments made with materials brought back by Apollo 11, 12, 14, and 15 may never have reached the Congressional Record, but they made the fact plain enough for all—no moon bugs.

The lunar quarantine procedure was abolished after the Apollo 14 mission was completed, to the relief of everyone connected with the space program, and especially Doctor Berry. The only time he had really enjoyed the quarantine was the time he put it in reverse, as it were, and quarantined the Apollo 11 astronauts the night before they took off. Richard M. Nixon had just been elected president, and wanted to take some part in the space program; he proposed that he hop down to Houston and have dinner with the crew. There had always been great concern that illness would develop in a space crew during their mission, so the crews of Apollo 7, 8, and 9 had been kept in pre-flight isolation. However, none of them had landed on the moon. Berry was absolutely positive the crew of Apollo 11 was not going to bring anything contagious back from the moon, and he made absolutely certain they didn't take anything contagious to the moon with them, either. He told the president "No."

In the three years and six months before the Apollo program terminated, four more spacecraft flew to the moon. Apollo 12, which began a ten-day mission on 14 November 1969, was struck by lightning twice during the launch—the first instance of any occurence during launching operations that could have caused a mission to be aborted. The electrical system checked out satisfactorily, and the mission continued. The lunar lander touched down in the Ocean of Storms, within 600 feet of where a lunar probe, Surveyor 3, had landed on 17 April 1967. A TV camera was recovered from the Surveyor, as well as sections of aluminum tubing, glass insulation, and cables. The surface crew set up an Apollo Lunar Surface Experiment Package (ALSEP) which included a passive seismometer, an atmosphere detector to determine the density of any atmosphere the moon might have, a lunar ionosphere detector to provide information on the energy and mass spectra of positive ions close to the lunar surface, and a device to measure the amount of lunar dust accumulated by the ALSEP. As in all moon missions, thousands of photographs were made, and rock and soil samples were collected.

The only serious operational casualty occured during the flight of Apollo 13, and resulted in its crew gaining the distinction of having returned from the moon without quite getting there. About 56 hours into the mission, an electrical short circuit in an oxygen tank set off an explosion that caused serious loss of oxygen. The spacecraft was already in lunar trajectory and had to slingshot around the moon before it could return to earth. But it was a 96-hour trip home, and the power, water, and oxygen supply had been cut to about enough for 38 hours. Through the efforts of a rapidly mobilized technical crew at MSC, and tight communications, the astronauts were able to "power down" all systems. They moved into the lunar module, which had all systems still complete, and could act as a lifeboat if necessary, until one hour before reentry. The lunar lander was then jettisoned and a routine splashdown followed, after a 6-day, 541,000-mile trip.

Apollo 14, the third successful lunar expedition, was commanded by the first American in space, Alan B. Shepard, Jr. The surface crew performed the usual scientific experiments and, using the first vehicle on the moon—a two-wheeled rickshaw-like affair—ventured almost a mile away from the lander to collect specimens.

The Apollo 14 crew was the last to be subjected to quarantine precautions. Because a member of the Apollo 13 crew had been exposed to a communicable disease, a special program was set up for Apollo 14, designed to strictly limit their contacts with outsiders before the flight; only wives and about 150 people considered essential to the mission had any direct contact with either prime or backup crews. Three weeks after Apollo 14 took off, the quarantine program ended.

Apollo 15 marked the fourth successful lunar landing mission, and the first in a series of three planned to fully utilize man's capability for scientific lunar exploration. The mission included extensive lunar surface activity, and was the first to use a wheeled, powered Lunar Roving Vehicle (LRV); the LRV moved on hollow wire-mesh wheels at a speed of eight miles an hour, and cost over twelve million dollars. It made three excursions, two for seven hours and one for six, and traveled 17.5 miles. Along with the usual photography and scientific experiments they obtained spectroscopic measurements of gamma ray, X-ray and alpha particles to provide a biochemical compositional map of the moon's

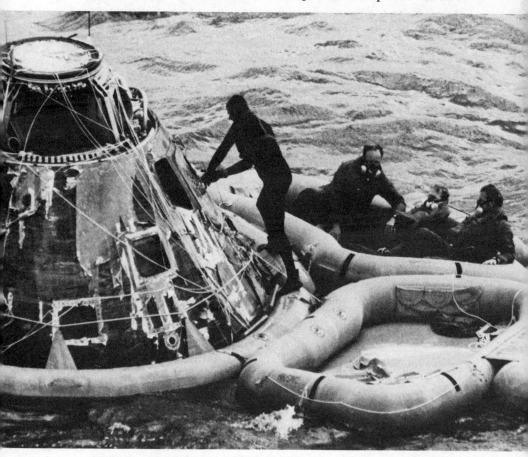

The Apollo 14 astronauts were the last men from the moon to be quarantined on their return to earth. Here their spacecraft is being sealed before pick-up by the recovery ship./*U.S. Navy*

surface. After returning to the command module, two more days were spent in lunar orbit, during which a sub-satellite was placed in its own orbit around the moon where it was expected to transmit data on the moon's environment for about a year.

Apollo 16, with some technical problems on the outward bound flight that kept the crew busy troubleshooting, carried another LRV which covered some 27 miles of the moon's surface, and carried out the usual TV photographic coverage of their activities, collected lunar material including deep-core samples down to a depth of 10 feet, and placed a second sub-satellite in orbit around the moon.

The last lunar mission, by Apollo 17, was the longest—14 days—and the surface crew spent more time on the moon—just over three days—than any other, and collected more material. It was also the first moon mission to carry a qualified geologist—Dr. Harrison H. Schmitt, who also served as lunar module pilot. The usual ALSEP was landed; this time it included a heat flow experiment, a lunar surface gravity experiment, instruments to detect micrometeorites and atmospheric composition, and instruments to detect seismographic activity, magnetic fields, and solar wind flow. While the surface crew was busy on the ground, the command module pilot conducted lunar atmospheric composition and density measurements, used an infrared radiometer to map lunar thermal characteristics, and used a lunar sounder to collect sub-surface structural data. Apollo 17 splashed down in the Pacific on 20 December 1972, just one day less than four years after Apollo 8 left the earth for the first flight to the moon.

The Apollo Lunar Landing Program, over a period of seven years put 17 spacecraft into space. Twelve men landed on the moon, where they spent a total of 672 hours. The 29 astronauts who flew in the program logged 7506 hours in flight. Aside from the vast store of scientific information brought back from the moon, the Apollo missions furnished engineers and scientists invaluable knowledge which over the next decades will assist in developing the biomedical and technical support necessary for men to carry out Tsiolkovsky's prophecy that eventually they would "conquer the whole space around the sun."

While a few crew members of Apollo flights experienced minor illnesses in space—motion sickness, nausea and vomiting, and viral gastroenteritis—their health in general was good, and very few of them experienced any psychological effects afterward. Since the Apollo crews had greater in-flight freedom of movement than the Mercury and Gemini crews, yet had the same problems, confinement had to be ruled out as a contributing factor.

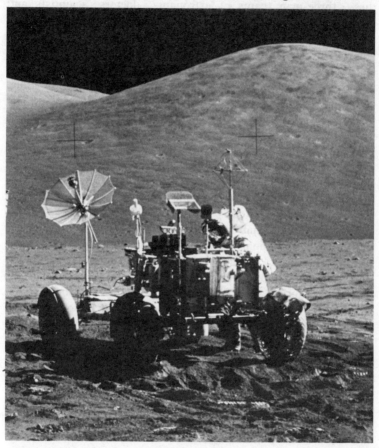

The lunar roving vehicle landed by the crew of Apollo 17. The hills in the background bound the moon valley known as Taurus-Littron. The Apollo 17 surface crew spent three days on the moon./*U.S. Navy*

With the termination of the Apollo program, it appeared that the men who had walked on the moon and others who had flown around it might be the last of their kind for many years. But this did not mean the ending of the space shots, those awesome moments at Cape Canaveral when Saturn rockets lifted in thundering clouds of fire to put more men in space. Four times in 1973 the rockets went up; first an unmanned launch, and then three, three-man teams of astronauts, doctors, scientists and engineers that went into space for a total of 12,000 man hours.

The launch of Skylab marked the beginning of a long term venture into the exploration of space from a permanent space station where trained scientists can direct their observations inward toward earth, outward to the sun, and out beyond the limits of the solar system, and the galaxy, to scan the universe. The equivalent of a small scientific complex on earth, Skylab held well-equipped laboratories for the study of physics, biology, astronomy, bacteriology, botany, geology, physiology, and zoology. Holding in orbit 235 miles above the earth, it had a zero gravity environment for the study of fluid surface-tension phenomena, free body inertial effects, biomedical and behavioral experiments, and test of the cardiovascular system.

The first three Skylab missions proved that men could function efficiently in conditions of weightlessness for long periods—the third mission lasted 84 days. Four of the men who took part in the three missions had never before been in space, but had no difficulty adapting. Said Navy physician-astronaut, Joe Kerwin, who had been in space, aboard Skylab. "You do have a sense of up and down...You just say to your brain 'Brain, I want that way to be up. And your brain says 'Okay, then that way is up.' If you want to rotate 90 degrees and work that way, your brain will follow you. I don't think it's vestibular at all. I think it's strictly eyeballs and brain. And it's remarkably efficient."

After the Skylab missions were completed, Skylab was put on hold, as it were—parked in orbit to wait for the inauguration of the earth-space shuttle. Although the first shuttle, named Enterprise, has been successfully test flown, the program has been delayed by engineering problems. Meanwhile, Skylab's orbit has been slowly deteriorating, and efforts to move it into a better flight attitude, late in 1978, were futile. It appears now that before the first Space

Shuttle goes into orbit—probably in late 1979 or early 1980, Skylab will make headlines once more as it loses orbital velocity, breaks up under the increasing pull of gravity, and returns to earth in a spectacular shower of rather expensive bits of assorted hardware.

The Space Shuttle, when it becomes operational, will not be expended in each flight, as the Apollo craft were. It is envisioned as a working vehicle, making a round trip—earth to orbit and return—in seven days.

After two weeks being serviced and reloaded, the Space Shuttle will be ready for the next flight. The "splashdown" days have ended. The Space Shuttle, although it will be boosted into space by rockets, will return to earth and land like an airplane, with the one exception that it will be a high-speed dead-stick landing. The shuttle's rocket engines are used only for maneuvering control during space flight, once it enters the atmosphere control is by conventional aerodynamic surfaces on the wings, and the vertical stabilizer.

When the Space Shuttle goes into service, flights will be launched from the Kennedy Space Center, and later from the Vandenberg Air Force Base in California, on a schedule that calls for from 40 to 60 flights a year. As each shuttle can carry from seven to ten people—crew and passengers—the next two decades will see hundreds of people journeying into space for periods ranging from days to months. Orbital flight will become mere "milk runs" for shuttle crews, field expeditions in one branch or another of scientific endeavor for researchers, and once-in-a-lifetime adventure for a chosen few who may make the trip for some extraspecial reason. Before the Skylab and Space Shuttle program winds down, men may have left earth for the first long voyage across space, to the red planet, Mars. No matter who goes where, everyone who leaves the earth for space will commence the trip in the same manner, riding a fiery chariot.

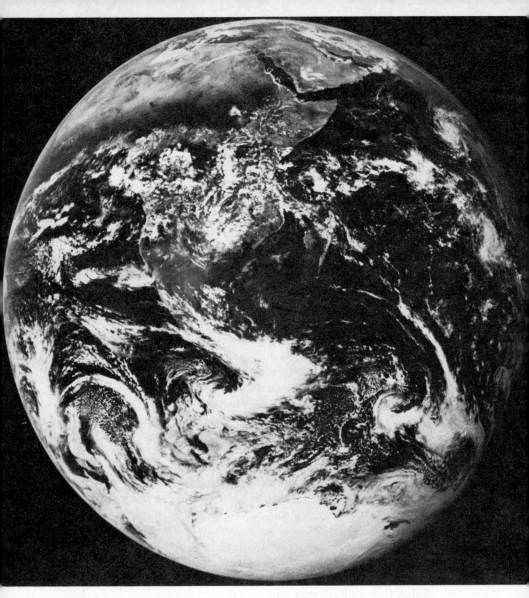

As the ancients watched darkness spread across the face of the moon, they finally
realized that they were seeing the shadow of the earth, and from the shape of the
shadow they deduced that the earth was round. Later, Copernicus proclaimed this,
and Magellan demonstrated it—to a certain extent. But not until the astronauts
headed out to the moon were men able to look down at the earth and *see* that it was
round—proof that Copernicus was right, after all. This photograph was made
during the Apollo 17 mission; only 26 men in all history have actually seen this
view, but it is one future astronauts will remember as they head out into space, and
the one they will most anticipate as they again return to earth./*NASA*

Epilogue

Thousands of years ago, before the dawn of written history, early man watched the stars and finally realized that they followed set paths across the sky and always made their appearance at the same time each season. Eventually they built monuments in which their understanding of celestial mechanics was preserved in everlasting stone—the Neolithic megaliths at Stonehenge, the Egyptian pyramids in the Valley of the Nile, and the intricate towers of lost civilizations in Yucatan.

After centuries of watching the stars, and studying them, man reached the stage in history when he was ready to take the first step on the way to reaching the stars. And in so doing, he has left modern monuments to his first venture into space that will outlast the ancient stonework of Stonehenge, Egypt, and Yucatan, and perhaps all the written records of the world. They stand in the Sea of Tranquility, the Sea of Serenity, and the Ocean of Storms, strange mechanical monster-like artifacts marking the places where space probes, and later manned spacecraft from earth, landed on the moon. In the silence and perfect vacuum of space, they will last as long as the moon does.

If visitors from outer space ever reach the moon, they will perhaps wonder at the plate proclaiming "Here men from planet earth first set foot upon the moon...We came in peace for all mankind." Those words marked the culmination of the American space program, the landing by Neil Armstrong and Edwin Aldrin in the Sea of Tranquility on 20 July 1969. The highly successful Apollo program terminated when Eugene Cernan and Harrison Schmitt landed in the Sea of Serenity on 19 December 1972. During that time 24 men went to the moon. The most sophisticated electronic communications system ever developed allowed the entire world to take part in every mission from countdown to splashdown. The tab for the entire program was set at about 25 billion dollars.

In a national economy requiring that practically every budgetary figure be expressed in megabucks, 25 billion dollars is a not uncommon sum. But justification of such an expenditure, on the basis of pork-barrel politics, can meet with carping objections: Where's the payoff? Critics point out that the space program left the moon littered with the most expensive wreckage of all time, and that the 800 pounds of rocks brought back by the astronauts—at about 30 million dollars a pound—were no bargain.

Against this, there is the fact that the spinoff from the space program has, during the past 20 years, been transferred to the fields of medicine, transportation, public safety, industry, pollution control, energy systems, construction, law enforcement, communications, home and farm, sports and recreation, and food products and preparation. It is difficult to find any facet of everyday life wherein the spinoff effect has not penetrated.

For medicine and health care alone, Americans spend some $83 billion each year. Developments in space medicine together with innovations in remote data acquisition, monitoring, and interpretation of physiological processes during flight, have generated numerous technical improvements in the quality and quantity of health care. Space medicine spinoffs range from cardiac pacemakers which can be recharged by short wave radio to cradle warmers for premature babies, and from electronic transmission of electrocardiograms of a heart attack victim in a speeding ambulance to a hospital miles away, to TV diagnosis of genetic effects while a baby is still in its mother's womb.

The ambulance-hospital hookup, enabling specialists to monitor the condition of a patient while he is enroute to the hospital involves the use of transmissions relayed from satellite in orbit about the earth. Diagnosing abnormalities in an unborn baby is made possible by a computer-enhanced image processing system developed from those which provided detailed views of the moon and, later, Venus, Mars, and Jupiter.

Many satellites, silent and invisible, orbit the earth in paths ranging from polar to equatorial orbits, at altitudes varying from a few hundred to over twenty-two thousand miles. There are dozens—hundreds—of them, and they have become essential to everyday life, although few of the people dependent on them realize it. Communications satellites relay two-way radio transmissions and television programs between various points of earth; land satellites monitor agricultural developments and ecological changes caused by forest fires, floods and mining, and help spot possible areas of pollution. Sea satellites report on ocean conditions, prevalence of ice, location of fish populations, threatening coastal disturbances, and developing changes in the scientific environment.

Magnetic satellites, to be launched in 1979, will map magnetic fields, help develop global resources maps, and identify areas for prospecting. Search and rescue satellites, scheduled to go into orbit in 1982, will monitor the locations of ships and aircraft at sea, and help to locate those in distress.

Earth orbiting satellites have become the work horses of the space age. But above and beyond them go the adventurers—the space probes that lift off from earth, never to return. Vikings, Pioneers, Surveyors—all have left this little world of tinkerers to cross into, through, and eventually perhaps beyond the vast realms conceived by Kepler, Corpernicus and Einstein.

The first views of Jupiter were sent back by Pioneer probe in 1973. In 1979, two billion miles in space, it will reach Uranus, and then leave the solar system on a voyage to infinity. The Voyager launched in 1977, will reach Jupiter in 1979; it will reach Uranus about 1986, and then it, too, will leave the solar system. Another Pioneer, which left the earth in 1972, will reach the orbit of Pluto in 1987 and then head toward the star Aldabaren, a voyage of some 300,000 years.

While these "purple pigeons"—a term for unmanned planetary exploration missions—are in space, advancing technology may make it possible to launch the first manned flight to Mars. Because

361

of the celestial mechanics involved, the flight will have to leave earth in 1986 or 1988, or be postponed until 2003 or 2018. By that time, the romatic age of the astronauts may be finished; the new space voyagers may be scientists, space age technicans, and highly specialized medical men, some of whom might have trained in the spacelabs which the Space Shuttle—Orbiter system may commence carrying into space in 1980.

The Orbiters, and their Spacelabs will take most biomedical research out of earth-based laboratories, and put it in space, where medical and scientific work will go on under actual, not simulated, conditions. The history of biomedical research will have come full circle: the physicians who first sought to study the physical and physiological aspects of flight spent their lives on the ground, with trips aloft measured in hours; the next generation of such people will adapt to weeks, even months, in space. For them, there may come times when they will have to adjust to life on earth.

This is the space age, and according to Dr. Hamilton S. Webb, it is the flight surgeons who represent space age medicine. Said Webb "...it is we who lay claim to a biological dominion in the cosmos." Undoubtedly, man is on the way. His medical achievements in the realm of flight began 200 years ago when the first balloons went aloft, taking physicians into a new environment. While the "purple pigeons" are still flying, those who continue the advance of aerospace medical research may well establish that claim.

Chronology

MAN IN FLIGHT
(selected events)

Balloon Flight in Open Gondolas

5 JUNE 1783—Montgolfier brothers, at Annonay, France, launched a balloon that reached an altitude of 6,000 feet in a 10-minute flight.

19 SEPTEMBER 1783—Montgolfier brothers, at Versailles, launched a balloon that carried a sheep, a duck, and a cock to an altitude of 1,700 feet on an 8-minute flight.

21 NOVEMBER 1783—Pilatre de Rozier and Marquis d' Arlandes made first manned balloon ascent from Bois de Boulogne, Paris. Flight lasted 25 minutes, covered about 2½ miles.

1 DECEMBER 1783—Jacques Charles and Aine Robert made first flight in a hydrogen-filled balloon, from Paris to Nesles, about 27 miles.

4 JUNE 1784—First ascent by a woman, Mme. Thible, who was accompanied by Monsieur Fleurant, at Lyons, France. Altitude, 8,500 feet. Duration, 45 minutes.

7 JANUARY 1785—First balloon crossing of the English Channel, by Jean-Marie Blanchard and Dr. John Jeffries, from Dover to province of Artois in France. Duration; 2 hours and 47 minutes.

15 JUNE 1785—Pilatre de Rozier and Pierre-Angle Romain became first casualties of air age when, on proposed flight from France to England, their hydrogen-filled balloon exploded.

9 JANUARY 1793—First balloon ascent in United States, by Jean-Marie Blanchard, from Walnut Street Prison in Philadelphia to Gloucester County, New Jersey. Altitude; 5,812 feet. Distance; 15 miles. **Duration;** 46 minutes.

22 OCTOBER 1797—Andre Jacques Garnerin made first parachute descent from a balloon, in Paris. Altitude; 3,000 feet.

17 JULY 1862—Henry Coxwell and James Glaisher took off from Wolverton, England, in first high-altitude balloon flight. They reached 26,200 feet, but both men experienced anoxia.

18 JANUARY 1871—A Frenchman, Vibert, took off from Paris and in 3 hours flew to Hynd, near the Zuyder Zee, a distance of 285 miles, for an average of 95mph.

22 MARCH 1874—Croce-Spinelli and Sivel, using oxygen-nitrogen mixture for breathing, reached an altitude of 24,300 feet during 2-hour 40-minute flight.

15 APRIL 1875—Croce-Spinelli, Sivel, and Tissandier, carrying oxygen-nitrogen mixture in goldbeater's skins, reached altitude of 28,200 feet. Croce-Spinelli and Sivel died of anoxia.

4 DECEMBER 1894—Arthur Berson, in Germany, used compressed oxygen in steel flasks to reach altitude of 30,000 feet.

31 JULY 1901—Berson, with Reinard Suring, took off from Tempelhof, Berlin, and reached altitude of 34,500 feet in 7-hour 30-minute flight.

364

4 MAY 1927—Hawthorne C. Gray took off from Scott Field, Illinois, and reached altitude of 42,470 feet. Exactly six months later, he again reached the same altitude, but died when his oxygen supply was exhausted.

Balloon Flight in Pressurized Gondolas

27 MAY 1931—Auguste Piccard and Paul Kipfer took off from Augsburg, Germany, and reached altitude of 51,775 feet.

20 NOVEMBER 1933—Thomas G. W. Settle and Chester Fordney took off from Akron, Ohio, and reached altitude of 61,237 feet before landing near Bridgeton, New Jersey.

30 JANUARY 1934—Three Russians reached an altitude of 72,182 feet, but were killed when balloon fell out of control.

10 JULY 1934—Explorer I, largest balloon built to date (capacity of 3,000,000 cubic feet, 310 feet tall), took off near Rapid City, South Dakota, with Army Air Corps officers Orvil A. Anderson, W. E. Kepner, and A. W. Stevens, and reached altitude of 60,613 feet when envelope began to tear. They bailed out at low altitude, and survived.

8 NOVEMBER 1956—Lieutenant Commanders Malcolm D. Ross and M. Lee Lewis set new world altitude record of 76,000 feet.

18 OCTOBER 1957—Ross and Lee reached altitude of 85,700 feet, record for two men in pressurized gondola.

2 JUNE 1958—Captain Joseph W. Kittinger, Jr., USAF, set new altitude record of 96,000 feet in Man High I balloon.

19-20 AUGUST 1958—Major David G. Simons, USAF, in Man High II, reached altitude of 101,516 feet.

8 OCTOBER 1958—Lieutenant Clifton McClure, in Man High III, aborted flight at altitude of 99,700 feet due to loss of temperature control in gondola.

365

Balloon Flight in Open Gondolas With Pressure Suits

16 NOVEMBER 1959—Captain Joseph W. Kittinger, Jr., took off in Excelsior I to test stabilized free-fall parachute in high-altitude descent. He bailed out at 76,000 feet and fell 65,000 feet before his chute opened.

16 AUGUST 1960—Kittinger bailed out from 102,800 feet.

4 MAY 1061—Commander Malcolm D. Ross and Lieutenant Commander Victor A. Prather, (MC), reached altitude of 113,700 feet. Their gondola landed at sea and Prather was drowned during the recovery. This is still the record altitude for manned balloon ascent.

Record Long Distance Balloon Flight

11 AUGUST 1978—Ben Abrozzo, Maxie Anderson, and Larry Newman, of Albuquerque, New Mexico, in Double Eagle II, helium-filled balloon, took off from Presque Isle, Maine, at 8:45 p.m. and headed for France. During their six-day flight, they flew as high as 24,000 feet. They landed near Misery, France, the afternoon of 17 August, having flown 3,120 miles in 137 hours to complete the first balloon crossing of the Atlantic. In 17 previous attempts by other balloons, seven liv u; had been lost.

Altitude Records For Fixed-wing Aircraft

18 JULY 1909—Louis Paulhan, at Douai, France; 492 feet in a Voisen.

29 AUGUST 1909—Hubert Latham, at Rheims, Germany; 508 feet in an Antoinette.

17 SEPTEMBER 1909—Orville Wright, at Berlin, Germany; 564 feet in a Wright aircraft.

20 SEPTEMBER 1909—Rougier, a Frenchman, at Brescia, Italy; 633 feet in a Voisen.

18 OCTOBER 1909—Charles de Lambert, at Paris; 984 feet in a Wright aircraft.

1 DECEMBER 1909—Hubert Latham, at Chalons, France; 1,486 feet in an Antoinette.

7 JULY 1910—Jan Olieslaegers, at Brussels, Belgium; 5,643 feet in a Bleriot.

8 DECEMBER 1910—George Legagneaux, at Pau, France; 10,204 feet in a Bleriot.

6 SEPTEMBER 1912—Roland Garros, at Dinard, France; 16,274 feet in a Bleriot.

23 DECEMBER 1913—Legagneaux, at St. Raphael, France; 20,080 feet in a Nieuport.

14 JULY 1914—Harry Oelrerich, at Leipzig, Germany; 25,755 feet in a D.F.W.

7 JUNE 1919—Jean Casale, at Issy-les-Moulineaux, France; 30,511 feet in a Nieuport.

5 SEPTEMBER 1923—Sadi Lecointe, at Villacoublay, France; 35,329 feet in a Nieuport.

25 MAY 1929—Willi Neuenhofen, at Dessau, Germany; 41,794 feet in a Junkers.

11 APRIL 1934—Renato Donati, at Rome, Italy; 47,352 feet in a Caproni.

8 MAY 1937—Mario Pezzi, at Montecello, Italy; 51,361 feet in a Caproni.

22 OCTOBER 1938—Mario Pezzi, at Montecello, Italy; 56,046 feet in a Caproni.

4 MAY 1953—Walter F. Gibb, at Bristol, England; 63,668 feet in an Electra.

29 AUGUST 1955—Walter F. Gibb, at Bristol, England; 65,889 feet in an Electra.

28 AUGUST 1957—Michael Randrup, at Luton, England; 70,310 feet in a Canberra.

14 JULY 1959—Vladimir Iljiuchin, at Podmoskovnoe, Russia; 94,635 feet in a T-437.

14 DECEMBER 1959—J. B. Jordan, at Edwards AFB, California; 103,389 feet in an F-104C.

28 APRIL 1961—Gueorgui Mossolov, at Podmoskovnoe, Russia; 113,890 feet in an E-66A.

6 JUNE 1962—Joseph A. Walker, at Edwards AFB, California; 246,700 feet in the X-15.

17 JULY 1962—Robert White, at Edwards AFB, California; 314,750 feet in the X-15.

22 August 1963—Joseph A. Walker, at Edwards AFB, California; 354,200 feet (over 67 miles) in the X-15.

Round-the-world Flights

6 JUNE 1924—At Seattle, Washington, a U.S. Army Douglas biplane under command of Captain L. Smith with a crew of 3 took off for the first circumnavigation of the world by air. Elapsed time; 5 months, 22 days; flight time, 363 hours.

7 AUGUST 1929—German dirigible Graf Zeppelin commenced the first round-the-world trip by a lighter-than-air craft. Elapsed time; 21 days, 7 minutes, 34 seconds.

2 MARCH 1949—U.S. Army B-29 commenced first non-stop, round-the-world flight using inflight refueling. Elapsed time; 94 hours 1 minute.

29 FEBRUARY 1962—John H. Glenn, first American to orbit the earth, made 3 orbits in Friendship 7. Elapsed time; 4 hours 55 minutes, 23 seconds. Time for one complete orbit, 98 minutes.

16 NOVEMBER 1973—Gerald P. Carr, William R. Pogue, and Edward G. Gibson, in Skylab 4, commenced the longest round-the-world trip made by Americans. They made 1,214 orbits (about 30 million miles) in elapsed time of 84 days, 1 hour, 16 minutes.

U.S. Spaceflights—Project Mercury

5 MAY 1961-FREEDOM 7—Alan B. Shepard made first suborbital flight. Duration; 15 minutes, 22 seconds. Recovery ship, USS *Champlain.*

21 JULY 1961-LIBERTY BELL 7—Virgil I. Grissom made second suborbital flight. Duration; 15 minutes, 37 seconds. Recovery ship, USS *Randolph.*

29 FEBRUARY 1962-FRIENDSHIP 7—John H. Glenn made first orbital flight around earth, completing 3 orbits. Duration; 4 hours, 55 minutes, 23 seconds. Recovery ship, USS *Noa.*

24 MAY 1962-AURORA 7—Scott Carpenter completed 3 orbits around earth. Duration; 4 hours, 56 minutes, 5 seconds. Recovery ship, USS *Pierce.*

3 OCTOBER 1962-SIGMA 7—Walter M. Schirra completed 6 orbits of earth. Duration; 9 hours, 13 minutes, 11 seconds. Recovery ship, USS *Kearsarge.*

15-16 MAY 1963-FAITH 7—Gordon Cooper completed 22 orbits of earth. Duration; 34 hours, 19 minutes, 49 seconds. Recovery ship, USS *Kearsarge.*

U.S. Spaceflight—Project Gemini

23 MARCH 1965-GEMINI 3—Virgil I. Grissom and John W. Young completed 3 orbits of earth. Duration; 4 hours, 53 minutes. Recovery ship, USS *Intrepid.*

3-7 JUNE 1965-GEMINI 4—James A. McDivitt and Edward H. White, III, completed 62 orbits of earth. Duration; 97 hours, 56 minutes. EVA, 20 minutes. Recovery ship, USS *Wasp.*

21-29 AUGUST 1965-GEMINI 5—Gordon Cooper and Charles Conrad, Jr., completed 120 orbits of earth. Duration; 190 hours, 56 minutes. Recovery ship, USS *Champlain.*

15-17 DECEMBER 1965-GEMINI 6—Walter M. Schirra and Thomas P. Stafford completed 16 orbits of earth. Duration; 25 hours, 51 minutes. Recovery ship, USS *Wasp.*

4-18 DECEMBER 1965-GEMINI 7—Frank Borman and James A. Lovell completed 206 orbits of earth. Duration; 330 hours, 35 minutes. Recovery ship, USS *Wasp.*

16 MARCH 1966-GEMINI 8—Neil A. Armstrong and David R. Scott completed 7 orbits of earth. Duration; 10 hours, 42 minutes. Recovery ship, USS *Leonard F. Mason.*

3-6 JUNE 1966-GEMINI 9A—Thomas P. Stafford and Eugene A. Cernan completed 44 orbits of earth. Duration; 10 hours, 42 minutes. Recovery ship, USS *Wasp.*

18-21 JULY 1966-GEMINI 10—John W. Young and Michael Collins completed 43 orbits of earth. Duration; 70 hours, 47 minutes. EVA, 39 minutes and 49 minutes. Maximum altitude, 478 miles. Recovery ship, USS *Guadalcanal.*

12-15 SEPTEMBER 1966-GEMINI 11—Charles Conrad and Richard F. Gordon, Jr., completed 44 orbits of earth. Duration; 70 hours, 17 minutes. EVA, 33 minutes and 2 hours 5 minutes. Maximum altitude, 853 miles. Recovery ship, USS *Guam.*

370

11-15 NOVEMBER 1966-GEMINI 12—James A. Lovell and Edwin A. Aldrin completed 59 orbits of earth. Duration: 94 hours, 35 minutes. EVA, three periods, total 5 hours 30 minutes. Recovery ship, USS *Wasp*.

U.S. Spaceflights—Project Apollo

11-12 OCTOBER 1968-APOLLO 7—Walter M. Schirra, Donn Eisele, and Walter Cunningham completed 163 orbits of earth. Duration: 260 hours, 8 minutes, 45 seconds. Recovery ship, USS *Essex*.

21-27 DECEMBER 1968-APOLLO 8—Frank Borman, James A. Lovell Jr., and William Anders flew to moon and made 10 orbits. Duration:147 hours, 11 seconds. Recovery ship, USS *Yorktown*.

3-13 MARCH 1969-APOLLO 9—James A. McDivitt, David R. Scott, and Russell L. Schweickart (command module "Gumdrop," lunar lander "Spider",) completed 151 orbits of earth. Duration: 241 hours, 53 seconds. Recovery ship, USS *Guadalcanal*.

18-26 MAY 1969-APOLLO 10—Thomas P. Stafford, John W. Young, and Eugene E. Cernan (command module "Charlie Brown," lunar lander "Snoopy,"), flew to moon and made 31 orbits. Duration: 192 hours, 3 minutes, 23 seconds. Recovery ship, USS *Princeton*.

16-24 JULY 1969-APOLLO 11—Neil A. Armstrong, Michael Collins, and Edwin E. Aldrin (command module "Columbia," lunar lander "Eagle") made third moon flight. First lunar landing in Sea of Tranquility. Duration: 195 hours, 18 minutes, 35 seconds. Recovery ship, USS *Hornet*.

14-24 NOVEMBER 1969-APOLLO 12—Charles Conrad, Jr., Richard F. Gordon, Jr., and Alan L. Bean (command module "Yankee Clipper," lunar lander "Intrepid") made fourth moon flight. Second lunar landing in Ocean of Storms. Duration: 244 hours, 36 minutes, 25 seconds. Recovery ship, USS *Hornet*.

11-17 APRIL 1971-APOLLO 13—James A. Lovell, Jr., Fred W. Haise, Jr., and John L. Swigert, Jr., (command module "Odyssey," lunar lander "Aquarius") aborted mission after oxygen tank ruptured. Duration: 142 hours, 54 minutes, 41 seconds. Recovery ship, USS *Iwo Jima.*

31 JANUARY—9 FEBRUARY 1971-APOLLO 14—Alan B. Shepard, Stuart A. Roosa, and Edgar D. Mitchell (command module "Kitty Hawk," lunar lander "Antares") made fifth moon flight; third lunar landing in Fra Mauro. Duration: 216 hours, 42 minutes, 1 second. Recovery ship, USS *New Orleans.*

26 JULY—7 AUGUST 1971-APOLLO 15—David R. Scott, James B. Irwin, and Alfred M. Worden, Jr., (command module "Endeavor," lunar lander "Falcon") made sixth moon flight; fourth lunar landing in Hadley Apennines. Duration: 295 hours, 12 minutes. Recovery ship, USS *Okinawa.*

16-27 APRIL 1972-APOLLO 16—John W. Young, Thomas K. Mattingly, II, and Charles M. Duke, Jr., (command module "Casper," lunar lander "Orion") made seventh moon flight; fifth lunar landing in Descartes Highlands. Duration: 265 hours, 51 minutes, 6 seconds. Recovery ship, USS *Ticonderoga.*

7-19 DECEMBER 1973-APOLLO 17—Eugene A. Cernan, Ronald E. Evans, and Harrison H. Schmitt (command module "America," lunar lander "Challenger") made final Apollo flight, eighth U.S. flight to moon and sixth lunar landing, in Taurus Littrow. Duration: 301 hours, 51 minutes, 59 seconds. Recovery ship, USS *Ticonderoga.*

USSR Spaceflights

12 APRIL 1961-VOSTOK 1—Yuri Gagarin made the world's first spaceflight. Duration; 108 minutes.

6 AUGUST 1961-VOSTOK 2—Titov flew in earth orbit for a duration of 25 hours and 18 minutes.

11 AUGUST 1962-VOSTOK 3—Nikolayev was in space for 94 hours and 22 minutes, and completed a dual mission with Vostok 4.

12 AUGUST 1962-VOSTOK 4—Popovich was in space for 70 hours and 57 minutes, and maneuvered to within 3.1 miles of Vostok 3.

14 JUNE 1963-VOSTOK 5—Bykovsky was in space for 119 hours and 6 minutes, and completed a dual mission with Vostok 6.

16 JUNE 1963-VOSTOK 6—Tereshkova, first woman in space, was aloft for 70 hours and 50 minutes, flew within 5 miles of Vostok 5.

12 OCTOBER 1964-VOSKHOD 1—Komarov, Feoktistov, and Yegorov completed a 24 hour and 17 minute mission first 3-man crew in space.

18 MARCH 1965-VOSKHOD 2—Leonov and Belyayev completed 26 hour and 2 minute mission, with EVA of 10 minutes by Leonov.

23 APRIL 1966-SOYUZ 1—Komarov was in space for 26 hours and 40 minutes, was killed on re-entry.

26 OCTOBER 1968-SOYUZ 3—Beregovoy maneuvered near unmanned Soyuz 2, in 94 hour and 51 minute mission.

14 JANUARY 1969-SOYUZ 4—Shatalov in 71 hour and 22 minute mission docked with Soyuz 5 and took on board two men from Soyuz 5.

15 JANUARY 1969-SOYUZ 5—Volynov, Yeliseyev, and Khrunov docked with Soyuz 4, as above.

11 OCTOBER 1969-SOYUZ 6—Shonin and Kubasov completed 118 hour and 21 minute mission, operating with Soyuz 7 and Soyuz 8.

12 OCTOBER 1969-SOYUZ 7—Filipchemko, Volkov, and Gorbatko completed 118 hour and 43 minute mission, operating with Soyuz 6 and Soyuz 8.

13 OCTOBER 1969-SOYUZ 8—Shatalov and Yeliseyev completed 118 hour and 51 minute mission, operating with Soyuz 6 and Soyuz 7.

1 JUNE 1970-SOYUZ 9—Kohayev and Sevastyanov made first nighttime launch, and longest mission to date—424 hours and 51 minutes.

22 APRIL 1971-SOYUZ 10—Shatalov, Yeliseyev, and Rukavishnikov joined up for 5.5 hours with Salyut in space. Mission was aborted early, ended in first nighttime recovery.

6 JUNE 1972-SOYUZ 11—Dobrovolsky, Volkov, and Patsayev were in space 570 hours and 22 minutes, but died of hypoxia and dysbarism due to hatch seal failure resulting in rapid decompression on re-entry.

18 DECEMBER 1973-SOYUZ 13—Klimuk and Lebedev completed mission of 188 hours and 55 minutes.

3 JULY 1974-SOYUZ 14—Popovich and Artyukhin docked with Salyut 3 and transferred to it, in 377 hour and 30 minute mission.

26 AUGUST 1974-SOYUZ 15—Sarafanov and Demin were aloft for 48 hours and 12 minutes.

2 DECEMBER 1974-SOYUZ 16—Filipchemko and Rukavishnikov were aloft for 142 hours and 24 minutes.

11 JANUARY 1975-SOYUZ 17—Gubarev and Grechko completed mission of 709 hours and 20 minutes, made first visit to Salyut 4.

5 APRIL 1975 (NO NUMBER)—Lazarev and Makarov aborted mission due to vehicle failure, landed in Western Siberia.

24 MAY 1975-SOYUZ 18—Klimuk and Sevastianov made second visit to Salyut 4, in mission lasting 1511 hours and 20 minutes.

15 JULY 1975-SOYUZ 19—Lednor and Kubasov aloft 142 hours and 31 minutes, docked with Apollo in joint US-USSR project.

6 JULY 1976-SOYUZ 21*—Volynor and Zholobor made a 49 day and 6 hour flight, transferred to Salyut 5 on 7 July.

15 SEPTEMBER 1976-SOYUZ 22—Bykovskiy and Aksenor completed mission lasting 7 days, 21 hours, and 54 minutes.

14 OCTOBER 1976-SOYUZ 23—Zudoz and Rozhdestvenskity were aloft for only 48 hours and 6 minutes; docking attempt with Salyut 5 failed.

7 FEBRUARY 1977-SOYUZ 24—Gorbatko and Glazkor docked and transferred to Salyut 5 on 8 February, returned on 25 February, duration of mission 425 hours and 23 minutes.

9 OCTOBER 1977-SOYUZ 25—Kovalenok and Ryumin were aloft for only 48 hours and 46 minutes; failed docking attempt with Salyut 6.

10 DECEMBER 1977-SOYUZ 26—Romanenko and Grechko spent 96 days in space; docked and transferred to Salyut 6 on 11 December and returned to earth on 16 March 1978 in Soyuz 27.

10 JANUARY 1978-SOYUZ 27—Dzhanbekov and Makarov spent 17 days in space, returned to earth in Soyuz 26.

2 MARCH 1978-SOYUZ 28—Gubarev and Remek completed mission lasting 190 hours and 17 minutes.

7 SEPTEMBER 1978-SOYUZ 29—Kovalenok and Ivanchenkov completed mission lasting 1911 hours and 23 minutes.

27 JUNE 1978-SOYUZ 30—Klimuk and Hermaszewski completed mission lasting 190 hours and 24 minutes.

26 AUGUST 1978 SOYUZ 31—Bykovskiy and Jahn were in space for 188 hours and 49 minutes. The spacecraft remained in orbit for 1,628 hours 14 minutes.

25 FEBRUARY 1979 SOYUZ 32—Lyakhov and Ryumin went aloft to man Salyut 6, which has been in space since late 1977.

12 MARCH 1979 PROGRESS 5—This was announced as a resupply mission to Salyut 6.

*There was no Soyuz 12
** Soyuz 20 was unmanned

U.S. Skylab Flights

25 MAN—22 JUNE 1973-SKYLAB 2—Charles Conrad, Paul J. Weitz, and Joseph Kerwin, completed 404 orbits of earth. Duration; 28 days, 49 minutes. Recovery ship, USS *Ticonderoga.*

28 JULY—25 SEPTEMBER 1973-SKYLAB 3—Alan L. Bean, Jack R. Lousma, and Owen Garriott completed 858 orbits of earth. Duration; 59 days, 11 hours, 9 minutes. Recovery ship, USS *New Orleans.*

16 NOVEMBER 1973—8 FEBRUARY 1974-SKYLAB 4—Gerald P. Carr, William R. Pogue, and Edward G. Gibson completed 1214 orbits of earth. Duration: 84 days, 1 hour, 16 minutes. Recovery ship, USS *New Orleans.*

***Skylab 1**, launched 15 May 1973, was unmanned.

Joint U.S. —USSR Project

15-23 JULY 1975-APOLLO-SOYUZ 19—Thomas P. Stafford, Vance Brand, and Donald K. Slayton completed 140 orbits of earth, docked with Soyuz. Duration; 9 days, 1 hour, 29 minutes.

Total U.S. spaceflights: 32. Astronauts participating: 49. Cumulative man hours in space: 23,083. Number of men to land on moon: 14. Lunar material returned to earth: 843 pounds.

Bibliography

Acosta, Jose de. *Natural y Moral de las Indias.* Seville: 1590. English translation, London: Blount and Ashley, 1604.

Armstrong, Harry G. *Aerospace Medicine.* Baltimore: The Williams and Wilkins Co., 1961.

....*Principles and Practice of Aviation Medicine.* London: Bailliere, Tindall and Cox, 1939.

Bauer, L. *Aviation Medicine.* Baltimore: The Williams and Wilkins Co., 1926.

Beaven, C. L. "A Chronological History of Aviation Medicine," *Flight Surgeons Topics*, 2:185-206, 1938.

Benford, Robert. *Doctors in the Sky.* Springfield, Ill.: Charles C. Thomas, 1955.

Benzinger, T. H. "The Human Thermostat," *Scientific American*, January, 1961.

...."Role of Thermoreceptors in Thermo-Regulation," in *Sensory Functions of the Skin*, vol. 27, ed. Lotterman, Y. Oxford and New York, Pergamon Press, 1976.

....ed. *Temperature, Part I, Arts and Concepts.* Stroudsberg, Pa.: Dowden, Hutchinson and Ross, Inc., 1977.

Bergaust, Erik, ed. *Illustrated Space Encyclopedia.* New York: G. P. Putnam & Sons, 1965.

Bergwin, Clyde R. and Coleman, William T. *Animal Astronauts.* Englewood Cliffs, N. J.: Prentice Hall, 1963.

Berry, Charles A., and Catterson, Allen D. *Pre-Gemini Medical Predictions versus Gemini Flight results.* Unpublished.

....*Biomedical Findings on American Astronauts Participating in Space Missions,* paper presented at Fourth International Symposium on Basic Environmental Problems of Man in Space, Yerevan, Armenia, 1971.

....*Medical Results of Apollo 14 - Implications for Longer Duration Space Flights,* paper presented at XX International Congress of Aviation and Space Medicine, Nice, France, 1972.

....*Space Medicine in Perspective - A Critical Review of the Manned Space Program,* read at 20th Clinical Convention of American Medical Association, Las Vegas, 1966.

Bert, Paul. *Barometric Pressure Researches in Experimental Physiology.* France, 1877. Translation, Hitchcock, M., et al. Columbus: College Book Company, 1943.

Blanchard, Jean Pierre. *The First Air Voyage in America,* 1793. n. p., 1793.

Bland, William M. Jr., and Berry, Charles A. "Project Mercury Experiences," *Astronautics and Aerospace Engineering,* Feb ruary, 1963.

Bond, Douglas D. *The Love and Fear of Flying.* New York: International Universities Press, 1952.

378

Booker, P. J.; Frewar, G. C.; and Pardoe, G. K. C. *Project Apollo.* New York: American Elsevier Publishing Co., 1971.

Boothby, W. M. and Lovelace, W. R., "Oxygen in Aviation," *Aviation Medicine,* 9:172-195, 1938.

Bourne, Geoffrey H., ed. *Medical and Biological Problems of Space Flight,* Proceedings of conference held in Nassau, The Bahamas, November 1961. New York: Academic Press, 1963.

Boyle, Charles B. *Space Among Us.* Washington, D. C.; Goddard Flight Center.

Burwell, Robert A. *Historical Review of Aircrew Selection.* Unpublished.

Caceres, Cesar A. *Biomedical Telemetry.* New York: Academic Press, 1965.

Campbell, Paul A. *Earthman, Spaceman, Universal Man.* New York: Pageant Press, Inc., 1965.

....*Medical and Biological Aspects of the Energies of Space.* New York: Columbia University Press, 1961.

....*The History of the Space Medicine Branch of the Aerospace Medical Association,* (section 1, from concept to Sputnik 1, 1950-57.) Unpublished.

Chambers, Randall M., Hitchcock, Lloyd, Jr., Gray, R. Flanagan, *Preliminary Considerations of Some Human Factors Problems for a Manned Orbital Laboratory Crew.* U.S. Naval Air Development Center, Johnsville, Pa., 1965.

....*Effects of Positive Pressure Breathing on Performance During Acceleration.* Produced jointly by Naval Air Development Center, Navy Bureau of Medicine and Surgery, and Navy Bureau of Weapons, 1963.

379

....*Psychological Problems in Disorientation.* Produced jointly by Naval Air Development Center, Navy Bureau of Medicine and Surgery, and Navy Bureau of Weapons, 1963.

....*Acceleration Training for Astronauts and Test Personnel*, presented at 22nd AGARD Aerospace Medical Panel Meeting G.A.F., Institute of Aviation Medicine, Furstenfeldbruck, 1966. Unpublished.

...."Isolation and Disorientation" reprinted from *Physiological Problems in Space Exploration.* Springfield, Ill., Charles C. Thomas.

...."The Psychology of Space Flight and Centrifuge Training," *Journal of the British Interplanetary Society,* vol. 21, 232-273, 1968.

...."Human Engineering Studies in Acceleration Environments," *Proceedings of Institute of Environmental Sciences,* April, 1965.

...."Human Engineering Studies in Acceleration Environments," *Proceedings of Environmental Sciences,* April, 1964.

...."Pilot Performance Capabilities During Centrifuge Simulations of Boost and Re-Entry," *American Rocket Society Journal,* November, 1961.

...."Problems and Research in Space Psychology," joint publication by Navy Bureau of Medicine and Surgery, and Bureau of Weapons, April, 1962.

Christy, Ralph. *Early Centrifugal Research.* Unpublished.

Collins, Michael. *Carrying the Fire.* New York: Farrar, Strauss & Giroux, 1974.

Cox, Donald W. *America's Explorers of Space.* Maplewood, N. J.: C. S. Hammond. 1967.

Dille, Robert. *Physical Standards - Their Development from*

Aeronauts to Astronauts. Unpublished.

Engle, Eloise. *Escape.* New York: John Day, 1963.

....*Sky Rangers.* New York: John Day, 1965.

Farmer, Gene, and Hamblin, Dora Jane. *First on the Moon.* Boston: Little, Brown and Company. 1970.

Gantz, Kenneth, ed. *Man in Space.* New York: Duell, Sloan and Pearce, 1959.

Gardiner, Leslie. *Man in the Clouds.* Edinburgh and London: W & R Chambers, Ltd. 1963.

Gerathewohl, Siegfried J. *Principles of Bioastronautics.* Englewood Cliffs, N. J.: Prentice Hall, Inc. 1963.

Glaisher, J., "Notes on Effects Experienced During Recent Balloon Ascents," *Lancet,* 2:559-560, 1862.

Greene, Ralph, "An Aviator and His Ears," *Industrial Medicine,* 5:669-671, 1938.

Hanrahan, James Stephen, and Bushnell, David. *Space Biology.* New York: Basic Books, 1960.

Henry, James P., Mosely, John D., ed. *Results of the Project Mercury Ballistic and Orbital Chimpanzee Flights,* NASA, 1963.

Holbrook, Heber A. *Civil Aviation Medicine in the Bureaucracy.* Bethesda, Md.: Banner Publishing Company, 1974.

Howard, Peter. "Aeromedical Research and the SST," The Harry G. Armstrong Lecture, RAF Institute of Aviation Medicine, Farnborough, England, 1977.

Hurtado, A., "Studies of Myohemoglobin at High Altitudes," *American Journal of Medical Sciences,* 194: 708-713; 1937.

Jastrow, Robert, and Thompson, Malcolm R. *Astronomy: Fundamentals and Frontiers,* 3rd ed. New York: John Wiley & Sons, 1977.

Jeffries, John. *A Narrative of the Two Aerial Voyages...1784 ...1785.* London: 1786. Reprinted, Institute of Aeronautical Sciences, 1941.

Johnson, Richard S., Dietlein, Lawrence F., and Berry, Charles A., ed. *Biomedical Results of Apollo,* NASA, 1975.

Kelley, Roy J. *The Human Centrifuge,* produced at School of Aviation Medicine, Randolph Air Force Base, Texas, 1957.

Kittinger, Joseph W., and Caidin, Martin. *The Long Lonely Leap.* New York: Dutton, 1961.

Lamb, Lawrence E. *Aerospace Medicine.* produced at School of Aviation Medicine, Randolph Air Force Base, Texas. No date.

Lambert, Edward H., "Comparison of the Physiological Effects of Positive Acceleration on a Human Centrifuge and in an Airplane," *Journal of Aviation Medicine,* vol. 20, Number 5.

Lavnikov, A. A. *Aviation Medicine* (translation of *Aviatsionnaya Meditsina.* Moscow: Voyenizdat, 1961.

Lewis, Richard. *The Voyages of Apollo: The Exploration of the Moon.* New York: Quadrangle, New York Times Book Co., 1974.

Ley, Willy. *Rockets, Missiles, and Men in Space.* New York: Viking Press, 1967.

Lindberg, Evan F., and Wood, Earl H., *Acceleration,* Prepared at Mayo Clinic, Rochester, Minnesota.

Link, Mae Mills and Coleman, Robert A. *Medical Support of the Army Air Forces in World War II.* Washington, D.C.; Office of Surgeon General, U.S. Air Force, 1955.

Mallan, Lloyd. *Men, Rockets and Space Rats.* New York: Julian Messner, 1955.

Marbarger, John P., ed. *Space Medicine, the Human Factor in Flights Beyond the Earth.* Urbana, Ill.: University of Illinois Press, 1951.

Marshall, G. S., "The Physiological Limits of Flying," *Journal of Aeronautical Society,* vol. 3, 1933.

Mason, Brian, and Melson, William G. *The Lunar Rocks.* New York: Wiley Interscience, 1970.

McFarland, Ross A. *Human Factors in Air Transport Design.* New York: McGraw-Hill Book Co., 1946.

Minners, Howard A. *History of Aviation Medicine up to 1930.* Unpublished.

Post, Wiley, and Gatty, Harold. *Around the World in Eight Days.* Garden City, N.Y.; Garden City Pub. Co., 1931.

Rickenbacker, Edward V. *Rickenbacker.* Englewood Cliffs, N.J.; Prentice-Hall, Inc., 1967.

Robinson, Douglas H. *The Dangerous Sky.* Seattle: University of Washington Press, 1973.

Rolt, L. T. C. *The Aeronauts.* New York; Walker and Co., 1966.

Ruff, Siegfried, and Strughold, Hubertus. *Compendium of Aviation Medicine.* Berlin: Medical Staff, German Air Corps, 1932.

Sass, Donald J. et al. *Effects of Breathing Liquid Fluorocarbons on Pleural Pressures and Other Physiological Parameters,* School of Aviation Medicine Technical Report 72-15, Brooks Air Force Base, Texas, 1972.

...."Liquid Breathing: Prevention of Pulmonary Arterial-venous Shunting During Acceleration," *Journal of Applied Physiology,* vol. 32, Number 4, April, 1972.

Schuon, Karl, and Pierce, Philip N. *John Glenn, Astronaut.* New York: Franklin Watts, 1962.

Sells, S. B., and Berry, Charles, A., ed. *Human Factors in Jet and Space Travel.* New York: The Ronald Press Co., 1961.

Sharpe, Mitchel R. *Living in Space.* Garden City N. Y.: Doubleday, 1969.

Slaagr, Ursula T. *Space Medicine.* Englewood Cliffs, N. J.: Prentice-Hall, Inc., 1962.

Sneath, P. H. A., ed. *Life Sciences and Space Research.* vol. IX Berlin: Akademia-Verlag, 1973.

Stehling, Kurt R., and Beller, William. *Sky Hook.* Garden City, N. Y., Doubleday Co., Inc., 1962.

Stevens, A., "Man's Farthest Aloft," *National Geographic Magazine,* 69: 59-94, 1936.

Strughold, Hubertus. *Compendium of Aerospace Medicine,* vol. 1. USAF School of Aviation Medicine, Brooks AFB, Texas, 1977.

Thomas, Shirley. *Men of Space.* 8 vols. Philadelphia: Chilton Co., Book Div., 1960-68.

Verne, Jules. *De la Terre a la Lune.* Paris: Montout, 1872. *From the Earth to the Moon.* London: Sampson Low, Marston & Co., Ltd., 1865.

Vishniac, W., and Favorite, F. G., *Life Sciences and Space Research.* Amsterdam: North Holland Pub. Co., 1970.

von Beckh, Harald J. *Multi-Directional G-Protection in Space Vehicles,* reprinted from VIII International Astronautical Congress, Barcelona, 1957.

...*Multi-Directional G-Protection During Experimental Sled Runs,* reprinted from X International Astronautical Congress, London, 1959.

von Diringshofen, Heinz. *Medical Guide for Flying Personnel.* Oberstabsarzt der Luftwaffe, 1939.

Williams, Alford, "Inverted Flight," *Aero Digest,* September, 1928.

Wilmer, W. H., "The Early Development of Aviation Medicine in the U.S." *Military Surgeon,* 77:115-135, 1935.

Wilson, Charles L., "Soviet High Altitude Pressure Suit Development," *Aerospace Medicine,* vol. 36, Number 9, September, 1965.

Wood, Earl H., et al. "Effects of Acceleration in Relation to Aviation." *Federation Proceedings,* vol. 36, Number 5, September, 1948.

...."Do Permanent Effects Result From Repeated Blackouts Caused by Positive Acceleration?" *Journal of Aviation Medicine,* October, 1948.

...."Effect of Partial Immersion in Water on Response of Healthy Men to Headward Acceleration," *Journal of Applied Physiology,* vol. 18, Number 6, November, 1963.

Publications by NASA, other government agencies.

Biomedical Research from Skylab, NASA SP 377.

Skylab, Our First Space Station, NASA SP 400s.

Space Medicine in Project Mercury. NASA SP 4003.

Chariots for Apollo, A History of Lunar Spacecraft. (Comment paper, not for release) NASA, 1976.

Apollo 11 Mission Commentary. (Unpublished transcript) JSC, NASA.

Bioastronautics Data Book. NASA SP 3066, 1973.

Smithsonian Annals of Flight, No. 8 - Wiley Post Pressure Suit. Washington, D.C.; Smithsonian Institution, 1971.

Smithsonian Annals of Flight, No. 10 - First Steps Toward Space. Washington, D.C.; Smithsonian Institution, 1974.

History of Research in Space Biology and Biodynamics at the Air Force Missile Development Center, Holloman Air Force Base, New Mexico, 1946-1958. Unpublished.

The Beginnings of Research in Space Biology at the Air Force Missile Development Center, Holloman Air Force Base, 1953-57. Unpublished.

Major Achievements in Space Biology at the Air Force Missile Development Center, Holloman Air Force Base, 1953-57.

History of Research in Subgravity and Zero G at the Air Force Missile Development Center, 1948-58. Unpublished.

Manhigh II. Air Force Missile Development Center Technical Report, Holloman Air Force Base, 1959.

History of Aero Medical Laboratory, Wright Field, Ohio. Unpublished.

Fourth International Symposium on Bioastronautics and the Exploration of Space. Aerospace Medical Division, Brooks Air Force Base, 1968.

"The R.C.A.F. Human Centrifuge and Acceleration Laboratory," *Journal of the Canadian Medical Services,* vol. 4 Number 1, November, 1946.

German Aviation Medicine, WWII. Department of the Air Force, 1950.

Foundations of Space Biology and Medicine, Joint USA-USSR publication, 3 volumes.

AGARDOGraph series, Advisory Group of Aerospace Research and Development, Neuilly, Sur-Seine, France.

Life Sciences and Space Research, 10 volumes, by Committee on Space Research (COSPAR) and USSR Academy of Sciences. Akademie-Verlag, Berlin, 1971-1975.

Encyclopedia of Space, Editions Rombaldi, Paris, 1968.

Principles of Biodynamics Applicable to Manned Aerospace Flight and Prolonged Linear and Radial Acceleration, AGARD, France, 1971.

Index

Barnstorming, 156
Barometric pressure, 318-319
Barr, Norman Lee, 18, 178-181
Bassett, Charles, 175
Bauer, Louis H., 46, 49, 51, 156
Baylor College of Medicine, 287
"Beanpole effect," 286
Bears, in research, 103
Bedrest studies, 271, 279
Beeding, Eli J., Jr., 103, 132, 210
Bell Aircraft Corporation, 112
Behnke, Albert, 114
Beischer, D., 114
Bends, 318
Benford, Robert, 125
Benson, Otis O., 112, 116, 125
Benzinger, Theodor H., 69-71, 114, 167
Berne, University of, 345
Berry, Charles, 143, 148, 149, 170, 171, 174, 177, 184, 282, 284, 292-294, 307, 331, 333, 341, 344, 349
Bert, Paul, 11, 34-37, 55
B.F. Goodrich Co., 221
Biological experts, 120
Biomedical telemetry, 174, 200, 331-333
Blackout, 195
Blanchard, Jean-Pierre, 9, 33, 133, 323
BLB oxygen mask, 64
Blount, Wilbur C., 103
Body armor, 229
Boeing 307 Stratoliners, 235
Boelcke, Oswald, 151
Bondurant, S., 132
Bosee, Roland, 231
Buettner, Konrad, 114, 116, 122
Boothby, Walter M., 64
Borman, Frank, 339, 341
Boynton, Mel, 76-77
Breakoff phenomenon, 303
Brewer, Walter E., 136
British Royal Aircraft Establishment, 247
Bronk, Detlev, 131
Brown, John L., 200
Bruno, Giordono, 268
Burgreev, Nikolai, 241

Bulbulian, Arthur H., 64
Bureau of Aviation Medicine, 157
Bush, William H., 133
Byrd, Richard E., 53
Byrnes, V.A., 306

Campbell, Paul, 116, 121, 122, 124, 138, 246
Cannon, R. Keith, 131
Cardiothoracic ratio, 315, 319
Cardiovascular system, 313-315; responce to g-force, 197-199
Carpenter, Malcolm S., 165, 174
Carr, Gerald M., 287-291
Carrying the Fire, 166, 282-284
Case Institute, 130
Casualties in aviation and space program, 151, 174-175
Cats, used in research, 98, 99; in weightlessness, 280-281
Centrifugal force, 192-195, 223, 224; centrifugal training of astronauts, 201, 202
Centrifuges, 77, 89, 91, 127, 178, 192, 195-196, 198-201, 200-203
Century of Progress, balloon, 15
Chaffee, Roger, 18, 175, 235
Chambers, Randall M., 200, 302
Charles, Jacques A. C., 2, 34
Charliere-type balloon, 3
Chief Surgeon, first 152
Chimpanzees, in research, 85, 87, 100-101
Christy, Ralph L., 199
Circadian cycle, 309-311
Clamann, Hans-Georg, 68
Clark, Brant, 303, 305
Clark, Carl C., 203
Clark, Dave, 229, 244
Clark, Robert T., 240
Cockpit and cabin development, 235-241, 244, 250-251
Colley, Russ E., 222
Collins, Michael, 146, 166, 282-284, 330
Concorde, SST, 250-253
Congreve, William, 326

Fruit flies, in research, 96-98, 104
Fordney, Chester, 16
Fordyce, George, 7
Franklin, Benjamin, 5
Free-fall tests, 25

Gagarin, Yuri, 136, 175, 188, 231
Galilei, Galileo, 268
Galloway, Wayne, 231
Garland, P. W., 132
Garriott, Owen K., 308
Gauer, Otto, 114, 196
Gauss, Karl Friedrich, 338
Geiss, Johannes, 345
Gell, C. F., 132
Generales, Constantine, D. J., 89, 90
General Mills Corporation, 17
George C. Marshall Spaceflight Center, 327
Gerathewohl, Siegfried, 112, 276, 280
German Aviation Medicine, World War II, 112
G-forces, 77, 194, 209, 212, 215
Gibson, Edward G., 287-289, 291
Giller, Edward B., 130
Gilruth, Robert E., 136, 143, 158, 337
Glenn, John, 165, 173, 203-204, 307, 343
Glennon, J., 130
Goddard, Robert H., 325
Goddard Spaceflight Center, 181
Goldfish, in research, 104
Gordon, Richard, 305
Graybiel, Ashton, 78, 126, 192, 303, 305
Graveline, Duane, 170, 276-282, 294, 297
Gravisphere, 340
Gravity, artificial, 270, 282, 297; force of, 267, 270
Gray, Hawthorne C., 14
Grayout, 195
Grechko, Greorgy, 244, 298
Greene, Ralph N., 46, 51
Grissom, Virgil I., 165, 235
Grow, Malcolm G., 59, 65, 112-113, 230
Guadalcanal, USS, 342

Guppies, in research, 91

Haber, Fritz, 271; Heinz, 114, 116, 117, 122, 271
Halberg, F., 311
Haldane, John Scott, 220
Hall, John F., 261
Ham, astrochimp, 83, 100
Hamsters, in research, 97
Hardy, James D., 130, 200
Hartmann, Hans, 55, 63
Hawkins, Willard, 240
Heat ablation, 336
Heaney, Robert P., 171
Heim, J. W., 61
Henry, James P., 91, 121, 128, 129, 133, 136, 272
Henschke, V. K., 114
Hess, Victor, 256
Hessberg, Rufus R., 87, 96, 132, 136, 192, 197, 209, 210, 280
Heatherington, Albert, 128
Hiatt, E. P., 132
High-altitude flight, 74; limits to, 15; Man-High II, 22; Man-High II, 24-25; Excelsior tests, 25-26, Stratolab, 27, 29; Etoile Polaire, 37; Preussen, 39
Holmes, D. Brainerd, 143
Homes, Robert H., 131
Homick, J. L., 312
Hoover, George, 17
Hordinsky, Jerry R., 290
Hornberger, Wilhelm, 71
Hornet, USS, 348
Howard-Dolman Depth Perception Apparatus, 156
Howard, Peter, 249
Human Factors in Air Transportation, 77
Human gradient calorimeter, 167, 168
Hunter, H. N., 132
Hunter, Robert J., 46
Hydrogen, in balloons, 3
Hynek, J. Alken, 128
Hyperoxia, 317
Hypobaria, 318
Hypodynamia, 315

Hypoxia, 218; first victims of, 11; symptoms of, 12-13; research on, 55

Illusory sensations of flight, 303
Information transmittal, 181, 187
Interagency Committee on Back-Contamination, 349
Isolation, effects of, 308
International Commission for Air Navigation, 156
Institute of Aeronautical Sciences, 125
International Astronautical Federation, 126, 128
Ivanchenkov, Alexander, 298
Ivy, Andrew C., 122

Jackson, C. B., 133
Jeffries, John, 9, 33
Jet lag, 310
Jet stream, 223
Johnson, Lyndon B., 135, 240, 323
Johnson, Richard, 245
Jones, Isaac, 153
Jones, I. H., 42, 46
Jones, Walton L., 200, 230, 231
Jongbloed, Jacob, 62
Jonson, Samuel, 7
Journal of Aviation Medicine, The, 49, 123, 125, 149, 198
Journal of Science, 59

Kamarov, Vladimir, 175
Karst, Samuel G., 240
Kelly, Oakley G., 219
Kennedy, J. F., 134
Kepler, Johannes, 268; "Kepler Regime," 331, 338; Keplerian trajectory, 271
Kerwin, Joe, 110, 170, 285-286, 287, 356
Kety, Seymour S., 132
Killian, James A., 129
Kind, Helmut, 71
Kipfer, Paul, 11
Kittinger, Joseph W., Jr., 19, 26, 213, 214

Knaut, George, 133
Knight, Pete, 327
Kovalynok, Vladimir, 298
Kraft, Christopher C., Jr., 81, 329, 340
Krasnoyarsk Institute of Physics, 240
Krebs, Hans A., 69

Lamb, Lawrence E., 170
Laika, Russian dog, 83, 94, 95
Lake Champlain, USS, 138
Lambert, Larry, 117
Lancaster, J. O., 118
Langham, Wright Haskell, 130
Lavoisier, Antoine, 14
Laughlin, C. P., 132
L. B. Johnson Space Center, 305
Lewis, M. Lee, 18, 19, 97
Lick Observatory, 345
Life sciences research, 139
Life support systems, 220
Light flashes in space, 304
Lilienthal, Joseph L., 77
Lilienthal, Otto, 40
Liljencrantz, Eric S., 79
Lindbergh, Charles A., 9, 54, 154, 340
Linear acceleration, 194
Liquid oxygen, 222
Lombard, Charles, 213
Longacre, Raymond T., 154
Long Lonely Leap, The, 214
Louis XVI, 3, 85
Lovelace, W. Randolph, 64, 74, 76, 130, 131
Lovelace Foundation, 163
Lovell, James A., 339, 341, 342
Lower body negative pressure (LBNP), 281, 315-316
Low-pressure chamber, 220
Lucia, Shannon W., 171
Lucian of Samosata, 322
Luft, U. C., 63
Lunar material, 347; lunar scientific experiments, 345-347, 353, 354; lunar surface, conditions of, 241
Lunardi, Vincenzo, 7
Lyster, Charles, 42, 46

Tsiolkovsky, Konstantin Eduardovitch, 269, 326, 329
Turtles, in subgravity, 98, 272
Tyler, Linda, 350

Udet, Ernst, 68, 70
University of California, 126
University of Houston, 305
University of Illinois, 122, 280
University of Minnesota, 311
University of Toronto, 193, 228

Valsalva maneuver, 319
Van Allen belt, 332, 335
Van Allen, James, 255, 258-259
Vera Historia, 322
Verin für Raumschiffahrt (VfR), 327
Verne, Jules, 97, 218, 325, 326, 339
Vestibular apparatus, 153, 154; functions of, 99; dysfunctions, 312, 313; visual illusions, 305
Vibration, 309
Visual acuity, 306; perception, 302
Voas, Robert, 149, 159
Vogel, John, 294
von Beckh, Harald J., 202, 223, 272
von Braun, Wernher, 89, 327, 343
von Diringshofen, Bernd, 66; Heinz, 66, 67, 68, 195, 223, 270
von Gerke, Henning, 114
von Greim, Robert Ritter, 49
von Karman Line, 331
von Richthofen, Rittmeister M., 151
von Schrotter, Hermann, 38, 40
V-2 rockets, 91, 93, 94, 112, 301, 327

Walker, A. D., 186
Walker, Joseph, 327
Walpole, Horace, 7
Ward, Julian, 240
Ward, William, 87
Warner, Edward P., 157
Washington, George, 9
Water immersion, 279-281
Webb, Hamilton, 276
Webb, James, 135

Weightlessness, 105, 313, 332; effects of prolonged duration, 282, 287, 296, 299; first experience of, 270; short term effects, 282, 293, 295, 299
Weightlessness, physiological effects; cardiovascular system, 271-272, 279-280, 281, 285, 297-298; diet, 276, 284-285, 289, 299; metabolism, 271, 276, 279, 283, 292, 293, 294, 296; musculoskeletal system, 271, 279, 285-287, 292, 294; orientation, 271-272, 276; red blood cells, 289; sleep, 283-284, 291; vestibular system, 272-281
Weightlessness, psychological effects of, 274, 281, 284, 289-292, 299
Wells, H. G., 325
Westover, O., 60
Whedon, G.D., 297, 192, 293, 294, 296, 297
White, Clayton S., 125
White, Edward, 18, 176, 235
Whitney, Raymond, 62
White, Stanley, 132, 133, 136, 147, 259, 174, 280
Wiener, Norbert, 121
Wiesman, Jerome, 134
Wilkinson Sword Co., 230
Williams, C. C., 175
Williams, W. C., 136, 138
Wilmer, William H., 42
Wilson, Charles L., 223, 226
Winnie May, 222, 223
Winzen; Otto, 17; Vera, 23
Women astronauts, 171-172; balloonists, 7; pilots, 53
WPW syndrome, 181
Wright, T. F., 157

X-1 aircraft, 116, 121; X-15 aircraft, 231, 327

Yeager, Charles, 113, 272
Yelisayev, Alexi, 299
Yellow Springs Instrument Co., 280
Young, R. S., 262

Zero gravity, 120
Zieglschmid, John, 180